PLAYFUL

APPROACHES

TO SERIOUS PROBLEMS

PLAYFUL

APPROACHES

TO SERIOUS PROBLEMS

Narrative Therapy with Children and their Families

JENNIFER FREEMAN

DAVID EPSTON

DEAN LOBOVITS

W. W. NORTON & COMPANY

NEW YORK · LONDON

Printed in the United States of America

3 4 5 6 7 8 9 0

For information about permission to reproduce selections from this book write to Permissions, W. W. Norton & Company, Inc., 500 Fifth Avenue, New York, NY 10110

The text of this book is composed in Weiss with the display set in Funhouse. Manufacturing by Haddon Craftsmen. Desktop composition and book design by Justine Burkat Trubey.

Library of Congress Cataloging-in-Publication Data
Freeman, Jennifer C.
       Playful approaches to serious problems : narrative therapy with children and their families / Jennifer Freeman, David Epston, Dean Lobovits.
          p.   cm.
       "A Norton professional book."
       Includes bibliographical references and index.
       ISBN 0-393-70229-4
       1. Storytelling—Therapeutic use. 2. Child psychotherapy. 3. Family psychotherapy. 4. Metaphor—Therapeutic use. 5. Fantasy—Therapeutic use. I. Epston, David. II. Lobovits, Dean. III. Title.
RJ505.S75F74   1997   96-52874
618.92'8914—dc21   CIP

W. W. Norton & Company, Inc., 500 Fifth Avenue, New York, NY 10110
   http://www.wwnorton.com

W. W. Norton & Company Ltd., 10 Coptic Street, London WC1A 1PU

For

Elana

and

Benny the Peanut Man

Contents

. . . .

Acknowledgments

· ·

We, Dean and Jenny, would like to thank our families and each and every person in our lives who has ever loved, supported, encouraged, mentored us, or laughed at our jokes. Sadly but wisely, our editor has advised that we restrict expressing gratitude solely to those who contributed directly to the generation of this book.

We want to voice our heartfelt gratitude to all the children and families who have enriched our lives through our work and play together, especially those who have generously lent their stories to this book.

We'd like to acknowledge Michael and Cheryl White. Michael is David Epston's brother in creation and Cheryl his sister in inception and publication of the ideas that guide and inspire this book. Just about every idea here could in some way be traced to their vision and compassion. We especially thank Michael for his personal contribution to this book, "The Bypass Operation."

To our co-author David, it has been an immense pleasure to bring each other's work to literary life, to craft sentences, argue over ideas, and be believed in by you. And to Ann Epston, thanks for keeping the faith alive!

We are very grateful to those who supported our writing efforts: Many thanks to Susan Barrows Munro for her editorial advice, patience, and humor. Hats off to Zeena Janowsky, Marcus Mann, Margaret Rossoff, and Adrienne Wolfert, who pored over the manuscript, enheartened us, gave us insightful feedback and editorial assistance. Davida Cohen, Wendy Davis Larkin, Sallyann Roth, Julie Searle, and Susan Andrea Weiner spent hours listening to readings, enjoyed finding the right word with us, and gave us good criticism and writerly advice. Cheers to Jill Kelly, who entered David's edits and then transmitted them across the virtual ocean between us, and Jane Hales, for fulfilling our requests for information and assisting us with Michael White's contribution. Thanks to Johannah Gray for the artful and fun photo sessions.

Kristy Sotelo, Jenessa Joffe, Clover Catskill, and Debbie Maxine gave generously of their time and energies to take loving care of Elana, and supported us in countless other ways so that we could write. Each of these people has a unique sense of humor and sharing laughter with them has been a big help. Without them, the completion of this book would have literally been impossible.

Darling Elana shared the same original "due date" as the manuscript and shared her parents' divided attention between her and this "twin" for her gestation and much of her first year.

Warm thanks to the many family members, friends, and colleagues who put up with the compromises to our social life and usual commitments. We appreciate that they humored us and did not roll their eyes when we groused about the demands of authorship.

Some wonderful communities of colleagues and co-conspirators have developed around this work. We appreciate those with whom we learned and collaborated in several study groups: Andrea Aidells, Erin Donahue, Sheila Jacobs, Anne Jauregui, Jane Lobell, Rick Maisel, Michelle Martin, Nurit Mussen, Susanne Pregerson, and Micheal Searle, as well as Lucia Gattone, Susan Shaw, and other members of a sister study group in Sonoma. We want to thank some others in the extended community for their encouragement and for their ideas and inspiration: Jennifer Andrews, Johnella Bird, David Clark, Gene Combs, Joanne DePetro, Vicki Dickerson, Jill Freedman, James Griffith, Melissa Griffith, Jeffrey Kerr, Stephen Madigan, John Neal, David Nylund, Sallyann Roth, Karl Tomm, and Jeff Zimmerman; and in the specific sense of also being Jenny's child therapy mates: Lisa Berndt, Cathy Lopston, and Kathleen Stacey, as well as expressive arts collaborators Pamela Barregar Dunne and Craig Smith.

Ronald Levinson and Keith McConnell supported Dean in his writing and his personal and professional growth at John F. Kennedy University.

Priscilla Caputo, John Carr, Karen Moore, and Emily Seidel were members of the Xanthos reflecting team that collaborated with Dean to develop many of the ideas he has presented.

For the ideas in this book on social justice and therapists' roles in the community we are beholden to: Warihi Campbell, Winnie Laban, Kiwi Tamasese, Flora Tuhaka, Charles Waldegrave, and the Just Therapy team from Lower Hutt, New Zealand; and for their social justice and cultural work stateside: Ram Gokul, Sheila Jacobs, Zoy Kazan, Linda Kuwatani, Ellen Peskin, John Prowell, Archie Smith Jr., Yvette Flores Ortiz, Mathew Mock, and Veronique Thompson.

To those we inevitably omitted from this list, we deeply apologize. If it takes a village to raise a child, it obviously takes one to write a book at the same time. Thanks to all of you.

David Epston would like to acknowledge Jenny and Dean's dedication in reigning such a wealth of material into a delightfully readable book. Much of this was done in tandem with a challenging pregnancy and Elana's first year. Without them, this book would be no more than a mess of transcripts and fondly remembered conversations from over the years.

David's friend and the co-director of the Family Therapy Centre, Johnella Bird, was one of the then-quartet of co-authors in the "talking stages" of this book. Regrettably, her circumstances did not allow her to contribute in a way that satisfied her and for that reason she decided to withdraw. We believe this book is the poorer for her absence. So much of David's work has developed through "What do you think about this, Johnella?" conversations over the last twelve or so years.

Introduction

. . . .

Her brown eyes sparkling and an expectant look on her face, eight-year-old Maria marched into Jenny's therapy office and announced, "I got a new idea to tell you about the Temper!" This was the second time Jenny was surprised in one short week. The first surprise came when Maria's mother Sarah phoned on Monday to say that, out of the blue, Maria had initiated this visit by asking her mother if she could "go see Jenny again." The second surprise came when Jenny saw Maria's uninhibited enthusiasm over her new idea about dealing with the Temper. Jenny remembered how shy and reticent Maria had seemed when they first met a year and a half before.

When Jenny had last seen Maria and her family, they had agreed that Maria was well on her way to becoming a "Temper Tamer." In their meetings that year, everyone had worked together to assist Maria to face up to the Temper and its companion, Misery, both of which had been dominating her life. Their collaboration was based on "fed-upness" with the way the Temper and Misery had been ruining family fun. Maria's family had initially described her as "exploding with rage, screeching, slamming doors, threatening everyone who comes near." One small upset over breakfast would grow to darken the rest of the day with arguments, sibling disputes, sulking, crying, and tantrums.

Maria had experimented with ways to take control of these problems, which had previously seemed so overwhelming of her. She discovered one of her very best anti-Temper techniques right off the bat: she could shake off the Temper by ducking out and taking a few minutes alone in a quiet room. Now, some eight months later, while practicing this anti-Temper technique, Maria had invented a new idea she felt certain Jenny would be keen to know about.

Striding into the playroom, smiling as she plunked herself down, she breathlessly began, "Last Saturday I was mad about a friend. She wouldn't share the bicycle with me. I was starting to have an angry temper day. Then I went to the bathroom to take a break. I just started tearing up toilet paper. Then I had an idea. I tored up the paper in the shape of the day's first letter, 'S' and flushed it down the toilet!"

Maria, grinning, looked up at Jenny, apparently expecting her to get the gist of it. Jenny guessed: "Did that help you shake off the temper?"

"Yes! I flushed the bad temper day down the toilet!"

"Did this good idea of yours open the door to a different kind of day?"

"Yep, then I decided I could have a happy new day!"

From her earlier therapy experiences, Maria guessed that Jenny would invite her to enter her latest story into the *Temper Tamer's Handbook: Cool Off and Be Cool*, a chronicle of children's accounts of their knowledges and ideas about taming temper. After she had dictated her entry to Jenny and illustrated it with a drawing, Maria talked about showing it to her family.

Jenny was not only tickled to hear about Maria's "flushing" practice, but intrigued by the concept Maria apparently had of therapy. Maria had sought a consultation with Jenny in order to tell her about an exciting breakthrough. Evidently, in Maria's mind therapy was a site for sharing her knowledge and competencies. Somehow, Maria no longer seemed to take the Temper and Misery so personally. In concert with her family, she approached these once shaming problems as interesting challenges, as an ongoing test of her mettle.

A challenge for us as family therapists is to find ways to motivate and inspire children in relation to the problems they face: How can children and adults each be fully engaged in family therapy? How do we invite children to bring forth their playfulness, imagination, and inventiveness in the face of serious problems? We consider in this book what attitudes and practices help a therapist to hold the most hopeful view, to evoke the child's capabilities, as well as restore a family's faith that a problem can be resolved. What makes it possible for young people's voices to be heard and for them to feel encouraged as they make their own contributions? How do we gain as responsible adults vis-à-vis a child, if we are light on our toes when confronting weighty problems? How is it possible to play, to maintain a sense of humor, and even have fun with children, while dealing effectively with distressing, frightening, or perilous situations?

We have joined a growing community of therapists around the world who are collaborating with children and families in ways that allow all of us (therapists, children, and parents alike) to be lighthearted, humorous, and creative—and yet surprisingly effective in resolving many of the problems that we face today. In our view, the developments collectively known as narrative therapy offer some unique and helpful perspectives to the field of child and family therapy. In the following pages we offer some approaches, guided primarily by the philosophy and practice of narrative therapy, that have cast fresh light for us on the questions above. We hope, by the end of this book, to have evoked your own questions and ideas.

WHY A "NARRATIVE" THERAPY?

The term narrative implies listening to and telling or retelling stories about people and the problems in their lives. In the face of serious and sometimes potentially deadly problems, the idea of hearing or telling stories may seem a trivial pursuit. It is hard to believe that conversations can shape new realities. But they do. The bridges of meaning we build with children help healing developments flourish instead of wither and be forgotten. Language can shape events into narratives of hope.

We humans have evolved as a species to use mental narratives to organize, predict, and understand the complexities of our lived experiences. Our choices are shaped largely by the meanings we attribute to events and to the options we are considering. A problem may have personal, psychological, sociocultural, or biological roots—or, more likely, a complex mix of the above. Moreover, young persons and their families may not have control over whether a certain problem is in their life. But even then, how they live with it is still within their choice. As Aldous Huxley once remarked, "Experience is not what happens to you. It is what you do with what happens to you."

WHY A PLAYFUL NARRATIVE APPROACH?

Narrative therapy employs a linguistic practice called externalization, which separates persons from problems. Separating the problem from the person in an externalizing conversation relieves the pressure of blame and defensiveness. Instead of being defined as inherently *being* a problem, a young person can now have a *relationship* with the externalized problem.

It has continued to astonish us how resourceful, responsible, and effective children can be in facing problems! Externalizing language allows a lighthearted approach to what is usually considered serious business. Playfulness enters into a family therapy when we narrate the relationship between a child and a problem.

When adults and children collaborate actively, play is a mutual friend. It inspires children to bring their resources to bear on problems and make their own unique contributions to family therapy. Playful approaches in narrative therapy direct the focus away from the child as a problem and onto the child-problem relationship in a way that is meaningful for adults as well as intriguing, not heavy-handed or boring, for children.

THE CONTEXT OF THIS BOOK

We would like to take a moment to clarify what this book is and what it is not. At first, in planning it, we thought we would present a history of the field of family and child therapy and offer a comprehensive survey of the work of many therapists around the world in the rapidly evolving field of narrative therapy. However, we have chosen a different path.

We see ourselves as part of and indebted to the broader fields of family and child therapy. What has brought us together is our mutual excitement about narrative therapy. This inspired us to write from our own clinical experience and offer our versions of the ideas and practices of narrative therapy as they apply to young persons and their families. It is for this reason that we seek your forbearance with the unabashed enthusiasm that may at times come across these pages. Not that we are condemning enthusiasm itself. Rather than arising solely from dedication to a theory, it has been evoked by deeply felt and intimately shared moments of community with children and families.

Every new approach develops within a certain context and at a particular point in history. And each paradigm, even if it is critical, owes much to those who came before. There has been a bountiful history of many waves of discovery and enthusiasm in the field of family therapy. We value those waves that came before us and look forward to those that are now forming way out at sea.

SOME NOTES ABOUT LANGUAGE

We in the text is used variously to mean we humans, we the authors, and we the authors and the reader.

The sticky issue of gender pronouns has been addressed by alternating their use by chapter, female for the introduction and even-numbered chapters and male for odd-numbered chapters.

When we use the term *sociocultural*, it should be considered inclusive of the sociocultural aspects of such factors as abilities, age, ethnicity, gender roles, race, sexual preference, socioeconomic status, and spirituality.

SKETCH OF THE BOOK

Part I lays out the basic rationale, ideas, and practices for facilitating playful conversations within the context of narrative therapy with children and their families. It is liberally illustrated with vignettes and longer case stories.

Part II gives an account of some particular interests of each of the authors: Jenny sees families in a playroom environment, with art materials, dollhouse, puppets, sandtray and shelves of miniature figures. She has been exploring play therapy and expressive arts approaches as a means of attending to both verbal and nonverbal communication. These approaches facilitate expressions often favored by children, expanding the possibilities for playful communication in narrative therapy. For David, children's special abilities are a unique means for them to contribute to change in their own and their family's life. His attention to "weird abilities" provides confirmation of some of the unique powers of children and families that are usually shunned, labeled, or disqualified by the culture at large. Dean's focus is on the social, cultural, and economic pressures that "divide and conquer" families. He has been developing ideas like "The Peace Family Project" for children, adolescents, and families caught in the crossfire of social and intrafamily conflict.

Part II ends with an essay on the rich world of children's imaginations. A young person's imagination can lead her into trouble, fear or disappointment; it can also generate ideas and solutions to problems. When a child's imagination works against her by creating or perpetuating a problem, she can strive to reclaim it for her own preferred uses.

In Part III we offer five extended case stories, inviting readers to immerse themselves in the particulars of narrative therapeutic conversation. Each story shows some variation of approaches that we are experimenting with. We have written them in a narrative form so as to reveal the thoughts and perceptions of the therapist.

This is not a book about recipes, formulas, or cases that represent a class of problem. The case stories in this book recount conversations with unique people facing particular problems. Our hope in choosing them is that collectively they embody something of the spirit of this work (or is it play?).

PLAYFUL

APPROACHES

TO SERIOUS PROBLEMS

1

. . . .

PLAYFUL

COMMUNICATION

CHAPTER 1

Playful Communication in Family Therapy

Problems tend to be grim. If they had a credo it might well be: "Take us seriously!" After all, serious problems demand to be taken this way, do they not? To the degree that a problem is oppressive, the gravity of our attention and the severity of measures taken to remedy it seem bound to increase. Inviting worry, despair, and hopelessness, weighty problems can immobilize families as well as the people who serve them. We wonder whether it is to the problems' advantage to be taken quite so seriously. By the same token, is their very existence threatened by humor and playfulness?

Given a choice, most children prefer to interact in a playful way. Serious discussion and methodical problem-solving may impose on children's communication, shutting out their voices, inhibiting their special abilities, knowledges and creative resources (Freeman, Loptson, & Stacey, 1995; Stacey, 1995). The price of choosing seriousness for us as therapists may be the dampening of our own resources, such as the ability to think laterally, remain curious, be lighthearted enough to engage playfully with the child, and have faith that the situation is resolvable. Lacking these, we may have our wits dulled, lose our appeal to kids, or become overwhelmed. Do we dare to be playfully creative in the face of worrisome problems? What happens when we engage our imagination, humor, and resourcefulness in opposition to the deadly seriousness of problems? We believe this leads to the rise of inspired problem-solving and the downfall of serious problems. As our friend Michael Searle (personal communication, August, 1995) mused, "Is play as repugnant to a problem as garlic is to a vampire?"

Weighty problems seem to have a knack for convincing caretakers that it's time to quit playing around and get down to business. Such concerns are very understandable. It is frustrating for adults when they are trying hard to address the situation at hand—and a child would rather play with miniature figures, bounce around the room, try to start a game, draw a picture, talk about a movie, or stare out the window. In family therapy, it is easy for the therapist and members of the family to get drawn into efforts to get children "on task," while concentrating on ways of problem-solving that are familiar to adults. To speak of light-handed, even playful approaches may seem trifling, pollyannish, or insubstantial in the face of concerns such as these. However, a serious approach may exclude or alienate children and work to the advantage of the problem.

It is one thing to be humorous and playful with a four-year-old child about the "Sneaky Pee" that causes her bed-wetting or about Temper taking over family mealtimes. But what about facing a frightening and perilous problem, such as an eating disorder, self-destructive behavior, the reckless running away of a teenager, family violence, a child's recovery from sexual abuse,[1] or a life-threatening illness?

Playful approaches should not be underestimated as a worthy challenge to serious problems. Like the twin masks of comedy and tragedy, play reflects both the mirth and pathos of the human experience. When children and adults meet, play provides a common language to express the breadth and depth of thoughts, emotions, and experience—in this way, we share a lingua franca. Moreover, playful communication isn't totally dependent on cognitive development, having the capacity of being highly contagious and inclusive of all ages.

In a child-focused family therapy, children's ways of being and communicating are appreciated and respected. When an adult enters into a playful interaction with a child, the child's competency and creativity expand. Adults in families are frequently surprised when playful communication allows children to take responsibility for problems and be resourceful in solving them. Children's interest in playful approaches involving games, imagination, fantasy, mystery, magic, symbolism, metaphor, and story-telling may initially appear irrelevant. But within these more elliptical realms of meaning-making we find treasures that are central to the child's motivation and ability to resolve problems.

Young people use their imaginations and their abilities in ways that are often unseen by adults; they may have special abilities that one would never guess. Jenny has been curious about how children who have never been in therapy work things out on their own. She decided to interview some children she knew, starting with a couple of open questions: Have you ever had a problem that you dealt with on your own? Was your imagination a help to you in this?

Jenny asked an eleven-year-old Australian friend, Annie, if she could interview her about "how young people solve problems on their own." Annie led her to a quiet spot, where they wouldn't be interrupted. They climbed up onto a lichen-covered rock looking out over paddocks of sheep, and Annie thought for a while as she and Jenny sat quietly together with the sun warming their backs. Then she told Jenny that when she was six she had been bothered by bed-wetting at night. She had found a way to make it go away.

Annie had gone outside in the evening to gaze at the stars and chanted a wish she had heard: "Star light, star bright, first star I see tonight, wish I may, wish I might, have the wish I wish tonight." Annie explained that it had to be the first star or it wouldn't work. This nightly ritual helped her decide, "I could stop myself if I really wanted to," and to "think it would work." She was pleased to find that after a while it did in fact work and she was able to enjoy waking up to dry sheets.

Asked about other times her imagination had been a friend to her, Annie went on to tell Jenny about an imaginary dog who had helped her at sad times. This imaginary dog required imaginary food and water on a regular basis, and slept by her bedside in his own basket. A great playmate, he could run around in circles to cheer her up, but he also could be "soft and sweet when you needed him." When Annie was sad, she would go for walks with him down in the back paddocks, where she could stop and cuddle him, or cry into his fur for comfort.

Megan, another child who was interviewed, had a boisterous imaginary friend named Julie who used to come with her to preschool and kindergarten. Julie used to get up on the racks on the school bus and jump around and wave. When Megan was mad at the teacher, Julie used to get on Megan's shoulder and make faces, which made Megan feel better about being in class. When Megan worried that Julie's rudeness would get her in trouble, she would whisper "get down quick." Luckily, the teacher never seemed to notice.

Eight-year-old Jane had an imaginary friend who used to help her with her homework. Her friend was a grown man, who came from a tropical island and was kind, clever, and quiet. He lived in a mask on the wall, and Jane could call him down to visit, to play, or to help out. She needed a lot of help with subjects like math and geography. Her friend would remind her about how to do sums, but then she had to go ahead and complete them by herself. However, sometimes, when pressed, he would even go so far as to supply particularly difficult answers!

It is a pleasure to experience the perceptions of a child who is free to express herself in a relaxed and natural way. For instance, in Laura Ranger's (1995, p. 22) poem, written at age six, she plays with the complexity of her feelings towards her little brother and her perceptions of the words he confuses when he talks.

Pete and Me

I love Pete
and Pete loves me.
Soon I'll be seven
and Pete will be three.

In our house
my mum and dad
let us skate up the hall.
Sometimes we fall.
I come scooting through
the kitchen door
and crash down on the wooden floor.

In the dark Pete says
there's a monster in the hall.
He imagines there is a dinosaur
in mum's work room.
We shoo it out with a broom.

Pete is cute
Now he is learning to talk.
He calls my uncle's dog 'Dirty',
but her real name is Gertie.
Pete says
'frocodiles live in a trailer'
when he means
'crocodiles live in Australia'.

Pete is very funny.
He got into mischief in the shed.
He found Dad's best paintbrush,
and painted engine oil
all over his bed.

In my room
I play with Eloise.
We say to Pete
'Get out please'.
I hate Pete
when he wrecks our game.
He hates me the same.

THE OVERLAPPING IMAGINATIONS
OF CHILDREN AND ADULTS

A child's mind is different from that of an adult, but is influenced to a large degree by adult imagination. Think of all the stories, songs, and fairy tales that children enjoy. Most were written by adults imagining worlds for children. *Alice in Wonderland* was written by a man with no children, Lewis Carroll (1989); *Winnie the Pooh* by a father (Milne, 1957) who felt awkward being with his son Robin, but wanted to find a way to reach out to him. Children are delighted by these stories. They listen, let loose their imaginations, and develop fantasies of their own. They take strands of adult input and weave them into continuous play and story-telling. Adult story-tellers provide a trellis on which children's imaginations and narratives flourish like vines.

We are interested in a relationship between adults and children in therapy to which each party brings unique resources. Children are surprisingly capable of resolving their own problems. Our aim is to access and collaborate with their imagination and knowledge. The interplay between adults and children allows for the enrichment of narratives. Instead of simply reflecting a child's language or listening and making theoretically based interpretations, we seek to be a welcomed and active participant in the child's worlds of meaning. Allowing our own imaginations to be sparked, we join children and family members in the generation of new choices and possibilities. Through having a different kind of conversation about a problem or playing with us in fantasy, the child often finds a "solution" we could never have anticipated.

We use questions to provide linguistic resources that the child may connect with his knowledge and imagination to expand possible meanings and open doors to novel ideas (Brunner, 1986). It is important that our contributions and questions be chosen in a way that is mindful of our influence. Loptson and Stacey (1995, p. 19) write:

As children are in a more malleable stage of development compared with adults, it is incumbent upon us that we exercise responsibility regarding the weight of our influence in shaping children's lives and the narratives by which they come to describe their lives. They, too, must be allowed to speak as subjects who have expertise about their own lives, rather than be spoken about as objects who are acted upon by others.

While young persons often appreciate attention paid to their abilities and knowledge, they are not likely to welcome attention to their problems. When asked, "Why did you do that?" "Can you tell me what's going on with you?" "What's the matter with you?" or "Why are you afraid?" children usually respond by saying "I don't know," averting or rolling their eyes, squirming, starting a fight with a sibling, or staring off into space. Young people often appear reluctant to take on self-as-problem descriptions; they prefer to communicate about problems obliquely, in metaphor or in play. Externalizing language is a help in this.

A PROBLEM IS A PROBLEM IS A PROBLEM

"The problem is the problem, the person is not the problem" is an oft quoted maxim of narrative therapy. The linguistic practice of externalization (White, 1989/1997; White & Epston, 1990b), which separates persons from problems, is a playful way to motivate children to face and diminish difficulties.

In a family, blame and shame about a problem tend to have a silencing and immobilizing effect. Moreover, when persons think of a problem as an integral part of their character or the nature of their relationships, it is difficult for them to change, as the problem seems so "close to home." Separating the problem from the person in an externalizing conversation relieves the pressure of blame and defensiveness. No longer defined as inherently being the problem, a young person can have a relationship with the externalized problem. This practice lets a person or group of persons enter into a more reflective and critical position vis-à-vis the problem. With some distance established between self and problem, family members can consider the effects of the problem on their lives and bring their own resources to bear in revising their relationship with it. In the space between person and problem, responsibility, choice, and personal agency tend to expand.

This practice also tends to create a lighter atmosphere wherein children are invited to be inventive in dealing with their problem, instead of being so immobilized by blame, guilt, or shame that their parents are required to carry the full burden of problem-solving. As White (1989/

1997, p. 6) has commented, externalizing conversation "frees persons to take a lighter, more effective and less stressed approach to 'deadly serious' problems."

Soiling was one of the first problems to be externalized by Michael White (1984/1997). In a straightforward externalization, encopresis was renamed "Sneaky Poo." Encopresis is a medical diagnostic term; in itself there is nothing wrong with it. However, the grammar that we use in speaking with and about young people has certain effects. To say that "Tom is encopretic" is to imply something about his identity. To say that "Tom's problem is that he soils his pants" is accurate, but it may be adding shame to an already humiliating situation. To say that "Sneaky Poo has been stinking up Tom's life by sneaking out in his pants" is a more gamesome way to describe Tom's relationship with the problem of soiling. It is more likely to invite Tom's participation in the discussion of his problem. It can also evoke a more sportive stance for Tom vis-à-vis the problem, as we can now talk about how "Tom can outsneak Sneaky Poo and stop it from sneaking out on him." Tom no longer has to be a different kind of person from the one he understands himself to be. In fact, revising his relation with such a problem as "Sneaky Poo" may very well confirm him as being just the right kind of person for the job at hand— "outsneaking Sneaky Poo."

Standing as an alternative to the diagnosis and treatment of pathology, the focus in an externalizing conversation is on expanding choice and possibility in the relationship between persons and problems. Roth and Epston (1996, p. 5) write:

> In contrast to the common cultural and professional practice of identifying the person as the problem or the problem as within the person, this work depicts the problem as external to the person. It does so not in the conviction that the problem is objectively separate, but as a linguistic counter-practice that makes more freeing constructions available.

When they enter therapy overwhelmed by a problem, members of the family may expect that the clinician will discover further underlying conflicts in their minds or relationships. Therapists take an active role in shaping the attributions that are used to describe young persons and families and to explain their problematic situations. When a therapist listens to, accepts, and then furthers the investigation of a pathological description of a child, the child's identity may suffer.[2]

When a problem is externalized, the attitude of young people in therapy usually shifts. When they realize that the problem, instead of them, is going to be put on the spot or under scrutiny, they enthusiastically join in the conversation. Relief shows on their faces. Their eyes light up, as if to say, "Yeah, that's it, that's how I look at it. It's not my fault." They are then in a position to acknowledge that the "problem" happens to be making them and others miserable and to discuss matters with, at times, remarkable candor.

Although in one sense it is a serious pursuit, we find this practice to be inherently playful and appealing to children. Maria, who appears in the introduction, sent Jenny a valentine card one year, with the caption "Poo Poo to Fear and Temper" and little drawings of each on the front. On the back was written "I like talking with you and I like calling fear and temper names. From Maria." Jenna, a nine-year-old whose story appears in Chapter 8, once wrote in relation to a mask she had made of "The Trickster Fear": "You're no longer nothing . . . being nothing made it hard to know you. Once you're named, you can be known and conquered!"

Aside from their understandable opposition to being blamed or shamed, perhaps children are showing common sense in resisting being defined by descriptions that imply that their identities are limited or fixed. Even adults do not find rigid negative descriptions of themselves particularly motivating toward change. Why shouldn't children resist a fixed adult-imposed definition or a normative characterization? After all, identity remains exploratory and relatively fluid well into adolescence.

Viewing the child as facing rather than being a problem is a helpful start to preserving the fluidity of identity formation. Externalization seems a natural fit for many children. It is compatible with the way they typically approach difficulties in the dynamic learning environment of play. In play, along with hats, costumes, and accents, multiple perspectives, personalities, and roles are tried on during "dress-up" and other games. This fluidity allows the child to explore variations of attitude, identity, and behavior—to try out the emotional flavor of the moment or day. In fact, when a child's play is repetitive, ritualistic, or confined in its range of roles and behaviors, we may wonder about abuse or other severe interruptions to developing identity.

For the child, externalization is like playing a game of "pretend." Implicitly, or sometimes even explicitly, we are saying to the child, "Let's pretend the problem is outside yourself and we'll play with it from there." As Paley (1990, p. 7) writes, "'Pretend' often confuses the adult but it is the child's real and serious world, the stage upon which any identity is possible and secret thoughts can be safely revealed."

As therapists, we have been especially trained in the use of words. But practicing the language of externalizing conversations is for us, as for many others, not so much about learning a technique as about developing a particular way of seeing things. As Roth and Epston (1996a, p. 149) write:[3]

> We do not see externalizing as a technical operation or as a method. It is a language practice that shows, invites, and evokes generative and respectful ways of thinking about and being with people struggling to develop the kinds of relationships they would prefer to have with the problems that discomfort them.

We have noticed some benefits for us personally. Focusing our attention on values, hopes, and preferences in relation to problems, rather than on pathology, we find ourselves less fatigued by the weight of the difficulties we encounter. Since we can now put the problem in the spotlight, we can be more forthright in our questions and comments. As well as allowing us to connect with children "where they live," this practice stimulates our creativity as well.

This approach is distinct from most open, unstructured play therapy, in that we collaborate closely with children in play that is actively focused on facing a problem. Children's sense of effectiveness as agents of change clearly increases when they experiment with possibilities in relationship to an externalized problem. In therapy with families the play is mainly with words, using humor wherever possible! But an externalizing conversation is easily enhanced with other forms of expression favored by children, such as play and expressive arts therapy.[4]

KEEPING THE FAITH

We may have sworn when we were kids that we would always remember what it was like to be a kid when we grew up. But how soon we forget! It may surprise us that we have to make a concerted effort to reclaim a knack for playful communication. It is easy to worry about being too playful—or not being playful enough—or to blunder over delicate moments in the therapeutic process by being overresponsible.

There is a certain dark realm where the serious problem reigns and, like Frodo the Hobbit looking up at the looming Mount Doom in Mordor (Tolkien, 1965), we find that it's tremendously hard to have faith that we will find a way out of the predicament with our young friends. But isn't this the way it is in most compelling stories?

Sometimes, like the trail of bread crumbs in Hansel and Gretel's forest, the thread of hope seems precariously delicate as we embark on our journey out of the problem's bleak territory. Moments of uncertainty or a lack of new ideas threaten our confidence. In the face of invitations to be despairing or serious, we take a deep breath and attempt to be present in the here and now. It can be hard to trust that the narrative trail will lead somewhere.

We try to remind ourselves that we don't carry the burden of invention alone. Most children are expert at creative play and will come forth with ideas of their own given half a chance. When we stay curious and open, our faith is rewarded by the mutual creativity that is generated in our relationships with children.

The linguistic bridges that reach between adult and child need to fit the child's developmental stage. If the adult's questions are too broad or abstract, or his ideas not fitting, the child will not connect with them. We clearly need to attend to individual narratives at differing developmental levels, being aware that "there is ample evidence to demonstrate that there are important differences in how children think, know, and understand and that children are not simply ignorant or inexperienced adults" (Garbarino, Stott et al., 1992, p. 41).

Sensitivity and respect are needed to appreciate the range of children's narratives, which are not always verbal and often use other forms of expression. When we are attuned to a child's cognitive capacity, the child will give us feedback by responding verbally and nonverbally to our conversation, connecting with our ideas and questions with ideas of his own.

A child can be invited to discuss the terms for a playful engagement: "What would be a more fun way of talking about this?" "Could we come up with a magic way of solving this problem you're facing?" "What about if we talked about it (or played with it) another way?" If we are considering moving beyond verbal conversation into other forms of expression, children usually have some idea about what they would prefer to be doing. If they don't, offering some choices usually works. For example: "Would you like to show it with a sand picture, or by writing a story about it, or would you like to talk about it with puppets?"

Possible ways to play with children in narrative therapy are endless. Sometimes the child or family comes up with an idea; other times the therapist has one that appeals. Whether approaches that work for the child tend toward the abstract or concrete, making a connection with the child's imagination is often central to this work.

André's Spy Pouch

Seven-year-old André's foster placement was threatened by his violent anger and frequent temper tantrums at home and at school. Jenny worked with André's foster family and supported André in telling his stories of pain about the traumas of his past, including the loss of his original family. For the sake of a placement he really cared about, it was somewhat urgent that the temper tantrums get resolved. Jenny had a conversation with André in which it was established beyond reasonable doubt that he was tired of Temper taking over and that he was interested in becoming a Temper Tamer (Durrant, 1989; Epston, 1989b/1997). André was asked if he wished to sharpen his skills at detecting Temper's appearance before it had it all over him. He was determined to practice stopping it in its tracks. He thought it would be a good idea to "spy on Temper."

During her work with André, Jenny was trying to think of some concrete ways to supplement the verbal play of externalizing language with younger children. Inspired by an idea of Davida Cohen (personal communication, June, 1993), Jenny went shopping for a Temper Tamer's Pouch and Kit. The pouch was one of those with several pockets that a child can strap around his waist. At their next meeting Jenny brought out the pouch. André's eyes lit up as he examined the contents. Jenny suggested that the small plastic spyglass could be used for spying on Temper and the whistle used for "blowing the whistle" on it when it was detected. The notebook and tiny pencil could be used for keeping track of his score against the Temper (times when he calmed himself down); there were also some stickers to put in his success column and a touchstone for remembering to be calm. André had the idea of adding a miniature Ninja figure to help give him strength to stop the temper. He decided that he could touch these objects if he needed to remind himself of his determination and his powers.

André couldn't wait to try using the pouch. The next week he reported that he had caught Temper out several times before it caught him. This provided an opportunity for Jenny to question André about the implications of his success and begin to develop a story around his temper-taming abilities.

Several months later, André made a drawing titled "the House of the Temper's"[22] (Figure 1.1) and dictated an account of his new relationship with Temper.

> The Temper's house is nice. He grows a temper flower. He's got people's hearts around his house. He's a thief and he stole them. Mine was around there somewhere.
>
> My friend doesn't want to be a Temper Tamer. I said, "You follow me, I'm going to the right place." The Temper says "you're my partner," then he sneaks in and steals your heart. He hugs on you and then he gets you in trouble. Then you have to come up and fight him. He wants me to jump on the teacher when she's talking about my friend. I told

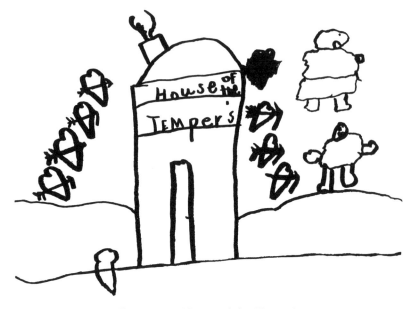

Figure 1.1. House of the Temper's.

him (Temper) he was lying to me. He tried to make me slap the teacher but I got mad at him and called him a jerk. I picked the Ninjas to help me tame him. I can show you how I can turn and walk away from the Temper.

A Day in the Life of Aaron

Listening to a child and family's narrative with an ear for symbolism and metaphor, we may come up with imaginative ideas. However, it is easy to make assumptions about what is happening in a child's experience and then jump into an externalization or come up with "solutions" that do not match the child's understanding of the problem. So we try to listen closely with an open mind to the meanings a child has ascribed to events. Sometimes, if a child's feelings about something seem mysterious or irrational, a detailed exploration will bring his version of the story to light. Having a child walk step by step through an event in words, actions, or art will tend to elicit important nuances and meanings of his account. We can "walk through" with the child in the literal context or in dramatic enactment (Chasin & White, 1989).

For example, six-year-old Aaron's teachers and parents were reporting his sudden rejection of school. Several hypotheses about Aaron were proffered, but his parents did not feel that there was really anything wrong with him. Nobody could get him to explain why his attitude toward school had changed. Dean tried to externalize Aaron's school worries and to get to his story about school through play, but all he could say was "I don't want to go."

Dean arranged to visit Aaron at his kindergarten. By meeting with his teachers and being with Aaron on site, Dean hoped that he would pick up some clues as to what was stressful for Aaron in his school life. Aaron and Dean met early before activities started so that Aaron could give him a tour of his school and walk him through a typical day. They started in the music room, where Aaron showed the instruments he enjoyed banging and rattling. He continued on, walking Dean through a "pretend day," showing where his various activities took place. As they passed the first-grade classroom, Dean noticed Aaron tensing up. Something about the tone of his voice when he said "that's our next room where we're supposed to be" made Dean suspicious.

When they sat down on a log in the playground, Dean asked Aaron what was going on in his mind as he walked by the first-grade classroom. Aaron explained anxiously, "Mrs. Mathews showed us in there; that's where we're going next year." "How come that's a worry to you?" asked Dean. "It's gonna be way crowded in there," Aaron exclaimed, "and some big boys are gonna fight me!" Dean was confused. "How is it gonna be crowded?" Aaron gave him a sideways glance and said, "Cause, you know, we're gonna be in with the first graders too." Finally it dawned on Dean what all the worry was about. He confirmed it with Mrs. Mathews. A month or two before, she had taken the kindergartners into the first-grade classroom and told them that this was where they would be the next year. Aaron's misapprehension was that when the kindergartners joined the first graders in the first-grade classroom it would be impossibly crowded. Not only that, but some of those scary bigger boys would be unavoidable. Aaron was very relieved to find out that the first grade class would be vacating the room and moving on to second grade, leaving plenty of space![5]

The Anti-Anti-Math Club: Math Lovers, Kind of

Unexamined sociocultural assumptions inform many problems that young people face; our therapeutic play includes reflection on these messages and their effects. The Anti-Anti-Math club was formed by two nine-year-old girls who had been struggling with their math grades. It all began when Jenny met with Shawna (who had worked with her before) to talk about the precipitous decline in her math grade. Questioning Shawna about the social context of the problem, Jenny discovered, not to her surprise, that there was an idea current in Shawna's peer group that high grades in math could lead to a girl being regarded as "un-cool." Shawna was asked to consider if boys were viewed the same way and, if not, how come? On reflection, Shawna became upset about the unfairness of such gender-based limitations of girls' abilities. She found it, in fact, discriminatory. As Shawna is biracial—Caucasian and African American—Jenny raised the question of racial discrimination, but Shawna said that the problem had more to do with her gender than her racial background.

During the following week, Shawna remembered that her friend Alice was also having trouble with math grades. Shawna invited her along to discuss the "unfairness of girls' getting a hard time for liking math." Alice readily joined in and quickly grasped the idea of considering their joint problem in terms of the limitation placed by their peer group on girls' expressing their math abilities.

Jenny inquired as to Shawna's and Alice's aspirations for the future. In response they drew pictures of their career choices. One wanted to be a doctor; the other a lawyer. Even before Jenny could form the question in her mind, both realized the relevance of math to their career choices. Alice argued that "It's not fair that we are turned off to math," considering that this might put an end to their dreams.

The pair then decided to stage a puppet play which they called "People That Dis Girls and Math and the Girls That Dis Them." The puppet play portrayed two female characters telling off other female and male characters for their "dumb" opinions about girls and math. Shawna and Alice declared a revolution against "dissing" girls for wanting to develop math skills and talked over the idea of starting a club in order to further their revolution.

At the beginning of their second meeting, Jenny's proposal of a name for the club, "the Anti-Anti-Math club" was met with curiosity. Shawna worked out that the name meant they were against the idea that girls should be against math just because they were girls. Shawna and Alice went on to produce revolutionary art and stories for their club. They also agreed to be available to other girls finding themselves in a similar dilemma.

The girls began collaborating on a series of nine drawings. In the first picture, titled "The Big Brown Pit of Math," a crying girl is standing next to a backboard with sums on it, saying, "I never knew math. I think the boys are better," while the teacher says, "not good!" (Figure 1.2)

Reflecting again on the impact that math might have on their careers, Alice drew a picture of herself as a lawyer working with a defendant before a murder trial saying, "The crime took thirty minutes. And to get to his house it took thirty minutes. So it's an hour." The defendant in the case joins this line of thinking: "So I'm not guilty, 'cause it's suppose to take an hour and a half" (Figure 1.3).

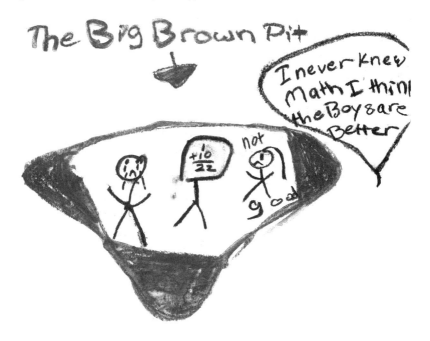

Figure 1.2 "The Big Brown Pit of Math"

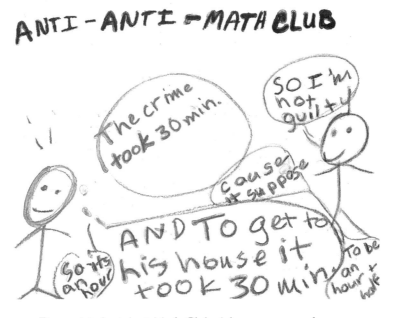

Figure 1.3 Anti-Anti-Math Club: A lawyer uses math.

In the next picture, the two girls are standing. One is saying, "We used to think that we were dum. But not now!" while her friend says, "We used to think that boys were better at math than us. But not no more!" (Figure 1.4). By way of finishing the series, the girls drew a picture together of some sums floating in a sea of color. They titled it "Math lovers, kind of."

Shawna and Alice decided in celebration of their club to make their own entries in a handbook Jenny had that related to school problems. They thought that their insights might perhaps be of use to some other girls. Here is a sample:

> *The problem of math: You see, some girls think that just because you get tricked, you don't like math. I mean, you say you do not like it and soon enough you don't like it. So don't be tricked like I was." (Shawna, age nine)*

> *"Don't listen to people who tell you some subjects don't count, cause they just want someone to be dumb with." (Alice, age nine)*

After two meetings of the Anti-Anti-Math Club, the girls arranged math tutoring and were able not only to catch up in math but to improve their grades.

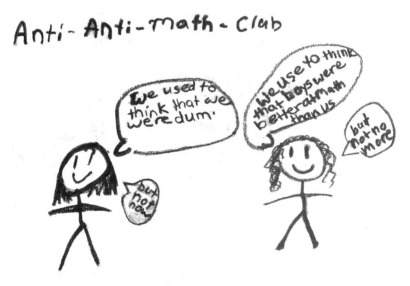

Figure 1.4 "We used to think that we were dum. But not now. We used to think that boys were better at math than us. But not no more!"

USE OF QUESTIONS TO GENERATE EXPERIENCE

In narrative therapy, children and families are invited to share accounts of past events and speculate about the future within the context of a new story in the making (Freedman & Combs, 1995; Tomm, 1987, 1988; White, 1988a/1997; White & Epston, 1990b). This approach is assisted by the therapist's curiosity and keen interest in the existing and possible worlds of children and families. Narrative interviews tend to move forward by way of questions and answers rather than by the therapist's statements, interpretations, or pronouncements. Karl Tomm has typed certain questions as "reflexive," because they are facilitative in intent; they tend to inspire inventiveness on the part of the therapist, and they generate reflection and choice for the child and family. Tomm (1988, p. 2) writes:

> In general, statements set forth issues, positions or views, whereas questions call forth issues, positions or views. Questions tend to call for answers and statements tend to provide them.

Narrative therapy questions are designed to reflect back to the child and family how they have embarked upon new paths or arrived at preferred destinations through the intentions or actions they have contemplated or taken. Freedman and Combs (1996, p. 113) write:

> As narrative therapists we think about questions, compose them, and use them differently than we did before. The biggest difference is that we use questions to generate experience rather than to gather information. When they generate experience of preferred realities, questions can be therapeutic in and of themselves.

Questions also provide important linguistic resources to a child by offering him possible ways of talking about a situation. Thus, the therapist develops, together with the young person and family, alternatives to the problem-saturated narratives that affect their lives adversely. If questions are not consciously used to co-author meaning with the young person, the child may lack the framework to develop a convincing alternative account of his or her relationship with a problem.

Although the use of questions goes hand in hand with a stance of active curiosity rather than professional certainty, our participation as therapists in the conversation inevitably moves it in certain directions. In therapy with children we have so much authority as adults, let alone as therapists, that we can easily take over and run the conversation. We need to stay close to the child's experience, using as much of his detail as possible in our questions. By doing so we will not miss out on the unique contributions children make, along with the synergy that occurs between us.

Questions and ideas may be placed on a continuum from reflective to directive (Tomm, 1988). Our usual guideline is that our activism increases in proportion to the degree of oppressiveness of a problem. In other words, when a child feels silenced and powerless in the face of the problem, we may need to take an active and even leading role in an inquiry that may lead to a alternative story. In doing so, we offer our imagination and energy, formulating ideas and questions that open space within which new possibilities can be imagined.

Ben and Puppy-Boy Talk

Ben's family had been terribly worried about Ben's problem with frequent and uncontrolled vomiting. He had suffered a gastric viral infection, the most obvious symptoms of which were severe nausea and vomiting. Everyone expected that after the infection was resolved the symptoms would follow suit. This, unfortunately, was not the case for Ben. If anything, the nausea and vomiting had increased, to the point where he had to be admitted to the hospital and his nutritional levels sustained by intravenous feeding.

When David first met Ben, he had not taken any food orally for over six months. Although Ben was quite feeble, he and his mother, Tessa, along with his constant companion, the drip, were able to make it into David's office for the first visit. Ben had a sickly pallor and found it hard to sustain conversation, seemingly drifting in and out of it. Tessa informed David that relations with her medical advisors had reached an all time low. The family was very frustrated with the hospital and the hospital staff was frustrated by Ben's condition.

David wanted first of all to contact their medical advisor, to confirm Tessa's take on Ben's medical standing. As Ben was still an inpatient at the children's hospital, David decided that his best option was to see if he could assist everyone involved in Ben's care. Here is David's letter:

Dear Ben's Parents & Medical Advisors:

I am writing to share my thoughts with you all. Situations such as the one Ben is experiencing are extremely difficult for him to deal with but equally difficult for loving parents and concerned medical practitioners. The current understanding—if I have got it right—is that Ben's nausea is left over, a kind of legacy that is starting to have a life of its own. Up until the current understanding, Ben was a "patient" and we all hoped that medical intervention would put things right. Perhaps, in fact, they have, despite the legacy living on.

As a "patient," a young person is expected to hand his life/body over to the medical consultants. In fact, as parents, you would have signed a consent form for this very purpose prior to Ben's hospital admission. To some extent, as a "patient" your job is to lie back and be "operated on." However, how does a young person come to understand that part of the solution rests with him? If our current understanding is right, only Ben, with our assistance, can bring to bear his imagination and abilities on his abdominal feelings, which now have meanings for him. I suspect they have come to mean for him the onset of vomiting and so naturally he must anticipate this. Given his experience over the past six months, to do otherwise would be folly.

The question I have for all of us is this: How do we assist a young person, made infirm by vomiting and whose will has been weakened, to repossess the problem, all the better to oppose it? It is quite reasonable on Ben's part to have arrived at the conclusion that this problem is either his doctor's problem or his parents' problem. And he is right in part. But if our current understanding is correct, no matter what his doctors do and no matter what his parents do, they are his abdominal feelings and his imagination.

I believe, too, that nothing is more distressing for loving parents than seeing their young children suffering in this way. It renders you quite helpless in the face of your children's suffering. I believe nothing is more frustrating for concerned medical practitioners than seeing their young patients suffering and feel helpless to intervene medically. At such times, the frustration of the doctors and the distress of the parents can lead to distrust of the other and to open competition. Such competition could rub out what both parties have to offer and reduce the respect and regard each of you have for the other. I have seen this happen so many times before that I consider it takes careful thought to avoid this trap. What helps is for the parents to realize the frustration of their medical advisors and the medical advisors to realize the distress of the parents.

How can you folks reach some common understanding and mutual regard and respect so some cooperative measures can be taken?

How can Ben be assisted to make the nausea problem his own, despite his infirmity, and invite his parents/medical advisors/nurses, etc., to support him in disowning the legacy of his illness?

Joint action is required and that can only emerge, in my mind, out of cooperation, a shared understanding of the current situation, and creativity. Creativity does not happen in conflict. Ben's situation is a confusing one and everyone will have to allow that the other has been confused up until recently.

I just hope I have made a contribution by drawing everyone's attention to the conditions for creativity and what might well work against that.

Yours sincerely,
David Epston

Several months later, David was called again by both the hospital personnel and Ben's family. Although better cooperation had prevailed, regrettably the symptoms that had overtaken Ben persisted. He was vomiting almost continually; in fact, just inhaling could trigger his slight body to be wracked. The situation had deteriorated so badly that he was on the point of death. The hospital had come up with a proposal for major irreversible surgery that would bypass Ben's stomach. Tessa, who remained with Ben in the hospital, was agonizing over this decision and had been unable to sleep for the previous three nights. The family decided to call on David again since it was the eleventh hour before the surgery was planned, and although no one wanted to take this option, there seemed to be perilously few alternatives.

David met with the family at the hospital eight days before Christmas. A week before, Ben's mother, father, and eight-year-old brother Jonathan had brought him a wonderful surprise—a playful puppy. It was there on the ward that David first met Renée, the most unlikely "dog-person" he ever expected to meet in a hospital. You couldn't help feeling joyous around her frisky puppy playfulness. Tessa, in the midst of her desperate concerns, provided a glimmer of hope. It seemed that Ben was responding well to the puppy and had for short periods been distracted from vomiting. David realized that this unexpected turn of events was full of potential meaning. The puppy just might be able to help Ben turn toward his playfulness and away from the vomiting problem.

Talking with Tessa, David decided right then and there to wheel Ben outside to the nearby park so that he could frolic with Renée. They all had a great time talking and playing together. David visited the next day, and again accompanied Ben in his wheelchair to play in the park with Renée. Already Ben's condition had improved enough so that he could get out of his wheelchair and chase the geese that waddled by the pond. Subsequently, David and Ben agreed to talk about what was happening and to make a recording for the hospital staff so that they could be apprised of the secret of Ben's improving condition. David insisted that Ben keep his options open to decide afterwards with whom he wished to share his revelations.

The interview presented below summarized the content of the first two meetings and sought to confirm and extend the story of Ben's recovery. David began by harking back to the surprise of the puppy; then he asked Ben to go over what had happened. "Can you tell how your Mum, Dad, and Jonathan came into the hospital and they had a surprise for you that you couldn't have guessed? What happened?"

"They came in saying 'Merry Christmas and a Happy New Year' with a basket and a puppy," Ben replied.

"Did you wonder what was in the basket or could you see right away what was in it?"

"I didn't see it but they let me know right away what it was."

"And when did you first realize that this was a live Christmas present? It wasn't a toy but a real dog-person?"

"When I first saw it."

"And do you think she fell in love with you right away?"

"Oh yes."

"And did you fall in love with her right away?"

"Yes."

"Why?" David wanted to know. "Why did you fall in love with her?" Ben thought about this question and did not have a ready answer. David was patient because he knew that the answer would come out of the excitement they shared about this wonderful present; he continued, "What name do you call your puppyperson?"

"Renée."

"Renée. Why did you give her that name?"

"I thought it was a nice name."

"Is it because it's a nice dog, you gave it a nice name?"

"Yes."

David felt this was an important judgment on Ben's part. If he could give a nice dog a nice name that meant he was a good judge of puppy-persons. David decided to test his theory: "If she was really a miserable dog, what name would you have called her? Would you have called her 'Grouchy' or 'Grumpy'?"

"Maybe," replied Ben.

"So you gave her a nice name because she's a nice dog." David continued, "What is the nicest thing about Renée? What do you like most about Renée?" Ben's answer was very important because it showed what his judgment of Renée's being "nice" was based upon.

"She's playful," said Ben. "Playful," repeated David. "Do you think Renée brought back the idea of fun and play into your life?"

"Yes."

"Did she give you fun and play back for Christmas?"

"Yes."

Always on the lookout for the chance to draw out a comparison between problem and the person, David then asked, "Do you think the vomiting problem had taken the fun and play away from you?"

"Yes," said Ben, ruefully.

This seemed to put the finger on the most painful part of the vomiting problem. David wanted Ben to contrast Renée's influence on his life with the influence of the vomiting problem. He asked Ben about his life before it had entered into it, "Now, remind me, because I didn't know you before this problem started to take the fun out of your life, what kind of boy were you before the problem started taking the fun out of your life?"

"A very good boy," Ben answered readily.

Deciding to cross-check Ben's opinion of the way he was before against the way he thought a best friend might have seen him then, David asked who Ben's best friend was. David likes asking children to look at themselves through their own eyes and then through the eyes of someone else, sometimes to reinforce their positive opinions of themselves, as with Ben, sometimes to offer them a more favorable opinion of themselves than they would usually risk stating, sometimes to connect them with a wise or caring adult person who might mentor them.

David's question to Ben was: "If I went and talked to your best friend, Daniel, and I asked him, 'Daniel, before the vomiting problem took away the fun from Ben, what kind of boy was Ben?', what would Daniel say?" Ben readily answered, "I was playful."

"A playful boy," repeated David. "Would he say that you can tell jokes and make him laugh? Can you make Daniel laugh?"

"Sometimes," Ben admitted.

David asked Ben to tell him one of his jokes and Ben did. In fact, Ben's original joke had even been put on Radio Lollipop, the radio station in the children's hospital!

Next David turned back to the subject of Renée and to something Ben had told him earlier, which still remained a secret. "You told me in secret . . . right?" David confirmed with Ben. "It's a secret and no one else has known this until now." Ben nodded conspiratorially. David revealed the secret they had agreed they might consider sharing with the others: "Renée has been talking to you in dog-boy talk!"

"Yes," Ben concurred.

David went on, "Renée has been telling you how to have fun again. And somehow or other, the more fun you have, the less your problem bothers you?"

"Yes," confirmed Ben, "Puppy-boy talk."

"That has been your special secret that you haven't told anyone? Just you and Renée?" David checked.

"Yes," said Ben.

"Do you think every boy should have a puppy or just a boy with problems?" David asked. Ben thought, "Any sort of boy should have a puppy."

"You know when you grow up and Renée grows up you are going to be a man and Renée will be an adult dog, do you think you will always be special friends?"

"Yes."

"If Renée ever had a problem and she got sad, grumpy, or angry with herself or the problem, would you do some boy-puppy talk with her?"

"Yes."

"Would you help her?" David asked.

"Yes."

"Well, that's a pretty lucky dog. And you are a lucky boy."

"Yep," agreed Ben.

"Do you think you've got a pretty good mother and a pretty good father and a pretty good brother to think up that idea?"

"Yep."

"Do you think they knew that Renée would do puppy-boy talk with you?"

"No."

"Was it just your idea and Renée's idea?"

"Yes."

"By the way, how old is Renée?" David wanted to know.

"Seven weeks old," Ben informed him.

"She's still got a lot to learn, hasn't she?" observed David to Ben's agreement. "Do you think because she knows so much already, she could learn more as she gets older?" David asked.

"Yes," Ben agreed.

David knew that Ben had suffered from some pretty bad dreams while he was sick and he now wanted to see if he and Renée could help Ben to sweeten them up a bit. "Ben, you know now that fun is coming back into your life and vomiting is going out of your life, does that mean you'll have good dreams?" To David's delight this was already occurring. "Does that make you have happier dreams?" David continued. "Did you have a Renée dream rather than a vomiting dream? What kind of dreams are you having now?"

"Nice dreams," said Ben.

"Were the vomiting dreams smelly and awful dreams?" David asked, making a safe guess that contrasted the two genres of dreaming. Ben agreed that the vomiting dreams were "awful."

"When did you start having nice dreams?" was David's next question.

"A few nights ago."

"What sort of dream do you think you will have tonight?"

"A good dream."

"Isn't it great to have good dreams?"

"Yes."

David then turned to the prospect of Ben's future without the problem: "Ben, would there be a time in the future when you are older and this problem is behind you, a thing of the past?"

"Yep."

David then checked to see if Ben might be willing to share his anti-vomiting expertise with some other kids in need. Not only would this aid other children, but Ben might learn more about what he knows by teaching it to others. "Would there ever be a time you would help other boys or girls who have problems like this?"

"Maybe," Ben answered thoughtfully.

"Maybe," David repeated, thinking that Ben might need to know more specifically what was involved. "So could I phone you, maybe in six months' time and say, 'Ben, I met this little boy about six and he's got this vomiting problem and it's really getting the better of him, would you help him?"

"Yes," Ben answered unequivocally.

"What advice do you think you would give him?" wondered David. He conjectured that if Ben were to speculate about this, he might be encouraged to distinguish his own knowledge.

"It's quite a long time to battle," Ben began.

"It's a long battle," David wrote as he repeated Ben's words.

"And once you get the hang of it, you start building up," Ben concluded.

"How long do you think it takes before you start battling until you get the hang of it?" asked David.

"If you are battling real good, it only takes about three weeks," opined Ben. "And then, some people won't vomit for a few days but the reason it took me so long was that I couldn't battle that good."

"So when can't you battle well?" David wanted to know.

"Just sometimes."

"Sometimes you can't battle good . . . sometimes you can?"

"Yah."

"What helps a boy battle good?"

"Umm . . . puppies."

"Puppies help you battle good. Anything else?" David asked, always ready to compile a list of helpful ideas.

"A cat," Ben added.

"A cat would do it? Is it love that does it, do you think?"

"Yes."

"And play?" David suggested, reminding Ben of Renée's most obvious quality.

"Yes," agreed Ben.

David wanted Ben to consult to himself about how he felt about his own battling: "When you started battling, did you feel pretty proud of yourself?" Then he contrasted Ben's feelings with the problem's opinions of its Renée-backed opponent: "What did the problem think about Ben? Did it think it couldn't push you around so easily? Do you think it started to know it was up against a pretty strong boy?"

"No," Ben answered, recalling that the problem thought it could have its way with him completely when he was first sick.

David got the idea. "Did you know when the problem had it all over you and was beating you pretty badly, do you think it thought you were a bit of a weakling?"

"Yes," Ben confirmed.

David contrasted the problem's opinion of Ben when he was so defeated with how it might view him now that he was battling back: "And what do you think it thinks of you now? Do you think it thinks you're a bit strong?"

"Yep!"

David sensed Ben's confidence about his renewed strength so his next query stretched the dialogue to a further prospect. "And do you think it is getting a bit scared of you?"

"Yes."

"Is that okay with you?"

"Yep."

"Are you a bit angry with your problem?"

"Yes."

"Why? Why are you angry with your problem?"

"Because I hate it."

"I don't blame you. Do you know that I hate it, too?"

"Yes."

"I like you but I don't like it. Is that okay with you?"

"Yes."

"Do you mind if I like you a lot but don't like your problem at all?"

"Nope."

David felt very reassured that Ben and his problem were on opposite sides of a very important fence. He liked seeing Ben oppose the problem but he wanted to check to see how Ben might handle a comeback by the problem—something that was very, very likely.

"If your problem scored the odd goal against you, would that be okay?"

"Oh, no," replied Ben, giving the problem no quarter.

David wanted to establish Ben's strategy before a comeback caught him by surprise and took the fight out of him. "Well, you can't win 'em all! So would you be upset if it got the odd goal? Or would it make you fight harder?"

"Fight harder," Ben stated resolutely. Now David had a measure of reassurance that Ben would be able to withstand despondency when contending with probable setbacks.

David ended the meeting with Ben with a short review: "Before this problem came into your life, were you sort of a boy who was pretty strong?" Ben explained to David that he was getting his old strength back, but that there was some new play in his life.

"Even though the problem took your strength away, do you think you are getting it back?" David checked again to see if he understood.

"Yep."

"Is it fun to be strong again?"

"Yep."

"Is it fun to have fun?"

"Yes."

David continued his review, composing his questions to address Ben's role as consultant: "I see. Say I met a boy who had this problem and he was feeling really miserable, and I said, 'Look, it could get better—in three days or three weeks—if you start battling.' But the boy said, 'It's hopeless! It's no good. I can't do it! It's too strong!' What would you say to that boy to encourage him?"

Ben did have some extremely pertinent advice: "It's hard but if you don't want to die, you have to battle. And I am doing it. I don't want to die."

"Are you fighting for your life?" David asked earnestly, sensing Ben's intensity.

"Yes," Ben replied unequivocally.

"Good for you. Isn't it funny that ever since you started fighting for your life, you are doing very well at it?"

"Yes."

"And isn't it interesting that you are getting your life back?"

"Yep," replied Ben, making the connection along with David.

David recalled an event from the day before when Tessa, Ben, and he went to the park: "Do you remember yesterday when you ran in the park and chased the geese, and they chased you? How long has it been since you were able to run and have such a good time?"

"I don't know."

"Quite a long time? When was the last time you ran around and had a good time?"

"I don't know."

"Was it a pleasant thing to run around like that?"

"Yes."

"Remember the day before yesterday when you went out to the park, I think you were enjoying yourself but you had to get around in the wheelchair. What happened yesterday? You left the wheelchair behind you and ran?"

"Yes," said Ben. "It's terrible that this problem was taking your fun away, wasn't it?" David asked, comparing Ben's playful day in the park with the day before when he was still wheelchair bound.

"Yes."

"And it tried to take your life; that's even worse."

David was happy to remind himself of what Ben was now looking forward to—a future without the problem. "Do you think Daniel will be glad to see you back at school?"

"Oh, yes."

"Do you think he will come over and play with you?"

"He could."

"Did you think it was a nice letter he wrote you yesterday?"

"Yes."

"What did you feel on the inside when you read that letter?"

"Good."

"Good . . . and did that tell you that you should live?"

"Yes."

"And that he wants you to come back and be his friend?"

"Yes."

"Do you think Daniel is proud of the way you are fighting?"

"Yep." Ben had no doubt.

"What happens when the problem gets hard?" David wanted to know Ben's policy here. Ben explained that the harder the problem gets the harder he would fight. He also turned down David's suggestions that someone could help him fight or do the fighting for him. He had to do it himself, he said. David thought maybe Ben had forgotten someone who could fight with him. Ben agreed he had—Renée. "I'm never forgetting Renée," David promised. "I know Renée is with you all the time. Do you think adults would believe a puppy could help a boy so much?"

"Some people don't."

"Do you think that you shouldn't tell some people your secret? Just tell trustworthy adults?"

"Yep."

"Are there any people here in the hospital you can trust or do you think you should just keep it to yourself?"

"All the nurses are trustworthy," Ben reassured David. "Dr. Webster, too," he added.

David finished off the interview with Ben by exploring what he might do with the tape they had made of their talking together. "Would you like to take this tape home to play on the weekends?" David asked. "It might be good to play before you go to sleep at night. It will give you good dreams and help you sleep. It's nice to have good dreams, isn't it?"

"Yep."

"I'll bet your problems have been spoiling your dreams. Do you think you will have a fun dream tonight?"

"Yes."

"Do you have any ideas of what you would like to dream about? Anything special? You know, if you want to watch a video, you go the shop and get the kind of video you want. What sort of dream would you like to watch tonight? Would you like to have a Ben versus the problem dream?"

"I wouldn't."

"You wouldn't. Ben beating the problem dream? Ben being happy dream?" David had been fishing in the wrong stream. Ben didn't want any dreams at all. "You don't want to have any dreams then? Just a peaceful sleep?" David said.

"Yep," Ben replied.

"Okay then. Well, 'sweet dreams' if you want to have dreams and 'sweet sleep' if you just want to have a sleep."

Ben was discharged not long after this meeting and was admitted only once more. Three months later, Tessa wrote:

I'm very happy with the way things are going. Ben is able to eat five times a day, achieving the time limits we set and even earning up to two nights a week off the nasal feeding tube! Plus regular school three times a week and just being able to do all the things that little boys like to get up to.

He's such a noisy delight to have back home, although we don't ever make forecasts when the end will be! The biggest hurdle I predict will be giving Ben responsibility for his eating. At the moment, we are having to supervise all meals as otherwise he would prefer to forget. Vomiting is still a small intrusion, usually initiated by a cough. On the whole we are happy to be enjoying the time together as a family, and are able to recognize the benefits that have come about from all of this, especially the changes in Ben. He's become a lot more affectionate and able to express his feelings more easily. And amazingly, his wonderful sense of humor has remained intact! So hopefully the news will keep getting better. Thanks for always staying in touch. By the way, if there's ever an occasion where our experience can be of help to another, please don't hesitate in contacting us. I'll sign off and let Ben have the rest of the page.

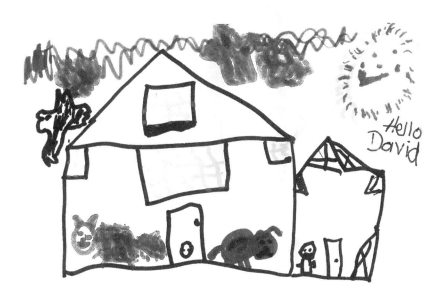

Figure 1.5 "A noisy delight to have back home."

Ben filled the rest of the page with a salutation, "Hello David!" and a drawing of Renée at home (Figure 1.5).

Almost a year later and quite out of the blue, David received a letter from Ben:

To David,

I am all better! And I am in the choir. We are learning Christmas songs. I am having a fight at school because kids say that I cheat on the game bottle tops and then I walk away because I don't cheat. And I am saving for the camp in December, Christmas presents, school books, shoes and the broken gutter.

Love by Ben

P.S. Have an awesome Christmas.

David replied:

Dear Ben,

What a wonderful Christmas surprise for me to learn that you are ALL BETTER! It almost could not have come at a better time for me. And I remember, too, that it is almost a year since Renée had that puppy-boy conversation with you that helped you so much. Do you still love Renée as much now that you are all better? Will you always be thankful to her for coming into your life just when you needed her? Is she growing up to be a special dog? Are you growing up to be a special boy? If so, do you think that has anything to do with getting yourself better the way you did? I am glad you don't cheat. I always thought you were a very honest boy. Are you looking forward to your Christmas camp? Why are you saving for the gutter? Did you break it?

Thanks for your suggestion of an awesome Christmas. You know I think I will have one. If you have the time, write back and tell me your answers to my questions. Say hello to Tessa and your dad and brother and give Renée some extra dog food tonight for me, if you don't mind.

Have a good 1994 without your problem,
    David

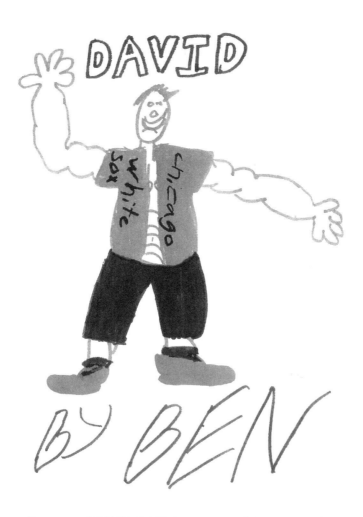

Figure 1.6 "HOW BEN IS. Ben is great! Oh, how HE IS."

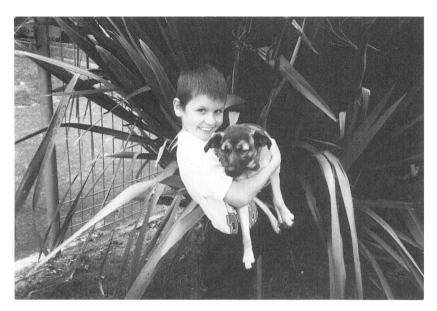

Figure 1.7 Ben with Renée.

A year later Ben sent David a card with a drawing of a well-muscled young boy on the cover wearing a Chicago White Sox jacket (Figure 1.6) and bearing the following information:

HOW BEN IS. Ben is great! Oh, how HE IS. He is playing soccer and dancing the mambo, cha cha, rock and roll and jive!

When contacted about this book, for further follow up Tessa and Ben offered a photograph of Ben and Renée together (Figure 1.7).

SUMMARY

Many problems invite an atmosphere of great seriousness, in which seemingly slender hopes and possibilities can be overwhelmed. However dire the circumstances seem, as in Ben's case, children usually welcome a playful spirit in which to express themselves and explore change. When a therapist can engage wholeheartedly in a playful relationship, even in the face of death, with the view to co-constructing a healing narrative, his courage will be rewarded. When a therapist trusts the creativity available in the mutual interaction of the imaginations of adults and children, their encounter will be fresh, exciting, and full of the unexpected.

. . . .

CHAPTER 2

Getting to Know the Child Apart from the Problem

Take a minute to imagine you are a child and you have come to see a stranger who your parents have told you is going to help with "your problem." After brief introductions, everyone sits down and your parents talk about how worried they are about you. "We just don't know what's wrong with her," they say. They go on to describe your bad behavior. The therapist responds by asking, "How long has this been happening?" What is it like to be in your shoes as this child, to be introduced to someone this way? How do you wish you could be introduced, described, and responded to in a coversation between your parents and a stranger?

A child is forming her impressions of what therapy is all about even as she walks through the door. When a parent or other adult introduces the child to a therapist, she usually has little control over how she is being described, let alone an opportunity to critique or protest those descriptions. She is potentially at the mercy of adults who will interpret her motivations and feelings through their eyes. Further, she may find herself being introduced to a stranger in terms of her putative pathology or problematic behavior. Following common protocol for presenting a problem to a professional person in family therapy, adults may worry or complain about the child in a way that is inadvertently embarrassing to the child.

A young person is likely to want to be seen favorably in the eyes of his parents and siblings, especially when being presented to a stranger like a therapist. How can we as therapists act so that the problem does not define the child's identity, dominate the agenda, and set the tone for the introduction of a young person to therapy? Well, for one, we can attempt to get to know the child apart from the problem. Opportunities arise or can be created from the start to develop a conversation about a child's interests, abilities, knowledge, and characteristics.

MEETING THE CHILD APART FROM THE PROBLEM

In narrative therapy, the therapist and family may start with an externalizing conversation about the problematic situation before the therapist tries to get to know more about the child. This may relieve the child's and family's sense of blame and guilt. However, the problem may be so internalized or merged with the child's identity that even beginning a session by discussing the problem may feel humiliating to her. It may be wise to start by inviting descriptions of the young person that exclude the problem. Because this approach is so unconventional, we seek the consent of parents first.

For instance, at their first meeting, Jenny noticed Patrick staring off into space with a sad face while members of the family busied themselves relating the various negative effects of his misbehavior both at home and at school. Jenny broke in, "I want to be respectful of your concern over the problem, but would it be okay with you if I took some time initially to get to know Patrick apart from the problem?" They were only too willing to tell about some of Patrick's interests and qualities. At the next session, Jenny asked Patrick what he remembered about the previous meeting. He recalled, "They said I'm smart and I can draw really well." Later Patrick confessed through the mouth of a puppet that he had a story about himself—that he was "real dumb." Needless to say, it took some time for things to change, but the foundation had been laid for Patrick to feel respected and learn to respect himself.

Focusing the spotlight on a young person's unique qualities and ideas for change creates a hopeful atmosphere. It is likely that this approach will break the ice and elicit the young person's attention, if not enthusiasm. Invaluable information may be discovered or rediscovered that connects us with the young person and gives clues to resources for dealing with the problem. Such discoveries can become the foundation upon which an alternative story is built, one based upon the child's and family's competencies and sufficiently compelling to stand up against the problem-dominated story.

WHEN A PROBLEM CLOUDS MEETING THE CHILD

If the family's description merges the identity of the young person with a problem or symptom, finding out more about the child's qualities may be hard work. Usually we persevere until we get past the cloud of the problem to see who this young person is when the problem is not over-taking her. It should be noted here that the family's worries and com-plaints must not be ignored. These need to be respected so that we do not appear to be minimizing the seriousness of the situation in a pollyannish manner. An externalizing conversation is invaluable here, as the problem can be referred to in a way that separates it from the young person's identity but does not ignore it.

Permission to proceed in a way that temporarily puts the problem aside can be requested from the young person and family, with a pro-logue such as, "I'm hearing that the Temper is very worrisome to you, and we'll certainly keep addressing it. Would it be all right if I took a little time here to find out more about who Kate is outside of the prob-lem . . . when she's not under the influence of the Temper?" "Can I take some time to get to know you all without the problem, so that I can first acknowledge and respect you as individuals, and within your relation-ships?" Or to the parents, "Do you think Kate might prefer to have me first get to know who she is when she's free of the problem or who she is when she's taken over by it?"

If the problem is already being discussed and is starting to dominate the conversation, these questions can be asked: "Would it be okay with everyone if I talked about the problem in a way that separates it from Kate and takes some of the heat or blame off her?" "Would it be okay with everyone if we all took a holiday from the problem to get some fresh air into the discussion?" "If we put the problem in a box and ig-nored it for a while, what would you tell me about her that's important?"

When there is a particularly dark cloud over the young person, ques-tions such as the following may be helpful: "Has the problem come over your lives like an eclipse that darkens your daytime? Have you been concerned for so long now that you find it hard to remember what you loved or appreciated about her? Have you even forgotten what you once found wonderful about her? Does it tend to rob you of your own self-respect as her parent?"

DISCOVERING ABILITIES

Having established agreement about proceeding along these lines, here are some opening questions: "What would you like me to know about you first?" "What are some things you enjoy doing most, or that you're most interested in?" "What have you been thinking about that you would guess that I, knowing that you are as old as you are, would be surprised by?"

Some questions for family members are: "Can you tell me about some of the abilities and interests Roxanne has that you appreciate about her?" "What makes Roxanne unique?" "What are some things you would like me to know about Roxanne aside from how the problem is affecting her?" "What are you each looking forward to returning to with her when the problem is out of the way?" "What are your hopes and dreams for her?" "If I were shipwrecked on a desert island with Roxanne, what would I come to respect about her? What would I come to depend on her for as time goes by?"

Some questions specifically for the parents might be: "At your proudest moment as her mother/father, what were you proud of?" "If I were a fly on the wall of your daughter's everyday life, what would I admire about her that only those who live with her could possibly know?" "What aspects of your daughter would you like me to know that make you feel you are a great mother/father?" "What should I know your daughter has got going for her to put against the problem, whatever it might be?"

When our focus is family relationships, we might ask, "What can you tell me about your father-son relationship that stands apart from the problem?" "What about the nature of your love for one another in this family is important for me to know from the start?"

Getting to know the young person apart from the problem can give us coordinates and set us on a playful adventure of change. Specific knowledge of her interests and abilities tells what a child might bring to put against the problem. Having this knowledge, the therapist then joins the child in conversation, providing linguistic bridges that enable her to tackle the problem in her own imaginative way.

The myriad abilities we locate are often surprising and delightful. An interest in juggling, drawing cartoons, creating science experiments, or an ambition to write a book on frogs and toads may be revealed. Finding out that a child is interested in martial arts, sports, or dance may lead to metaphors for dealing with the problem. Mental karate, for example, may be used to "fight" an externalized problem. A child may bring to light an active visual imagination and rich fantasy life. Sometimes unusual abilities or resources emerge, such as an uncanny perceptiveness or a child's relationship with an imaginary friend. (In Chapter 10 we focus on these "special and weird" abilities.)

Leon's Game

During a first meeting with Dean, nine-year-old Leon seemed humiliated by his family's discussion of his "lack of self-control," "being a major distraction in class," and "getting in trouble all the time," even though these

problems were being externalized as the "Squirmies." Leon wriggled behind the couch or hit himself over the head with a pillow as they told of
the effects of the Squirmies, which included the embarrassment he experienced during school when he was taken out of the class that was full of
his friends and made to go to the vice principal. The school was now
considering placing him in another class with students he didn't know. It
seemed to everyone that whenever Leon was "acting up with his friends,"
he would lose track of what he was supposed to be doing in class.[1] Before
assuming that Leon's behavior should be tailored to the expectations of
the school, Dean explored the possibilities of expanding acceptance of
Leon's energy and spiritedness by himself, his family, and the school, and
planned a letter to this effect. "The Squirmies" were then carefully re-
sorted to include a list of behaviors that were unacceptable to Leon in
terms of their effects on his school life and friendships.

Dean focused a good part of his interest on getting to know Leon
apart from problem-oriented concerns. Leon spoke proudly of his ar-
chery and fishing abilities and, in particular, his special ability as an
inventor. His parents said that he was always in his room or out in the
backyard inventing new games and scientific experiments. They described his active imagination and determination in pursuing his inventions. The squirming lessened as they spoke in this vein and Dean was
able to see Leon's face for the first time as he leaned forward to clarify or
add a point or two to his parents' descriptions. Following this, Leon
seemed unabashed when a discussion of the problem resumed. Dean
wondered out loud if the Squirmies wanted Leon to lose his friends as
well as his self-respect in class. Would Leon rather put his attention to
school first—and leave the Squirmies outside the classroom on the playground—so he could enjoy being in the class with his friends, instead of
being sent to the office? How could he outwit the Squirmies so that
they didn't keep embarrassing him?

"Have you ever used your talent of inventing games to put the
Squirmies in their place?" Dean inquired. Like other children with abilities such as being able to invent games and experiments, Leon jumped
at the opportunity to put his talents to work. Sometimes invitations
such as this lead to an unexpected inspiration. Leon surprised everyone
at the next session by announcing that he had come up with an invention of his own to deal with the Squirmies.

Dean asked Leon to let him in on it. Instead of inventing a game that
let the Squirmies out, Leon had taken aim at the Squirmies. He had
made a drawing of himself inside the classroom. There were concentric
circles starting from the limits of the classroom to the playground outside. Here was how the game worked. If the Squirmies "got me in the

classroom," ten points went to the Squirmies and zero to Leon. If Leon held off the Squirmies in class (practicing the "calming skills" he had identified with Dean), he got more and more points, up to a maximum of ten, for putting the Squirmies where they belonged—on the playground during recess. His mother chuckled on hearing of Leon's ingenuity. She now understood why his teacher had told her, just the day before, that Leon raced headlong from the classroom, careening past her into the school yard. "He must have been trying to score a ten!"

Wonder Boy

In the following example, David (the therapist) learned from nine-year-old Gregory's mother, Maggie, about some of Gregory's special abilities. These abilities did not fit with the account of the school that Gregory was depressed and needed to be kept back a year. Gregory's ability to imagine, in particular, had an unexpected effect on his story of himself as a student and changed his reputation at school.

Maggie had moved to a different city with Gregory and his younger sister, aged eight, after her divorce. Gregory's new school invited her to a meeting to express their concern over what they referred to as Gregory's "depression." It seemed that they had reached this conclusion because Gregory was disinterested in schoolwork and Gregory's mother had told them that she was recently divorced.[2]

On first meeting Gregory, David inquired about Gregory's abilities. Maggie told him that Gregory was "into wondering, thinking, and working things out. He has a good mind for certain things, especially dreaming." To David, Maggie's description seemed at odds with the perspective of the school, which was that Gregory needed to be put back a grade.

David asked Gregory if he was "more of a play person than a school person." He agreed wholeheartedly, "I just sit there and think." "Does that mean you have more of a mind for anti-work than work?" David continued. Gregory grinned his agreement. "What kind of anti-work is your mind into?" David wanted to know. "Imagining," Gregory shot back. "How do you go about your way of imagining?" David asked. Gregory responded, "I'm looking at other people and looking through their eyes. When I'm watching TV it's as if I know what they're going to say next."

Gregory's excitement about his imagination was palpable. This made David curious about how Gregory's imagination worked: "When you are doing this, do you have to close your eyes, or can you do it with your eyes open?" Immediately bending his head down and pressing it to his knees, Gregory began, "I can put my eyes into my knees. I can see a lot of colors and a streamer." "Oh, really!" exclaimed David. "Can you show me how you do it and I'll write down what you say?"

Gregory continued confidently, "A big blurry three, a big blurry green three."

"Mmhmm," murmured David, writing. "What else?"

"A missile and a truck."

"A missile and a truck. You've got a great knee there!"

Gregory almost interrupted, "Oops, I can see a box."

"A box of what?"

"A lot of boxes."

"Boxes. What's in them, do you think?" asked David.

"Jack in the boxes, two are open. Oh, a motorcycle is coming out of it, and like a little bridge for the motorcycle."

"What color is the motorcycle? Red or what?"

"Silver."

"Is there anyone riding it?"

"Not really."

"It's a riderless motorcycle?" wondered David.

"Yeah."

"Is it going fast or slow? Has it got its motor going or is it rolling?"

"It's got its motor going."

"Who started it, do you think?"

"Probably just started up and pushed it up."

"The Jack in the box did it, do you think?" David guessed.

"Mmhmm," Gregory paused. "I can see a car as well. Yellow."

"Car as well?"

"And I can see a plane—jets!" exclaimed Gregory.

"Jets?"

"It just blew up!"

"Oh dear, it just blew up."

"Yep. Someone just blew the jet up. And I can see the blob. It's a little blob and you can see things in it."

"It is a blob that scares you?" David asked.

"No, it's a friendly blob."

"Mmhmm. Can you put yourself in there?"

"Yeah. I'll try," Gregory giggled. "Oops, I just squashed something."

"Was it a worm or a beetle?"

"No, it was something round, probably a piece of fruit."

"Fruit?"

"No, a soccer ball."

David was inspired by Gregory's vivid descriptions to invite him into collaborative imagining. "Okay, you have just entered a dream," he suggested, "and you have squashed a soccer ball." Gregory nodded.

David wondered to himself if Gregory's imagining skills could con-
tribute to turning around his school problems. With his next question
David put his own imagination to work: "Do you want to be Wonder
Boy in this dream?"

"Okay, I'll try," said Gregory and continued, "I just went into a phone
box and came out."

"Did you change your clothes into a Wonder Boy outfit?"

"Yeah. I was flying along and hit my head on a lamp pole."

"You had better go back for some more Wonder Boy training!" David
said with a grin.

David invited Gregory to enter the mind and use the extraordinary
abilities of Wonder Boy: "Now this Wonder Boy has a bit of a problem
with school. He's a very bright boy."

Gregory caught on and raced forward: "He's sitting at his desk, playing with his pencil. The teacher is angry with him for playing around
too much. He's looking around watching everyone else doing their work."

David asked Gregory how Wonder Boy would go about dealing with
the school problem. Gregory described the wonder tactics Wonder Boy
would use in writing class: "If he was writing an adventure story, he
could stop and imagine he was in the story, then stop and write that
down. Then he would go back into imagining himself into the story and
keep going back and forth until the adventure is over. This would take
Wonder Boy about three-fourths of an hour."

Next they turned to reading. Gregory told David what Wonder Boy
would do with that: "To improve your reading, once you've read the
story through, you could stop and dream the story through, all the way
through, like any TV program. Go back and check to see if your dream
is right, for at least a chapter."

By this time Gregory was so inspired that he imagined Wonder Boy's
tactics being applied at home. "You could even do it at home," he said.
He dictated to David: "Try to turn dishwashing from work to fun. Pretend the dishtowel is a mine in a mine field. But instead of the mine
blowing up, it blows the dishes dry."

Maggie's eyes were wide and unblinking as she heard Gregory apply
his special abilities to various problems. But Gregory had a larger surprise in store for her: "I feel sad for people my age who all they can see
is what they are looking at. And I thought I couldn't do anything at
school. But sometimes I get into dreaming when I can't be bothered
doing work. I just look at something until my eyes can't blink and I start
dreaming. But I can pull out of it when I need to," he explained.

When David asked if it would be wise to "spread this knowledge
around," Gregory told him that "only one friend might get it and an-

other might listen." He added that "adults don't listen at all, but Mum probably would listen."

By this time Maggie had caught her breath again and said, "I had no idea he had such a visual imagination."

Not surprisingly, Gregory responded, "I do it in secret."

"I'd love to be able to take my dreams where I want them to go, like you can!" Maggie marveled.

David's final question to Gregory was, "Has it been worthwhile for you to know that your special abilities can be put to many uses?" Gregory let David know that he had gained a new impression of his abilities and of himself as a student: "I know I can help my problems at school. Before, I didn't know I could do it or be bothered thinking about it. It will help!"

Several months later Maggie contacted David to let him know that the school had gained a new impression of Gregory as well. She told him that the principal had called to inform her that Gregory's "depression had lifted" and that he was doing well in his studies. She added that she thought he was "a very imaginative boy."

GROWING UP AND GROWING THE PROBLEM DOWN

Sometimes we ask about developmental shifts, growth and readiness for change, as well as abilities, interests, and qualities. Many children are keenly interested in "growing up." This idea provided inspiration for four-year-old Andrew to tackle a Temper that had him tantrumming and sometimes smashing his head, leaving him marked with bruises.

Andrew's family was worried. It was hard for Jenny to imagine this charming wide-faced boy, who sat peacefully on his mother's lap playing with his truck, being so taken over by Temper. After Jenny reviewed with his parents, Jean and Brian, some of the effects of the Temper, she turned to Andrew and asked, "Would you like to be the boss of the Temper or should the Temper be the boss of you? Does it make you feel younger than you really are?" Andrew replied that he would like to be the boss and that he was sick of the Temper "bossing me around and giving me bad things."

Jenny then addressed an open question to the family: "I'm wondering, can you tell me about a time in Andrew's development when he was proud of himself for taking a big step with something that he wanted to master?" She paraphrased this for Andrew in four-year-old language: "Andrew, can you think of something you did that grew you into being a bigger boy? And made you proud of being the boss in your own life?"

Brian volunteered an amusing tale about the time Andrew toilet trained himself. Andrew could hardly contain his pride and excitedly chipped in his own comments. There had been very little pressure around toilet training, and Andrew decided on his own that it was time. One day he trailed after Brian into the bathroom and, with a flourish, dropped his diapers on the floor. He exclaimed that he was sick of them and asked his father to give him a peeing lesson. As he listened, Andrew giggled with delight at the denouement of the tale—he never wore diapers again!

Jenny interviewed Andrew and his parents about his general readiness to tackle the Temper, as well as any specific signs that he was ready to take it on. She asked Andrew whether he thought he was old enough to become a "Temper Tamer." Jean and Brian thought he was ready, and Andrew said, "I want to be a big boy boss of my life." Andrew's interest in doing "big boy things" moved him toward feeling that he could stop, or at least "boss" the Temper when it arose. In the face of such enthusiastic determination, the Temper began to make itself scarce within a week or two!

STICKY BEGINNINGS: INVITATIONS TO GET SERIOUS

Invitations to get more serious and rigid instead of playful can occur at the outset of therapy. Remember, it is to the advantage of problems to throw helpers off a relaxed, playful approach from the start. If we were to personify problems as a group they would probably be described as dour, sour creatures, whose main goal in life is to get people to conform to unreasonable sociocultural norms—to keep people enslaved in dark caves with a limited view of things, to entrance them so that they forget their wonderful potential, and to keep a soggy damper on their creativity, confidence and good humor.

To compound the difficulty of staying loose and playful, any child and family therapist or caretaker knows that a child's presence in an unfamiliar place is, by definition, unpredictable, and sometimes unsettling. There are times, probably familiar to every child and family therapist, where one's efforts to engage and enchant the child seem to fall flat. Wild cards can turn up even in the first few minutes of therapy.

A therapist may have tried to get to know the child apart from the problem or to relieve embarrassment or avoidance through an externalizing conversation. She may be pleased with her own verbal dexterity, yet the child is still ignoring the adults, looking off into deep space, or buzzing around the room creating multiple distractions. These moments can be quite embarrassing for parents, who feel responsible for the child, cajoling "you need to sit down and listen," remonstrating "please stop banging the cabinet door and answer the question," and finally pleading or losing their tempers. The following describes an example of how we might connect with a child at such times of initial awkwardness.

Swimming with Ellie

A four-year-old girl, Ellie, came with Tanya, her sole lesbian parent, to a first meeting with Jenny (the therapist). The problem was recurrent "out-of-control behavior." Introductions were made, but as soon as Tanya and Jenny began to turn their attention to defining the problem, Ellie responded with unintelligible silly talk and began to throw herself around the room with abandon. Her mother commented that Ellie often became wild and silly when they were trying to deal with problems. Tanya asked her daughter to please "settle down" and talk to this nice person in "more grown-up language." She wanted her to contain the silliness, she explained, since this was the problem in the first place and they needed to talk about it. She explained that she was worried that Ellie might get even wilder and beyond control. But requests to "speak clearly," "calm down," or "come over here and talk" resulted in rapid escalation of the tension and embarrassment in the room. Ellie muttered something about "who's a doo-doo head" and gyrated around, knocking a vase of flowers over onto the floor.

As she helped mop up the water, Jenny reflected on why so many children wouldn't sit and "cooperate," instead immediately challenging the adults, creating such awkwardness in the consulting room. She thought of all the disruptions of her best-laid therapeutic plans: scenes of children fighting in the waiting room, children playing wildly, children throwing toys at the windows, children interrupting and changing the subject or running about when the adults were trying to get somewhere sensible with them. Jenny sighed. She wished Tanya had come in alone so that she could have just given her some good advice on ways to deal with wild behavior!

The silly talk got sillier and the wild behavior got wilder. Jenny initiated an externalizing conversation. She asked Tanya if it seemed like "Wildness and Tension" fed off each other and whether she found herself getting inadvertently caught up in power struggles with Ellie. Tanya said she was sad that this happened all too easily.

The grown-ups talked over the current challenge and decided to try a more playful way of interacting with Ellie instead of trying so hard to get her to sit still and talk. Jenny asked Tanya about ideas she had experimented with that led to the kinds of communication between mother and daughter that suited Tanya better as a parent and that seemed to work for Ellie. Tanya suggested that they both get down on the carpet so they would be at Ellie's level. Jenny liked this idea and wondered aloud to Ellie, "Can we join you on the floor and in your game too?" (Younger children are more likely to be comfortable playing on the floor than sitting still in a chair, which invites a more adult style of conversation. However, playful communication is not bound by place. Either the chair or the floor might work, depending on the child and the culture of the family and child.)

"Do you like to play pretend games with Ellie?" Jenny asked Tanya, who nodded in response. "Would you like to try one now?" "Okay," said Tanya. Jenny invited herself and Tanya into Ellie's game: "Can we join you? What are you being right now? Are you a fish, a cat, a car?" she wondered. Ellie made a fish mouth by pursing her lips and made silly gurgling sounds. Jenny gurgled back a little. Tanya laughed and joined in. "Is the rug a pond, a river, or the ocean?" she asked. "An ocean," Ellie replied. "It looks pretty wild and stormy in this ocean," Jenny noted. "How does a fish swim in a storm?" she asked. Ellie showed how a fish would thrash around. Jenny and Tanya joined her to make waves and wind with their arms and sounds. After watching Ellie have a good thrash, Jenny noticed some calm developing in Ellie's swimming motions. "Is this how a fish would swim out of a wild storm?" she wondered. Ellie smiled as her body relaxed further. "It looks like the storm is passing. How does a fish have a quiet swim?" Ellie made slow, steady, sweeping movements with her joined palms. "When a fish is swimming calmly, does she find other fish to swim with?" Jenny wondered.

Tanya and Jenny talked about how relaxation and calm had come into the ocean to replace stormy wildness and tension. Jenny wondered if it was more fun for Ellie to use play-acting and movement to calm the wildness, instead of letting it take her over and wreck their talking. She asked Ellie if "Wildness" sometimes made her feel bad, like she was out of control. Did this make her feel alone and tense? Ellie nodded with a sober face and slightly down-turned mouth. "I see you know how to find your way out to calmness," Jenny observed. She continued to interview Ellie about her "self-calming skills." Tanya helped Ellie make a list of these on a chart in different colors, for Ellie to take home as a reminder and as the beginning of a longer list of skills they might remember or discover later on.

Jenny sought to work collaboratively with Tanya and Ellie, to restore and confirm their knowledge of how they got along together in a relaxed way. Tanya reviewed other times when the family had found their way out of Wildness and Tension without a struggle. Noticing that Wildness seemed to take over when Ellie was anxious, Jenny asked whether they might like to "spy" on the Wildness some more, to see what conditions could cause a storm to brew up.

Tanya reported during the next session that she noticed Wildness often grew out of anxiety or disappointed expectations. This lead to brainstorming about ways of helping Ellie to express her expectations about upcoming events and encouraging her to relax into novel situations.

"Wild behavior" had presented itself right away at the first meeting, challenging the adults to deal with it. The shift in communication from an adult-centered model to a playful one eased the tension for everyone. Ellie's exuberant energy was included instead of becoming an awkward barrier to the conversation. She became more willing to talk about the things her mother wanted to address and to explore her own good ideas and knowledge. The metaphoric play gave Tanya a fresh way of seeing how Wildness and Tension brewed up and how they could be transformed. Tanya later commented, "It was useful to see how the tension and anxiety worked against us and remember that we could relax and get our way out of it faster by playing than we could by fighting."

CHAPTER 3

. . . .

Stories of Hope

Stories both describe and shape people's lives. In this chapter we talk about stories—why they are important and how they are conceptualized in narrative therapy. First we offer some perspectives on the shaping of narratives. Next we consider that personal narratives are inextricably embedded in sociocultural, political, and economic contexts. Lastly we discuss the language of externalization, including its grammar, and the use of metaphors to describe person-problem relationships.

When referring to stories, we don't mean fairy tales or even storytelling by way of therapeutic metaphors. People tell stories in their internal dialogue and in social communications about themselves and others. Personal and relational stories come in many forms: some are tragic, comic, or romantic; others are mundane or repetitive. Some are startling. Some inspire; others accuse or degrade.

Meaning is shaped and characters are construed in narrative form. The way we interpret events affects how we behave and interact with others. While no one story can hope to completely capture the complexity of lived experience, what we emphasize or omit has real effects on the teller or the listener.

PERSPECTIVES ON SHAPING NARRATIVES

Problem-saturated stories

Problems tend to be taken very personally. Suffering is magnified when the problem implies something negative about a child or family's identity, describing it as inadequate, helpless, bad, or intentionally negligent. A young person may say, "I'm hopeless, I'm dumb, I never get anything right." "I deserve to die." Others may pronounce: "He's lazy, he doesn't care about anything." "He's a bad seed." Or they may diagnose: "He is conduct disordered," or "She's an hysteric." Relationships may be characterized: "My son and I have incompatible temperaments. We just don't get along," or diagnosed: "They're a dysfunctional family." Problem-oriented descriptions may define a relationship with a physical problem: "He doesn't have the strength to deal with the asthma." Such descriptions seem deceptively simple, but they come with a story (character, plot, circumstance, and intentions) and tend to be backed up by historical "evidence."

When they come to therapy, family members are focused on the problem and its surrounding narrative. When they pay attention to what is going wrong, their stories become saturated by the problem. A problem-saturated story (White, 1989/1997; White & Epston, 1990b) exerts a powerful influence on perceptions. It engenders selective attention and memory, leading family members to lose track of information that doesn't fit the dominant story while noticing information that confirms it, that seemingly proves its fixed suppositions. A story that describes a person in a negative way tends to shape thoughts and behavior unfavorably. The longer attributions of defect or dysfunction are entertained, the more intractable the negative focus becomes.

The problem-saturated story limits perspective, edits out threads of hope and positive meaning, and precludes refreshing possibilities and potentials. Change may then seem impossible in spite of a person's best efforts to take control of a problem or to change others. Finding himself unable to manage his own "defect" or powerless to affect the negative behavior and attitudes of others, a person may experience the problem as overwhelming.

When a young person or other members of a family are trying to tell us their story and convey how burdensome a problem is, we might feel the urge to solve or normalize it. However, if we jump too quickly into searching for solutions or try to put a positive face on the situation prematurely, family members are likely to feel that we have not appreciated the depth or quality of their struggle. An externalizing conversation offers a way to listen closely and join with the family, without confirming limited or pathologizing descriptions. The effects of the problem are mapped in detail, along with the family's preferred way of being and its success in constraining the problem. As we attend to and explore the nuances of their experience of the problem in our dialogue, the effects of a problem-saturated story on family members lives and relationships become evident.

Externalizing language needs to be flexible and continuously matched to the ongoing conversation. It only serves us well to the extent that we stay closely connected with the experience of the young person and family. As Sallyann Roth and David Epston (1996a) write:

> Does the conversation leave people feeling that their unique experience in living is being fully, complexly, faithfully, and poignantly described? Do they feel that the conversation is bringing forth descriptions, observations, feelings, and perspectives that seem very close to their experience as they live it? Does the conversation illuminate the obscure and overshadowed; that is, does it go just a step beyond what has previously registered in their consciousness? Do people feel that they are sharing an experience—not a theory—of what is, what has been, and what might be? Are their experiences being storied rather than deduced and explicated? (p. 152)

Problematic stories as restraints

Rather than attending to problems as symptoms of underlying dysfunction, we focus on the life experiences people would prefer. We can then view the problem-saturated story—undergirded by normative expectations about how people should relate, behave and what beliefs they should hold—as standing in their way (White, 1986a/1997). When we separate a person's or family's preferred experiences from the confines of a problem-saturated story, we find ourselves oriented toward inspiring histories, present strengths, and future dreams and hopes. The way a problem works as a restraint to these is then brought to life.

Let's say that a problem-saturated story described a family in terms of endless misery and strife. We might begin by asking each member of the family, "Can you describe what it is like when you are relatively free of the problem?" or "What exactly would be happening if you waved a magic wand and woke up tomorrow with the problem resolved?"[1] or "When family life is no longer eclipsed by the Fighting or Misery, what experiences will shine through again?"

We ask how the family's choices are being limited by the problem-saturated story. What choices are in harmony with the values that are important to the family and lead in preferred directions? What story might these choices tell about the family and how does that story contrast with the problem-saturated version?

The parents might express a preference for peaceful and close family life and the children might agree that peace would be more fun than squabbling. Then we might ask, "How is the Fighting destroying peace and turning people away from each other? How does the Fighting make you forget what is really important to you? Does it overshadow your love for one another? What would happen if family members united against Fighting instead of being divided by it? How does Fighting get in the way of fun? Is it stopping you all from being able to enjoy going out on adventures together? How does it prevent you from trusting your daughter to go visit her friends and stay overnight?" Such questions get at the influence of the problem (embedded in its story) over the young person or family.

As the effects of the problem-saturated story are being examined, exceptions to its influence are concurrently sought and recovered. These exceptions (sparkling moments) or "unique outcomes" (Goffman, 1961; White, 1989/1997; White & Epston, 1990b) consist of thoughts, motives, intentions, feelings, or actions that are at odds with the problem-saturated story. The family's influence over the problem is now being explored. Attending to outcomes that stand apart from the problem-saturated story, we weave with the family a new story that is encouraging and confirming.

Alternative stories

This brings us to the alternative story. We are keenly interested in the strengths, special abilities, and aspirations of the young person and other members of the family. Woven with events and descriptions that run counter to the problem-saturated story, this information leads to an alternative story—one that reflects both the richness of their lives and their preferred ways of being known. An alternative view develops, one that contrasts with the problem-saturated picture of the child or family.

For example, in Ben's story (in chapter 1) David noticed that something beneficial was happening between Ben and his new puppy Renée. Ben's happiness in communicating with his puppy ("puppy-boy talk") distracted him from the out-of-control vomiting and provided a slim hope in what appeared to be a tragic story of continuous misery and of Ben's body being out of his (or anyone else's) control. Wanting to help a potential new reality take hold, David drew out in careful detail the story of Ben's relationship with Renée, with all it could imply and had to offer. The linguistic work of building bridges of meaning helped healing developments flourish instead of being overlooked and forgotten. Language shaped this event into a narrative of hope.

A heroic element is often present in the emerging alternative story, particularly in therapy with children. A young person can develop the sense of being the protagonist in a story of change and hope, while the problem is considered an antagonist. Against the child's qualities of courage, determination, and ingenuity, for example, the externalized problem is vilified in terms of its "unfair" effects. Not surprisingly, the child, sensing an injustice, is highly motivated to test his mettle and challenge this relationship with the problem. We call the problem's story the plot. The alternative story often develops an heroic counterplot, in which the protagonist conspires to undermine the problem or contests the matter directly with his antagonist.

The child and problem do not always engage as adversaries; that is just one metaphorical way of describing a person-problem relationship (Freeman & Lobovits, 1993; Roth & Epston, 1996a). The resolution of the story is often complex and usually evolves along with the parallel narratives of other family members. A discussion of alternative metaphors for the person-problem relationship comprises the final section of this chapter.

SOCIOCULTURAL CONTEXT OF NARRATIVES

Now we turn to a core dimension of narrative therapy, the sociocultural context of narratives (Freedman & Combs, 1996; Lobovits, Maisel, & Freeman, 1995; Madigan, 1991; Pinderhughes, 1989; Tamasese & Waldegrave, 1993; Tapping, 1993; Waldegrave, 1990, 1991; White, 1991/1992).

By the time they come to therapy, families are usually well steeped in problem-saturated narratives that are influenced by sociocultural assumptions. Just as there is a complex relationship between a family and a problem, there is also a complex relationship between the problem and wider social forces (Rosenwald & Ochberg, 1992). These forces can be both external to the family and internalized by them. It is important to keep track of the social context in which a problem occurs, so that we won't naively assume a problem is solely based in the individual or the family when other factors are at play. Freedman and Combs (1996) write:

> As we work with the people who come to see us, we think about the interactions between the stories that they are living out in their personal lives and the stories that are circulating in their cultures—both their local culture and the larger culture. We think about how cultural stories are influencing the way they interpret their daily experience and how their daily actions are influencing the stories that circulate in society. (pp. 16–17)

Since problem-saturated stories are nested in social, cultural, economic, and gender assumptions about roles and behavior, we inquire about these factors and strive to be aware of how they are affecting different family members. Factors such as racism and sexism that affect children and their families need to be acknowledged and sometimes acted upon. This involves both identifying social conditions and challenging taken-for-granted assumptions that narrow a person's choices. Thus, we include in our therapy narratives about aspects of problems that have their roots in social injustices, such as structural unemployment, housing problems, or discrimination against single parents (Waldegrave, 1990, 1991, 1992).

Martha, Super-Mom

Twelve-year-old Franklin, a Filipino American, was diverted by the police to a youth services agency, where he and his mother met with Dean. Martha, a sole parent, seemed to face Hobson's choice. She could change her career-track position to one with little advancement potential and lower pay so that she could be home with Franklin after school hours. Or she could keep her existing job and find herself unable to "properly" monitor Franklin, thereby confirming her "failure as a mother."

The conversation about social pressures evolved into placing the stereotypes about single mothers and women of color in the workplace in a dialectic with an alternative narrative about Martha. Dean asked Martha what social messages she felt pressured by. She and Dean articulated the ways in which a sole-parent who is the provider for her family is subject to stereotypes about women who pursue their career and "emotionally abandon" their children. "How can a woman and especially a woman of color maintain her career track without being considered a disloyal employee or a neglectful mother?" Martha named her fear that her loyalty as an employee was placed in question when she attempted to mediate between job and family and talked of how she felt this was amplified for an Asian woman. The pressures she felt as a mother were also articulated with questions such as, "Is a stay-at-home-mother the role model I have to live up to? Is it the best or only hope for my child?"

In conversation, Martha recognized that living under these biases had convinced her "that she was only half a worker and half a mother." This had resulted in her feeling that she had to give increasingly of herself to her job and her parenting, more than male or white women workers or parents with partners. Consequently, she had adopted the notion that she couldn't ask much of her employer or her son without feeling that she wasn't "doing enough."

Franklin sat quietly through the discussion. When Dean asked his opinion of the matters at hand, Martha made an interesting discovery. She was surprised to hear Franklin's "nonsexist" view of women. It turned out that he appreciated his mother as a "person" because she had an important job and he saw her a "parent" because she was caring for him.

Choices became available to Martha that had been eclipsed by single mothering stereotypes. She now felt entitled to bring her concerns to her employer in order to seek a reasonable solution. She also asked Franklin to give. She was again surprised that Franklin was interested in signing up for an afterschool sports program at the Boys Club. After some time, Martha obtained approval to go on flex time and a transfer to a corporate site closer to home, which didn't compromise her career.

Supporting family members in recognizing and revising their relationship with these problematic sociocultural effects is one step. The Just Therapy Centre in New Zealand (Waldegrave, 1990, 1992) gathers information about the effects of unemployment, inadequate housing, and racial discrimination on family mental health. They then take the extraordinary step of bringing this information to the public eye through white paper research reports and press releases. Some of those with whom they work also become involved in social action and advocacy for other families.

Hear No Evil, Speak No Evil, Be No Evil

An overt articulation of the sociocultural context of problem-person relationships enables the family and therapist to critically examine the effects of problem narratives and to choose and develop person-affirming narratives. Family members can then team up to free themselves from the limitations placed on their lives by these influences.

Sociocultural issues formed an integral part of twelve-year-old Emma's dilemma. This is the story about how she came up with an experiment to address these issues, along with her "reputation" problem at school.

Emma, who is Caucasian American, had recently moved to a new school. Her teacher complained to her parents that competitive and loud arguments with other students kept getting her into trouble and preventing her from making friends with her classmates. Emma complained that she hated the other kids, saying, "Take one of my enemies, Gloria—nobody likes her, she's annoying, she's violent, she has a bladder problem, and she smells bad a lot."

Her parents felt that she had a part in developing a bad reputation at school, but that it did not really fit with the kind of person they knew her to be. Since Emma is a very bright, engaging, and multi-talented person, they could only speculate about how she had contracted this reputation. Her stepmother Daria took a stab at guessing why. In addition to her nervousness at being a new kid, perhaps it had something to do with Emma's being a dramatic, outspoken girl and a leader. Jenny offered a sociocultural perspective on Emma's difficulties, discussing with Daria the pressures on girls Emma's age to conform to gender roles that discourage them from continuing to develop their spontaneous and lucid voices.[2] Emma listened with interest.

Daria and Jenny then talked with Emma about her attitudes toward girls who are leaders and have strong, clear voices. Jenny wondered, "Can a girl have a strong voice and still make friends?" This hit a nerve with Emma, who felt that she had gotten caught up in power struggles with other girls. Jenny continued along these lines, "Can a girl demonstrate her leadership qualities without being considered overly competitive by her friends, 'unfeminine' by the boys, and troublesome by her teachers?" Emma looked at her quizzically. Jenny continued, "What other possibilities are there for girls to work things out?" Daria articulated the bind she was in another way: if Emma expressed herself in a strong voice she risked attracting negative attention and getting into trouble. On the other hand, if she toned down, she risked losing some of her natural leadership ability. What to do?

At the next session Emma just wanted to play marbles. "I don't want to talk about it," she announced, "except I decided to try an experiment. I'll tell you more next time," she added mysteriously.

Several weeks later, when they met next, Jenny told Emma she was waiting with bated breath to hear what had happened. Emma was ready to reveal the experiment, which she called: "See no evil, hear no evil, speak no evil, be no evil." She drew Figure 3.1 while she explained what she had discovered. It turned out she had decided to see what would happen if she ignored "loud trouble" wherever she saw or heard it. She had deliberately tried "staying out of other people's business," which helped her to take a break from getting in fights and trouble. Jenny was concerned that Emma felt required to tone her voice down and repress her vibrant personality. Luckily Emma had discovered through her experiment that she could still be herself and be admired for her ideas. She found this out in her theater class, "a good place, "she said, "to get your drama out." She had auditioned for a lead role in the school play and made friends with another girl who had a "dramatic personality and a voice." A different story line was now developing, one that she felt reflected more of who she wanted to be.

Jenny proposed that she and Emma write a "reputation-changing letter" to the teacher about these discoveries. "It might be a good idea,"

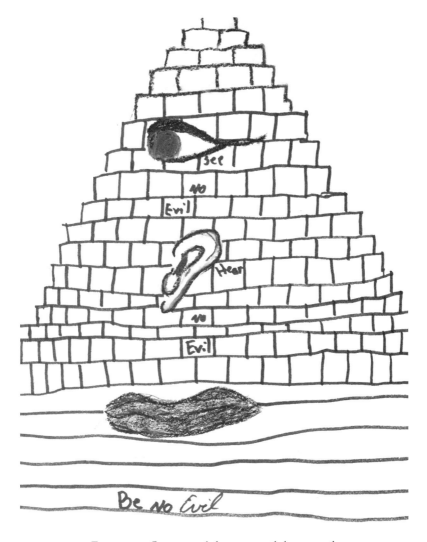

Figure 3.1 See no evil; hear no evil; be no evil.

Emma agreed, but when they sat down to draft a letter together she casually tossed her pen down, saying, "It's okay, I think my teacher's already noticed."

Therapist responsibility

As therapists we rarely stop to examine how narratives are shaped by sociocultural biases and stereotypes and how these encourage us to take a particular point of view, to select some facts as important and give some experiences meaning while others are ignored.[3] The point of view we take as a "reader" of another person's story profoundly influences what we consider noteworthy and meaningful. Following a psychotherapeutic/psychiatric recipe based on the diagnosis and treatment of individual or family pathology, a therapist may identify who needs to be fixed, what is to be diagnosed as pathological, and what expert-guided treatment is in order—all subject to the underexamined cultural, class, and gender biases of the professional and his profession. Such biases affect how the therapist selects from clients' narratives which events are meaningful subjects for "therapeutic" attention and which should be excluded.

When the reference points of a narrative are taken for granted, there is usually little or no opportunity to dialogue, choose, share observations, or comment. Thus we may find ourselves in the position of inadvertently supporting unexamined stereotypes that support narratives of pathology. As therapists we need to examine our own biases, agendas, and values and make them available for comment by our clients, colleagues, and ourselves. Our collaborative aim is to expose the dilemmas that silence and separate us.

When we experience sociocultural issues such as racial or gender prejudice in our consulting rooms, we feel we have a responsibility to address them. For example, Joellen, a fourteen-year-old Caucasian girl complained bitterly about "those black bitches" when discussing the fights she was getting into at school. Jenny felt an ethical responsibility to address the racism; in fact, she couldn't feel comfortable proceeding with the conversation unless she did. At the same time, she knew that if she came across as moralistic she might turn this girl off.

Jenny invited her young client into a discussion about social groupings and racial tensions at school. Jenny wondered what experiences Joellen had had that led to such bitterness. They began by exploring her personal feelings of misery and isolation at school. Did Misery and Isolation promise her company by joining a group that shared "us and them" attitudes?

It turned out that Joellen was feeling uncomfortable about the racial tension, as well as left out and insecure. This generated further questions: Was interracial group rivalry infecting the school with tension? Was she happy and satisfied with her membership in a group that was brought together through hurt and fear? How did she feel about Misery leading her into a group that was brought together by putting down another group? Was her insecurity helped or hurt by Racism and the attitudes it encouraged? Did she think that Racism used a divide-and-conquer strategy to bring insecurity and alienation into young people's lives? What stereotypes did it use to do its dirty work?

Questions such as these invite reflection on the personal effects of prejudicial attitudes on the young person and invite her to identify the problematic relational requirements that maintain such attitudes. Instead of lecturing about right and wrong, we can externalize the effects and operations of "isms" so the personal misery and social alienation they promote can be seen more clearly.

THE LANGUAGE OF EXTERNALIZATION

How do words make a person?

We now turn to an exploration of the effects of grammar and metaphor on a therapeutic narrative. Externalizing conversations are conducted with an externalizing grammar. To experiment with listening to the effects of this grammar, first read the following description of eight-year-old Samuel by his parents and then consider the questions that follow:[4]

> *Samuel is very self-centered. He has no patience. When he can't have just what he wants, exactly when he wants it, he throws a fit.*

How do you feel when you read this? What does this description say to you about Samuel? What does it say about his parents? What does it say about why his parents have brought him for help? What does it suggest in terms of helping Samuel and his family? Who should provide that help?

Read the following description of Samuel by himself and consider the questions that follow:

> *I hate school. The stuff they want me to do is boring, I'd rather play my own games. The teacher and the other kids don't like me because I won't pretend to be interested. If they get in my face, I get in theirs.*

How do you feel when you read this? What does this description say to you about Samuel? What does it say about his school experience? What does it add or subtract from his parents description? How would you feel about helping Samuel? What treatment strategies does it suggest? By whom?

Read the following diagnostic description of Samuel by a therapist and consider the questions that follow:

> *Samuel has an abbreviated attention span. He should be further evaluated for attention deficit hyperactivity disorder. Samuel cannot contain his anxiety well for his age. Samuel*

regresses to a narcissistic and grandiose stage of development in social situations that require age-appropriate cooperation.

How do you feel when you read this? What does this description say to you about Samuel? What does it say about his character and development? What does it add or subtract from his parents' description? What treatment strategies does it suggest? By whom?

Finally, here is an externalizing narrative, with some questions to follow:

Is Samuel the type of young person who can be very clear about what he wants and expects? Do Temper and Impatience get the better of him when he perceives an injustice, or when events don't follow the lead of his vivid imagination? Has this interfered with his peace of mind? Has it affected his reputation with the teachers and other kids? What do his own games offer that elicit his interest?

How do you feel when you read this? What does this description say to you about Samuel? What does it say about his character and development? What does it add or subtract from his parents' and therapist's descriptions? What kind of treatment strategies does it suggest? Who will be an effective agent of change—Samuel, his parents, his therapist?

Each of the above descriptions contributes a different perspective to understanding Samuel, and there is narrative power in each. The externalizing questions are not intended to replace the description of Samuel by himself, his parents, or the therapist, or to describe a new whole "truth" about Samuel. Rather it invites consideration of the effects of viewing the problem from various vantage points on Samuel himself, his parents, and any well-intentioned "helpers."

For example, consider for a moment combining all the different descriptions to see Samuel's situation from multiple perspectives. Now consider removing the externalized description. What has been lost? What has been emphasized? What possibilities are evoked by the externalized description that are not there without it? Who is empowered to make changes in Samuel's life with it or without it?

Crafting person-problem metaphors

The commitment to separate problems from people's identities usually takes us on a conversational journey through several metaphors of externalization, as different features and effects of the problem-person relationship emerge and are named and discussed in a reflective way.

Metaphors describing a relationship between person and problem are chosen or crafted with a child or family using their own language as much as possible. In attempting to name the problem, we usually ask the family or child something like "If we were to give this problem we're talking about a name, what could we call it?" Sometimes a name springs easily to someone's mind. If the child or family is having difficulty thinking of an apt metaphor, we may offer ones other families have come up with. We might ask, "Would you like to hear some ways of describing your relationship with the problem that other kids and families have used, or would you rather keep thinking about it yourself?"

To avoid imposing our own preferences regarding metaphors and the relationships implied by them, we check carefully with the young person and family: "Is this way of talking about it working for you?" "If not, is there another more fitting description we could come up with?" "What would suit you best?" "If this name for the problem is warm, what would make it hot?" "If this metaphor is about at arm's length to what you mean, what would bring it into sharp focus in your mind's eye?"

Problems come in many guises and forms and there are many ways to work—or, rather, play—with them. Some problems can be captured as characters, some named as partners in dynamic duets, others seen as mutating or having several other problem partners in crime. Let us start here by focusing on some relatively straightforward externalizations.

Melanie's mom and dad brought her to see Dean because they were concerned about her "constant sourness" and "grumpy moods." Whenever Melanie was asked a question, no matter how gentle it was, she would look away. Dean guessed that she was embarrassed, perhaps assuming that the problem was deemed to be all her fault. Dean asked her parents what they thought it was like for her to be dealing with "the Grumpies." As the conversation proceeded in this manner of speaking, Melanie began to join in. Instead of responding to every question with "I don't know," she began to talk about how the Grumpies had "messed up" both her fun and friendships.

Melanie's openness to discuss the Grumpies will be helpful in exposing the conditions that support them; perhaps they are related to grief or depression, perhaps they lie in her external environment (abuse or something she is unhappy about at school), or in relationships (tensions with peers or at home), or in internalized sociocultural stereotypes that foster low self-esteem in girls.

A problem such as a child's anger may invite a relatively simple externalization. But what if the child is living with chronically bitter divorce proceedings and has legitimate cause for such anger? Perhaps the family is undergoing the hardship of unemployment and splitting apart under the consequent economic pressures. In such circumstances, a simple externalization such as "getting rid of Temper" disqualifies the child's experience of family distress and leads us astray. Including the family in therapy reminds us to address the context of everyone's suffering.

The social context needs to be named and brought into an externalizing conversation in terms of exploring, for instance, the "effects of unemployment" on each person in the family. The family's "warring," "tension," or "broken apartness" can be discussed in the light of the economic issues they face. The economic conditions that displace them, the cultural practices that support their devaluation, and the accompanying feelings of humiliation can be identified and named. Demographics that show the increased incidence of divorce and family dissolution under these conditions can be shared with the family. Simultaneously, we may look at how the child's feelings of anger and helplessness assist his emotional survival, on the one hand, and how they do not serve such purposes, on the other.

Interactional metaphors

Some problems may be described metaphorically as existing in the space between people. Not only are the problems that come between people externalized, but the relationship may also be externalized. Thus, the problem "Fighting" may be discussed, for example, in terms of its effects on a mother-daughter relationship, as in the following case.

Delia, a mother who was separated from her partner, sought therapy for her ten-year-old daughter, April, because, as she put it, "she seems to hate me these days." April's responses to her mother were scathing. She kept threatening to go live with her father. Delia lamented that communication with April had so broken down and she found herself so angry and tired of the tension that she wondered whether she wanted to continue to live with her daughter.

Since Delia and April hadn't spontaneously offered a metaphor to describe what was coming between them, Jenny shared some that other families used, including, "the Uncommunication", "the wall of hurt," "the gulf," "the history of unresolved resentments," "the rejection dynamic," "the push aways." April thought for a moment and picked "the wall" to describe what was coming between her and her mother. Delia accepted this name. Both April and Delia found it relatively easy to respond to Jenny's questions as to the effects of "the wall" on their mother-daughter relationship. They pinpointed some building blocks of "the wall," such as "tension about Dad's new girlfriend" and Delia's "feeling of rejection" and "fear about being a single mother."

The escalating cycle of hurt and rejection created by miscommunications over where April would live was revealed. April was able to acknowledge that "the wall" was hurting her and that she wished their relationship could "go back to how it used to be." April and her mother cried together and talked about what each of them needed to break through the feelings of rejection. Before long "the wall" was dismantled. The love that had been obscured by "the wall" returned to its rightful place in the center of their mother-daughter relationship.

Dual externalization

Simple externalizations of this kind are often effective and to the point; however, it is important not to get fixated on finding one externalization to sum up the problem. Often a family faces multiple complex problems. It is better to be flexible and prepared to externalize various problematic situations that arise in the course of the conversation.

An especially useful practice for us has been to analyze vicious cycles with families and to look for and support more virtuous cycles. In the next example, a complex dual externalization in a vicious cycle is used to explore a hurtful way of relating between two teenage siblings.

Fourteen-year-old Lauren was so incensed with her younger brother, John, aged twelve, that she couldn't find a kind thing to say about him. John felt desperate and tried to stay as far away from her as possible, in order to salvage his self-respect. Every interaction was dominated by Lauren's negativity and John's silent retreats. These ways of relating formed the basis for their "not being able to get along." From her side of the relationship, Lauren saw John as "acting like a baby," while John saw her as "mean."

When Dean opened up an externalizing conversation by asking Lauren about "the negativity," she told him, to his surprise, that "I can't be openly angry with John." To Dean's "why is that?" she responded that, if she were, he would "just dig a hole for himself." She felt frustrated because this meant she couldn't give him any real feedback about her needs or concerns in the relationship. Due to these frustrating limitations, she kept slipping into "negativity," even though, she said, she did not intend to be mean to her brother.

When Dean asked about the "hole digging" side of things, John was able to allow that "as soon as she opens her mouth, I go dig a hole to hide." This way, a fight would start up before he heard what it was she wanted to say to him. They ruefully admitted that these fights were ruining a brother-sister relationship they both had valued before becoming teenagers. Both felt sad and bitter about what was happening to them.

When Lauren's negativity and John's hole-digging were externalized, they were able to step back from the emotional tangle and reflect on how "negativity" and "hole-digging" were connected in fomenting the bitterness viciously cycling through their relationship. This permitted them to recall times when it was relatively friendly. Memories of a mutually supportive relationship encouraged them to break through the vicious cycle and reestablish a virtuous one. Perhaps, Dean remarked with a wink, they were digging a hole together to pitch the negativity into.

Relationship metaphors

In the early days of narrative therapy metaphors used for approaching problems tended toward the competitive or aggressive. They often captured the idea of expelling a problem from a person's life; for instance, we would speak of "fighting," "kicking out," "winning over," or "beating" a problem. We now believe that these aggressive, "power over the problem" metaphors need examination, as they draw on and may even serve to support tendencies toward domination, competition, and aggressiveness in social relationships. They may also, through their heavy-handedness, discourage a lighter or more playful approach (Freeman & Lobovits, 1993; Roth & Epston 1996a).

As an alternative to metaphoric power struggles, we have explored metaphors of "power in relation to the problem." A metaphor describing an ongoing relationship with a problem can be chosen instead of one describing the effort to defeat it or drive it away. It is important to consult with family members as to their preferred metaphors, since these are rooted in culture and gender. For example, when Karl Tomm (Tomm, Suzuki, & Suzuki, 1990) was presenting the idea of externalization in Japan, it was explained to him by his Japanese colleagues that metaphors of confrontation and struggle were inconsistent with "the basic Japanese orientation of compromise and coexistence with problems" (p. 104).

We may need to learn how to come into harmony with certain emotions and life circumstances, rather than assuming we can get rid of them permanently. It may be a more useful to think of coming into harmony with or balancing bipolar disorder than of banishing it. If a person experiences depression, an externalizing conversation is useful in looking at what "feeds" or supports it and what can be done about it. As Christian Beels (in Cowley, 1995, p. 74) says:

> The question is how you want to face the experiences you're stuck with. What kind of relationship are you going to have with depression? What

have you found effective? It's not an either-or situation, where you're cured or defeated.

Isn't it setting young people up for disappointment to introduce the idea that they can expel human emotions such as anger or fear forever? As clinicians we deal with what meanings persons make of the conditions they face and how these very meanings shape experience. Since we humans have an immense capacity to reflect and to make choices, we can create a conscious relationship with our evolutionary inheritance (Freeman, 1979; Wilson, 1993). For example, we may explore in detail with young persons their complex relationship with fear, in terms of how it might be adaptive and problematic at the same time. We might ask: "When is Fear a friend to you and does you a favor or two? And when is it an enemy that takes over and does you a disservice or three?"

There are certain biologically-based disorders, such as autism, that at this time are not generally amenable to anything approaching a "cure." But this does not mean that a family's relationship to the illness cannot vary and change in terms of how they make meaning of it and deal with it. A young person may not be able to get rid of eczema or asthma; however, these can be negotiated with, leading to greater conscious control of their runaway negative effects. For example, an eight-year-old boy suffered from a rare genetic skin disorder that required his parents or others to bandage his wounds daily. The concern over the problem was so pervasive that it had spread into every corner of their lives; bandaging was taking up to six hours a day and the family could talk and think of little else. He and his parents came to an arrangement whereby their attention and concern for the problem would be limited to a special "bandaging room" where the problem now "resided." They agreed to restrict all conversation about the problem and any remedies for it to its quarters. The family repossessed the rest of the house and the rest of their lives. In doing so, by their estimate, his skin condition improved by 80 percent.

In choosing an appropriate metaphor, we begin by reflecting with the child or family in an open-ended way about the best description of the relationship to the problem. Is the problem "tying them up," "keeping them in prison," "tricking them," or "limiting them"? Describing the problem is a collaborative process, part of the fun as we play with words and symbols.

With children, it is often helpful and fun to personify the problem which is seen as a character, occasionally even a monster. Even an amorphous character can be brought to life by being named, drawn, located in space, etc., in ways that make it simultaneously fantastic and concrete (Figure 3.2). A note of caution here: it is tempting for beginners to turn every problem into a monster. Monsters sometimes backfire. A monster can be an overwhelming image, one that ends up intimidating or even scaring the child. It can also lead to an oversimplification of a family's experience by a therapist.

Depending on the nature of the problem and the family's preferred relationship to it, a multitude of different metaphors can be created (Roth & Epston, 1996a). While some problems invite being tickled with wit and humor, others deserve to be killed off, kicked out, or vanquished from a person's life.

One useful guideline is that the appropriate metaphoric relationship correlates with the degree of oppression of the problem. Some particu-

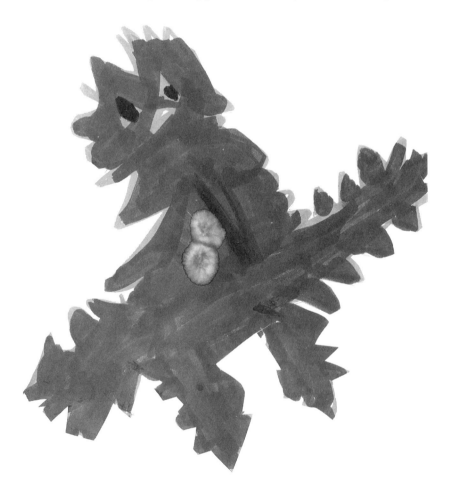

Figure 3.2 "Bad Feelings" externalized.

larly oppressive problems, such as anorexia nervosa, warrant a combative approach, in which the problem is labeled and opposed. For example, imagine a hospital counseling room where the therapist, David, is meeting with an emaciated sixteen-year-old young woman near death. Instead of trying to persuade her that she must keep her drip in, David reads her archival material from the Anti-Anorexia League,[5] in which women speak of their resistance to and struggles against anorexia. He then proceeds with questions such as the following:

"Kirsten, when you are talking to me, are you talking for yourself, or is Anorexia talking for you? If Anorexia starts talking for you or stops you from speaking for yourself, would you consider that you were being gagged? Is Anorexia, in a manner of speaking, talking you into punishing and torturing yourself? Why do you think this Anorexia has forbidden you to have life, liberty, freedom, and happiness? On what grounds is Anorexia denying you your freedom? What are its charges against you? Were you given an opportunity to defend yourself? Do you consider that justice is being done in your case?"[6]

Other problems may be befriended, tamed, or employed for more worthwhile purposes. For example, Temper can be playfully tamed without the expectation that the young person will never feel angry again. A young person may prefer to "turn her back on a problem," "trick it," "tame it," "overthrow it," "soothe it," "prune it back to good stock," as opposed to "stand up to it" (See Figures 3.3 and 3.4), "talk back to it," "stage a revolution against it," "send it to prison," "set a trap for it," "throw it out," "use my imagination to 'transmogrify' it," "send it off into outer space!" or tell it to "go get a life!" For some people, metaphors that relate to spiritual practices may be suitable, such as "rising or climbing above," "letting go of," or "balancing oneself in relation to a" problem. We may also discuss ideas of "turning away from" or "seeking other options to" the externalized problem.

Life-cycle concepts may be a source of metaphors as well; consider "growing out of a certain phase and moving into a new one" or "embracing this transition." With younger children, metaphors of "readiness for a change" based on signs of maturity may be particularly helpful. With this age group, we also use the idea of "you growing up" rather than letting the problem "grow you down." We also might ask: "Have you grown on the inside while the problem has shrunk?"

When people feel that the problem is a "part of" them or decline to participate in externalizing the problem, we talk about "how to have this part come into alignment with what you want for yourself," or "sort out any useful part of the problem that you want to keep from parts you wish to throw away," or even "how to make friends with this part."

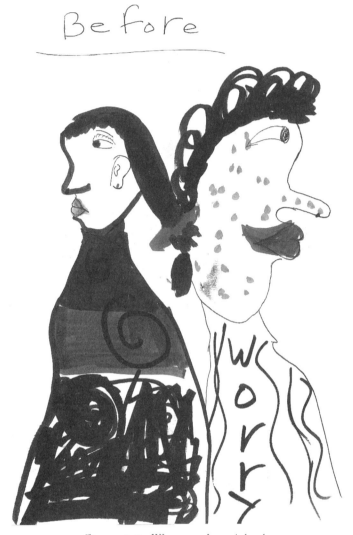

Figure 3.3 Worry on Jenna's back.

Of course, a person's perspective may shift as things progress. As the relationship to the problem changes over time, so might the metaphor. For example, a person may learn to stand up to an overbearing (internalized) "critic," regain self-respect, and then find that the critic has some wisdom to offer when self-respect renders it "bearable." With such a metaphor, gender considerations come into play. For young women, for example, the relationship to an internalized critic or to self-doubt is likely to have roots in gender prescriptions to monitor the self in certain ways.

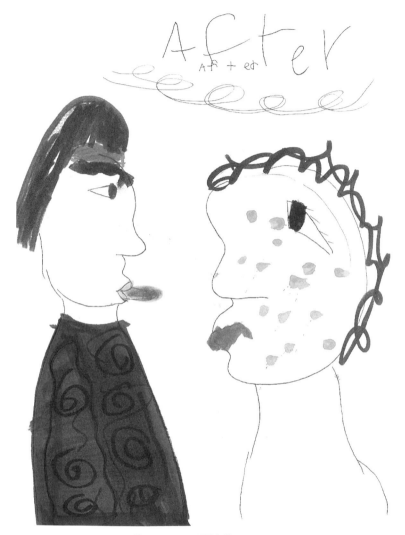

Figure 3.4 "Phhfft" to Worry.

SUMMARY

Externalizing conversation serves to make problem-person relationships available for revision. This practice enhances our ability to provide a safe space in which to critique the taken-for-granted assumptions that constrain us and our clients from leading the lives we prefer to live (Parker, 1995). We encourage the reader to experiment with the ideas presented here with a playful, lighthearted, and inclusive spirit. At the same time, we caution against considering these ideas solely as therapeutic techniques devoid of the sociocultural responsibilities that we have described.

· · · · · · · · · · · · · · · · · · · ·
Parents in Child-Inclusive
Family Therapy

In family therapy, both children and their caretakers[1] have relationships with the problem at hand. This chapter is about parents' participation in a child-focused narrative family therapy. We offer three parallel perspectives to discuss this: (1) the roles parents take as they participate in playful approaches focused on the child's relationship to the problem; (2) the mutual influence of parents and children, but especially the significant influence children have on parents—presenting growthful challenges for them that a therapist can help name and support; and (3) the effects of sociocultural stereotypes and expectations on the self-perceptions and actions of parents. Finally, we present a specific approach to the feeding problems of young children that illustrates how the concerns of the parents and sociocultural issues are addressed while they ally with their child in playfully resolving the problem.

We are open to meeting with parents and children in flexible configurations. Frequent consultation with the family guides us in deciding which members or concerned others attend particular sessions.[2] Moreover, throughout the therapy family members are asked where they wish the focus to be. Family therapy is complex; streams of various concerns about particular problems and individuals converge, flow apart, and reconverge. For example, in the story about Ben in Chapter 1, his parents' concerns about interacting with hospital staff were addressed while Ben gained control over his vomiting problem with the help of his puppy, Renée. In Chapter 11 we discuss a child who became a Temper Tamer and inspired his parents to renounce what they referred to as "multigenerational histories of rageaholism" as a way of family life, as well as to examine and oppose glorification of violence by the media.

Some problems are understandably very onerous to parents. Their own stories of pain and struggle need to be heard and addressed while the child's difficulties are approached on her level. For example, in the story of Tony and his family (Chapter 14) his mother and grandmother discuss the difficulties of raising an African American male in an unjust society, while Tony is assisted in his escape from Trouble. In another example (Chapter 11) a couple faces economic pressures while their son, Evan, takes a stand against fighting in the family.

PARENT PARTICIPATION IN PLAYFUL APPROACHES

Many problems that bring families to therapy center on the child, such as school issues, fears, coping with bed-wetting, or a physical illness like asthma. Many of the case stories in this book show a child or children playing a central role in problem resolution, while his or her parents join the endeavor in various ways. It is especially gratifying for parents to see their child applying her knowledge and ability to the problem. Parents are not just bystanders to their children's ingenuity—they catch the spirit and participate actively. Parents often enjoy getting drawn into and contributing to more lighthearted ways of communicating.

Parents can take many roles in a narrative therapy:

- They brainstorm ideas and solutions with the child (e.g., Marina and Robert sending Zoe to school with a pocket full of kisses for her separation worries in Chapter 8).
- They may become co-conspirators, spying on or opposing a problem (e.g., Paul's family backs him in outwitting Sneaky Poo in Chapter 5).
- Similarly, sometimes the family acts metaphorically as a team, with the problem on one side and the family on the other. Each member makes a contribution to dealing with the problem.
- Parents add meanings that contribute to the child's narratives as they emerge in play or in conversation (e.g., Jason's mother in Chapter 15, who looks at his sandtray and contributes to the symbolic meanings he is making).
- They may participate in a ritual or game or "rite of passage" (e.g., the bypass operation in this chapter, the honesty party in Chapter 7, or Jonathon's nightwatching venture in Chapter 13).
- They supply details and examples that develop promising nar-

ratives or exceptions to problem-saturated stories (e.g., provide instances of past success with the problem or a list of the child's accomplishments during the week).

• They form an audience to a child's restorying, corroborate that the child's behavior has changed, and celebrate change with her (e.g., Zoe's parents, in Chapter 8, form a puppet reflecting team to reflect on her story of change).

DESPERATION CAN BE CONTAGIOUS

Often parents tell us that they are at their wits' end by the time they arrive for therapy. The child's communication may have included evasion, avoidance, procrastination, or hostility. A parent may have been provoked to anger, frustration, or withdrawal. We have noticed our own temptation while practicing therapy to be upset or distance ourselves from a parent when she is expressing intense frustration, skepticism, desperation, or hopelessness. We find, however, that when we welcome parents and their feelings, both good and bad, they engage fully and revelations occur. When we are not afraid of the intense negativity that accompanies serious problems and don't pathologize caretakers for it, hopeful narratives begin to emerge.

Lyle and Shane

When Dean witnessed Lyle harshly telling his truant teen-aged son, Shane, "Go ahead and be a failure. What do I care?" he resisted his initial fear that the young man was being rejected by his father. He was just barely able to retain his composure and his faith in Lyle's parental concern. When he did so he began to hear the intense disappointment that this father was expressing. Lyle despaired that his desire that his son get an education had not been transmitted to Shane.

When Dean heard, "He's got no discipline. He's given up on school. He only cares about his so-called friends, who aren't going anywhere either," he moved closer to Lyle's hurt and frustration to help him articulate his concern. He discovered that this father had a unique understanding of the obstacles that Shane had to overcome to face Truancy. It seemed that Shane had given up on his view of himself as a student who could succeed.

From Lyle's statements that, "He'll never get anywhere with his attitude. He thinks the world owes him something. He hasn't had to really make sacrifices to get what he has," Dean learned to appreciate that this father knew his son well. Lyle knew his son was a person who was spurred on by pragmatic challenges. He understood that Shane was finding these on the streets when he was out being truant with his friends. He also knew that his son felt the academic challenges he faced "weren't real" and that he wanted to quit school and get a job.

Dean also perceived Lyle's estimation of what would be a meaningful measure of change for his son when he said, "If that's the way you feel, the least you could do would be to look your teacher in the eye and tell him that you don't understand the relevance of what's being taught instead of just running away. You've gotta face up to people and tell them when you don't understand something, even if you're afraid you'll look stupid. This problem won't go away if you leave school. It can happen on a job."

Dean learned an important lesson about parenting from Lyle when he told Shane at the end of their meeting, "If school isn't the right place for you to learn how to speak up for yourself and you need to quit and get a job in order to find out who you are and how the world works, I'll support you. I want you to have the education I didn't have but it doesn't look like that's in the cards right now. I don't want you to be someone you're not, but I do want you to be all you can be."

When Dean listened to Lyle's pain and respected him, instead of shielding himself, he came to appreciate the full complexity of this father's struggle. He appreciated Lyle's desire to love and accept Shane for who he was, while at the same time not wanting to collude with his son to avoid the effort to become "all you can be."

CHILDREN'S INFLUENCE ON PARENTS
IN FAMILY THERAPY

It is much easier for family therapists to articulate the influence that parents have on children than vice versa. One of the most obvious times when a child can become very influential is when a problem takes the family to therapy. This opportunity for parental change should not be missed by excluding children from the therapy. A family therapist can unite with the parents to identify their aspirations and provide a forum for personal and family change.

For example, Ray and Nicole and their six-year-old son Kevin struggled successfully to recover emotionally from a racist incident where Kevin was assaulted and nearly smothered to death by three white boys at his school (Lobovits, Maisel, & Freeman, 1995). They met the challenges that faced them by defining "standing up to prejudice" as a positive family legacy, they asserted their unique cultural identity as African

Americans in a predominantly white school situation and therapy, and they tapped the wellspring of their spirituality to endure and persevere in spite of obstacles. Needless to say, it is unfortunate that this family should be faced with such a challenge at all.

In other cases, when children have suffered abuse or have perpetrated abuse themselves, we have seen parents take up the task of bringing an end to multigenerational patterns of their own, such as abusive rage, alcoholism, prejudice, or rigid gender role expectations.

We have found it very heartening to witness parents who are willing to take the same "medicine" they are prescribing for their children. We have seen parents become inspired by their children to tame their own tempers, face their own fears, or become more influential in their own lives vis-à-vis an illness or disability.

At times we are asked by family members to focus on difficulties in family communication, such as arguing, "not minding," power struggles, and so on. We find that difficulties in parent-child communication improve when the child not only becomes an active participant in the family dialogue about the problem at hand but also finds that her concerns are granted a valued place in the wider forum of family interests. As Chasin and White (1989, p. 5) aptly put it, "Each child brings to the session not only a separate viewpoint, but also uniquely evocative and contributory modes of communicating, often characterized by immediacy, spontaneity, and refreshing candor." To this we would add humor, laughter, and opportunities for parental growth and change.

SOCIAL EXPECTATIONS OF PARENTS

Conventional helping strategies may involve isolating the child from the parents in therapy in order to remediate "inadequate parenting" and provide "corrective" experiences for the child or translating the child to the parents through expert interpretations. Walters, Carter, Papp, and Silverstein (1988) have commented that, in some psychological theories and in the culture at large, parents (particularly mothers) are often viewed as wholly responsible for their children's emotional distress. As a result of internalizing these generalized convictions, many parents report feeling blameworthy when their children suffer from problems that bring them to the attention of a helping professional. We try to expose the effects of assumptions about "bad parents" causing children's problems. Once these assumptions are externalized they can be made available for comment and critique. This reduces the corrosive effects of external parent-blaming and internal parental self-blame.

Moreover, we choose to assume that most parents hold their children's interests in mind and heart. Most of the time, we feel, parents are trying to do their best in difficult situations and intend to be helpful and loving toward their children. We try to keep in mind that we, faced with a similar situation, might not cope as well.[3]

This is not to imply naively that at times parents have not taken on attitudes and behaviors that do not serve them or their children well. These can be externalized and a parent's relationships with them explored and revised. If we do not specifically address negative presumptions about parents in our society and in our helping theories, negative attitudes toward parents are bound to be felt by us and conveyed to them.

When we question whether parental behavior is abusive or neglectful, we choose to face those issues with the parents in an externalizing conversation where our concerns are transparent. The problematic behavior is externalized in a fashion that encourages a full and frank discussion. For example, if abusive behavior on the part of the parents is instrumental in a child's fears or temper, the abusive behavioral practices and their sociocultural backing are externalized and discussed. Issues of personal responsibility and collusion with those practices become available for comment and choice-making (Jenkins, 1990).[4] Then, for example, where abusiveness on the part of men is concerned, as White (1991/1992, p. 39) puts it, these men must be "engaged in the identification and performance of alternative knowledges of men's ways of being."

Cultural differences can also play an influential role in our perceptions of parents. It is unreasonable to assume that we completely understand the diverse sociocultural and economic influences that shape parental attitudes and behavior. This is especially true when a family from a different class or cultural group comes to us for help. Families have an existing ecology of thoughts, emotions, and behaviors, based on their unique history and traditions. Assuming that we automatically know what constitutes "good" or "bad" parenting in a family from a different culture than our own shows disrespect for these ecologies and can do more harm than good. Therefore, therapists working with families from different cultures should develop practices that honor cultural differences and hold their judgments and decisions accountable to members of those cultural groups (Lobovits, Maisel, & Freeman, 1995; Madigan, 1991; Tamasese & Waldegrave, 1993; Tapping, 1993; Waldegrave, 1990).

The most loving family can be adversely affected by the stereotypes that feed parent-blaming and constrain their attempts to improve matters. This can cause parents a great deal of distress. In spite of caretakers' best intentions, the presence of guilt and or perhaps ignorance may exert a strong influence, leading them to participate inadvertently in the life of the problem that adversely affects their child. By this we mean that parents can find themselves colluding with a problem when their options for change are restricted to those that conform to the sociocultural expectations and prescriptions placed on them. For example, for parents dealing with a young child who is refusing adequate nutrition, the prescription for a "good" parent requires a parent's increasing preoccupation with the child's food intake and responsibility for changing the child's eating habits. Unfortunately, the more the parent conforms with this expectation the less opportunity the child with the "feeding problem" will have to recognize her appetite and the more the child's sense of responsibility for feeding herself will be diminished.

In another example of inadvertent participation in the life of a problem, a vicious cycle occurs with adolescents when discourses about kids "being out of control" invite parents into feeling that they are bad parents if they don't exercise increasing control, in response to which the adolescent gets into more trouble. This vicious cycle is likely to close off other avenues like remaining curious, talking with the young person about her thoughts, concerns, and interests, and negotiating more or less workable solutions for everyone.

Through externalizing conversations, aspects of the problem-parent relationship, including pressures to conform, are revealed and discussed. For example, in the case stories presented below, several notions are ferreted out for examination as the feeding problem is externalized: (a) very young children have a "disorder" and thus cannot solve it for themselves, (b) poor parenting (especially mothering) is to blame for such early childhood feeding problems, (c) parents have the responsibility to solve the problem, and (d) if they fail they must submit themselves, their failure, and their child to a "helping professional" who will do a better job of it.

Externalizing the problem of parental guilt or blame can take parents out of the hot seat of self-blame, free up their creativity, and motivate change from within their unique ecology of parental attitudes and behavior (White, 1991/1992). When this happens, parents no longer experience the problem as emanating from themselves or their relationships with their spouse or children. Furthermore, they remember that they have aspirations for their children, values to transmit, and cultural identities to preserve that are independent of the problem and its requirements. It is within those hopes, ideals, and traditions that the child-affirming qualities and skills of a parent are nourished.

THE BYPASS OPERATION: AN APPROACH TO FEEDING PROBLEMS IN YOUNG CHILDREN

Our theoretical foray having come to its end, we offer an extended example of Michael White and David Epston's playful approach to feeding problems with young children. We hope to illustrate:

- how the sociocultural context of both parent-blaming and the problem of the child are externalized;
- how a playful approach "bypasses" the problem and parent-blaming and encourages the creative experimentation of the children and their families;
- how the inadvertent participation of parents in the "life" of the problem is made available for their review and critique in a nonpathologizing manner and with an attitude of respect for their best intentions and efforts.

The following description of the "bypass" approach is based on an unpublished manuscript written by Michael and David about ten years ago. We were concerned that it would be left to collect more dust and eventually become lost to the passage of time. This would be unfortunate, since some ideas that we believe to be precious would be forfeited. With Michael's agreement, we have dusted it off and reworked it for this volume.

This approach evolved from Michael and David's being consulted by families on numerous occasions about feeding problems of young children—problems such as refusal of food and inadequate nutritional intake. By the time the parents met Michael and David, these feeding problems often had out-survived various professional interventions and folk remedies.

Parents reported histories of (a) continuing reflux and gastric disorders, (b) childhood illnesses or medications that had suppressed the appetite, and (c) diminishing food intake and body weight. In all of the initial consultations with these families, it was discovered that there was a history of attempts to address the problem through medical workups and through behavioral/psychological practices. Despite this, the feeding problems had not only persisted but worsened over time.

Although there were various presentations of the feeding problems,

David and Michael recognized some common features in their histories. They observed that family members, particularly the parents, were engaged in all kinds of measures to try to get their child to accept food. The parents had usually internalized strong cultural assumptions and social expectations that had them attributing fault to themselves. They believed, sometimes secretly so, that the feeding problem reflected their inadequacy and failure as parents, and they experienced considerable guilt on this account. The children who were the objects of these "helping" efforts had little or no sense of themselves as agents who could effectively act in relation to matters that concerned their own lives.

This central engagement of parents in measures to try to feed their children is totally understandable. If children's nutritional intake is minimal and they are suffering for this, parents will take increasing responsibility in their efforts to modify this nutritional intake. However, as an outcome of this development, children often experience less competence at recognizing their own appetite and assume less responsibility for satisfying it, gradually becoming less able to care for their nutritional needs. David and Michael considered that these developments were reinforced by a socioculturally informed vicious cycle that engages all family members in inadvertent participation in the "life" of the problem. Family members become increasingly organized around the problem, binding themselves together in a repetitive and self-defeating cycle. The real effects of this on all concerned are self-blame, desperation, and burnout.

When the situation became sufficiently desperate for the parents of these children, they all consulted health professionals about the feeding failure. Although most felt shame as parents at this point, this mostly went unrecognized and was not subsequently addressed. The outcome for the parents was a sense of "being judged wanting," regardless of whether or not this was the intention of the health professionals who were initially consulted (some of these parents had been explicitly and powerfully pathologized in their interactions with "mental health" professionals, who had ferreted out exotic accounts of parental responsibility for the etiology of the feeding problem, thereby confirming the parents' worse fears). In response to this sense of shame, and to the explicit expectations and exhortations of neighbors, friends, and relatives, most of these parents had lost touch with the successful stories of their own histories and had withdrawn considerably from their social networks.

Upon meeting with these families and reviewing the various forces at work that were in league with the maintenance of the feeding problems and with the construction of the stories of parental failure, Michael and David found parents and children enthusiastic to step into a novel solution. In response, and with the encouragement of these parents and children, Michael and David developed an approach to feeding problems that they call the bypass operation.

Moratorium on guilt

The bypass approach begins with a moratorium on guilt. It is important for a therapist to encourage a moratorium on guilt and self-blame in order to provide relief for the parents, particularly for mothers. This frees parents of a burden that can be paralyzing and readies them to engage in the exploration of, and participation in, novel approaches to resolving their children's feeding problems. David and Michael have developed a number of ways to initiate this moratorium.

One tack is to predict or preempt the guilt and self-blame of family members through a series of seemingly presumptuous questions generated by information collected from other families. A prologue provides a rationale for the questions. The therapist might begin, "Because I have been involved in many consultations around feeding problems like yours, I have collected a wide range of self-accusations from your predecessors. Can you tell me which, if any, you have been subscribing to? Please listen to them carefully so you can determine which fit your experience. I would also be interested to discover which you have managed to avoid, and whether you could add some original self-accusations to this list that would usefully expand the collection." The therapist then works through the list. For example:

- "Have you accused yourself of breastfeeding your child for too long?"
- "Have you accused yourself of not breastfeeding your child long enough?"
- "Have you accused yourself of having a child too soon?"
- "Have you accused yourself of having a child too late?"
- "Have you accused yourself of being too close to your child?"
- "Have you accused yourself of not being close enough to your child?"
- "Have you accused yourself of contributing to this feeding problem through ambivalent feelings?"
- "Have you accused yourself of contributing to this feeding problem through a lack of ambivalent feelings and through total acceptance of your child?"
- "Have you accused yourself of going back to paid work too early?"
- "Have you accused yourself for experiencing insecurity in your decision about not going back to paid work?"

- "Have you accused yourselves of not being united enough as a couple?"
- "Have you accused yourselves of not being independent enough in your relationship with each other?"

And so on.

This provides just a small sample of the options for self-accusation. The possibilities for this seem limitless (although most parents can identify with some or all of the above). Parents are usually relieved to have their self-accusations not only acknowledged but subtly undermined at the same time. With the use of irony, the therapist and parents can join in the pathos of suffering from taking into themselves the freely available guilt and blame that circulates around parenting, particularly around mothering, in our culture.

It is also possible to engage families in selecting facts that more directly contradict specific self-accusations, for example those that are informed by "mother-blaming." To accomplish this, questions are asked of family members that give rise to stories of events that undermine parents' problem-saturated definitions of themselves and their relationships. Attending to such stories leads to the formulation of further questions that engage family members in detailed conversations about how they have, on these occasions, managed to escape the influence of the powerful self-accusations featured in problem-saturated definitions of themselves as parents. Also, this review puts therapist and parents in touch with various self-accusations that they could have embraced but have managed to avoid so doing.

For example, when Michael was asking Elise and Byron which of these self-accusations were familiar to them and which were not, it became evident that, in spite of their familiarity with these accusations, they had managed to resist the trap of pathologizing their relationship with each other as parents. He asked how it was that they had managed to avoid this despite the despair and desperation they had gone through. What did this achievement reflect about their relationship with each other? In the ensuing reauthoring conversation, Elise and Byron found themselves redescribing their relationship through the identification of its "solidarity," its capacity for "understanding," and according to the important values that provided a foundation for this. As this conversation progressed, and as Elise and Byron experienced the honoring of their relationship in the therapeutic context, they ceased to be so powerfully under the thrall of many of their self-accusations and their sense of failure and hopelessness was attenuated.

Challenging isolation and social vulnerability

Many parents become increasingly isolated in response to unsolicited and conflicting advice offered by friends and strangers. As their children look quite sickly, they often feel obliged to defend themselves against overt or covert accusations of "bad mothering," "child abuse," etc. When they tire of this, they often withdraw from their social networks and isolate themselves from extended family, friends, and acquaintances. To disrupt this, David and Michael found providing the mother (parents) with a "To Whom It May Concern" letter to be very effective. For example:

To Whom It May Concern,

Steven has had a feeding difficulty almost since birth and for this reason is small for his age. He is under the care of Dr. Adams, consultant pediatrician, and is involved with this agency to overcome the behavioral problems associated with a history of feeding difficulties. In our professional opinion, Mr. and Ms. Norman are extremely capable and loving parents coping with an extremely difficult situation. We request that you respect them.

Sincerely,

David Epston

Below is an excerpt from an interview that David conducted with these parents to explore the effects of the letter. It shows not only the ways the letter was used to circumvent guilt and blame but also the pain of isolation.

"Did you think it was important that we gave you that letter? Did you show it to anyone?" asked David. "Yes, I did," replied Alaine. "Good. Under what circumstances?" queried David.

Alaine thought for a moment and then began, "Well, I used to get quite a few people saying to me, 'Oh, what's wrong with him? Doesn't he look sick?' and I would say, 'Well, he doesn't eat and he doesn't grow.' 'Don't you feed him?' they'd ask. 'Aren't you looking after him?' I know these people probably didn't say it the way I took it but at the time that's the way it felt."

The pain in her statement was palpable. "I don't blame you," empathized David. "And what would people say when they read the letter? Did that solve the problem from your point of view?"

"Yes, it would actually," Alaine answered. "They wouldn't utter another word." She laughed. "I showed my doctor, my GP. He was marvelous and he said he thought it was really good. I even showed it to Dr. Adams. If you've got a healthy, bouncy baby, you're a wonderful parent."

David appreciated the irony of her maxim and added, "Yes, right. And if it's sick, there's something wrong with you."

"That's right, it's your fault," Alaine added knowingly. "But it's not at all," she added emphatically. Morris, her husband, added, "Of course, I think that letter was good for us as well, because just a week or so ago we got it out and actually read it again for ourselves."

"If I had known, I would have written a longer letter," David joked. Morris continued, "It's probably the reassurance for what we are doing that made it good for us read it again. Because I never really let people talk to me about it—it has nothing to do with them. But the pressure of neighbors and friends—you know we have lost a lot of friends through Steven, because we just couldn't tolerate their attitudes toward what was happening so we just separated from them all."[5]

Naming the child's inner strength

Along with or subsequent to the work with parents described above, the therapist playfully discovers and engages the child's strength of purpose and responsibility to eat. This type of discovery is usually achieved as an outcome of an externalizing conversation in which there is a detailed exploration of the effects of the "eating problem" on the child's life:

- "What does this eating problem talk the child into about herself?"
- "How does it leave her feeling a lot of the time?"
- "How does it interfere with her physical abilities?"
- "Does it sap her energy?"
- "Does it try to interfere in making friends?"
- "Does it plan to throw the spanner in the works of her connection with mom and dad?"
- "Has it been attempting to ruin her hopes for having more fun?"
- "Has it been trying to wreck her chances of going to playschool or kindergarten, or maybe sleeping over at a friend's house?"

This is just a small sample of some of the questions that might be asked. It is important that they be rendered in an age-appropriate form. With very young children, parents can assist in engaging them in such conversations.

In the course of these externalizing conversations, unique outcomes or exceptions soon become apparent in various domains of the child's life. Eating problems are never totally successful in their attempts to dominate children's lives. There are always going to be examples of the child's strength of purpose prevailing in certain situations, and there will even be examples of physical prowess despite the eating problem's efforts to entirely sap the child's strength. For example, children are often described by their parents as "strong willed" in many respects, including their refusal of food. When this occurs, the therapist expresses curiosity about the whereabouts of the child's "strength" when it comes to solving the problem. Then therapist and the family may jointly puzzle over this anomaly.

Examples of the child's strength of purpose are pooled together, and an inquiry is begun as to the nature of these:

- "Where did the strength come from?"
- "What sort of strength is it?"
- "What would be a good name for this strength?"

Various identities are evoked in the naming of this strength. With young children these are invariably animal identities: "Tasmanian Devil Strength," "Elephant Strength," "Whale Strength," and so on.[6] But for some reason, with these children, more often than not, the strength is named "Tiger Strength."

The naming of the strength in this way provides options for therapist-generated questions that shape extended narratives on the child's "tigerishness" (or "Tasmanian devilishness," or whatever) and the historical importance of this to her survival. As these narratives unfold through the engagement of the parents and the child, the problem-saturated story of the child's life and identity is overshadowed. This sets the scene for the child to develop a stronger alliance with her tiger and to support the tiger's efforts to rid her life of the feeding problem. This also sets the scene for the institution of a far more playful approach to this deadly serious problem, which is a very substantial relief to parents who have suffered so much anxiety and who have experienced their efforts to resolve the problem to be just so much fruitless work.

Whenever we want to call on the young person's strength of purpose we mention its "tigerishness." Questions are asked of the young person that relate to his or her strength of purpose through the tiger metaphor:

- "Do you think you have a tiger inside of you that makes you so strong?"
- "Are you pleased to discover you've got a tiger inside of you?"
- "How did you get such a tiger inside of you?"
- "Have you tamed the tiger inside of you or does it run wild?"

- "When I first met you, do you think I would have been able to guess that you had tamed the tiger inside of you?"
- (To the parents) "Had either of you realized this or is it news to both of you too?"

The moratorium on self-accusations and associated guilt, the erosion of the parental sense of isolation and social vulnerability, the reauthoring conversations that parents and child have stepped into, and the specific naming of the child's strength ready everyone for the bypass operation.

Applying for the bypass operation

Many families have a history of having once been playful together. Even if they have not been playful before, they usually relish the possibility. After a conversation about this past experience or future desire, the therapist highlights the family's expectations of either the return of the long-lost playfulness or the delightful emergence of such an unfamiliar state. In a lighthearted way, the therapist then introduces the application for the bypass operation. The application consists of questions to ratify a family's readiness to proceed playfully. Application questions articulate the family's two options: to further cooperate with the seriousness of the problem or to oppose it and engage in a playful solution.

We provide some examples of these questions here. The responses to these questions invariably constitute a turning point for parents and for children.

Application questions for parents:

- "Right now, do you feel further inclined to explore theories about your culpability for the eating problem, or do you think that now would be the right time to invest your energies in a solution that is entirely different from what has been attempted so far?"
- "In view of what you have been through, do you think it would be wise to continue some of the heavy problem-solving tactics that you have been introduced to in the history of this problem, or would you be more inclined to choose a lighter and playful approach to solving this problem if this were available to you, one that is more in line with some of the fun ways that you can be together as a family?"

Questions for the young person around his/her relationship with "the tiger inside of you":

- "Thank you for teaching me about your tiger strength. What is it that makes tigers strong? Does feeding tigers make them strong, or does starving them make them strong?"
- "If feeding makes tigers strong, do you think you should get in the way of your tiger, or do you think you should step aside and let your tiger feed itself?"
- "If your tiger is your friend, do you think you ought to feed it or starve it?"
- "Do you think you should get in the road of your tiger at meal times, or do you think it would be best to let it past so that it can eat?"

In response to these application questions, parents invariably opt to break from further investigations of culpability and burdensome approaches to the eating problem and express a strong preference for lighter and more playful options. Children decide that it would only be fair to let their tigers feed themselves. They usually express a keenness to step aside to let their tigers feed, so long as this doesn't directly implicate them in eating. Now the family is ready for the operation.

The bypass operation

The bypass operation takes the form of a playful eating ritual. An odd days/even days schedule is drawn up, and parents and children are informed that on every second day only the tiger is to attend meals. On these days the child will make herself scarce so that she can be true to her agreement not to interrupt the feeding of the tiger. On the interim days, the child can attend the meal table as usual, but without any expectation that she will eat.

Parents are asked to make a tiger costume that the child is to wear on tiger feeding days only. After discussing with us some of the options for the development of such costumes, they usually put together wonderful creations. A tigerish persona is brought to life by the introduction of tiger apparel, tiger practice, tiger adventures, tiger menus, etc. Some examples are tiger tails fabricated of plaited yellow and black wool, cut-out paper bags for tiger heads, and screen printed tiger t-shirts. A tiger menu is developed with the help of the child, who is assisted in this task by the parents. Because tigers are "not fussy eaters," the menu is usually selected from a wide range of foods rather from an exacting dietary regime.

Parents are also asked to create a "Tiger Album." The tiger menu can be incorporated in this album, as well as details of different tigerish feats engaged in by the tiger on its feeding days. These details can include photographs that capture on film tigerish stealth, endurance, and vigor. The parents and the child can also go in search of tigerish memorabilia and paraphernalia, and this can also be included in the album. It is recommended that this album be brought to the next meeting to be shared with the therapist.

The costumes, albums, and other paraphernalia encourage a playful ambiance, in contrast to the spirit of deadly seriousness that has pervaded previous efforts to modify the child's eating behavior. This further contributes to a suspension of the parents' anxiety in relation to the child's nutrition. In this approach, the introduction of the tigerish persona makes it possible to bypass the requirement that the child eat or, for that matter, that she have an appetite. The appetite is identified with the tiger, not the child. This externalization of and objectifying of the child's appetite also make it possible for parents and children to bypass their customary anxious interactions in relation to food: It makes it possible for them to unite in a cooperative effort, one that is based on a shared concern for the tiger's adequate nourishment, instead of being pitted against each other in their effort to solve a vexing problem that has everyone at a loss.

Case examples

The bypassing approach is illustrated by two case stories. In the first the therapist, Michael White, follows the above protocol. In the second, David Epston and his co-therapist Phyllis Brock modify the protocol when the family makes a serendipitous and creative suggestion.

Fred

Fred, four years of age, a small, thin boy with poor speech development, was distinctly pale and had large black rings under his eyes. He had been referred to Michael by a pediatrician who had exhausted numerous conventional avenues to ameliorate Fred's self-starvation and was now very concerned about significant growth hormone deficiency. The conventional avenues had included several hospitalizations and various behavioral programs.

Fred had experienced poor health from ten months of age after developing a gastric infection, one that was initially misdiagnosed. As a result, Fred became seriously ill and required emergency admission to the intensive care ward of a city hospital. Since Fred's family lived in a remote area, he had to be transported to the hospital in an air-ambulance. Unfortunately, because this ambulance carried several intensive care specialists, there was no room for either parent to accompany Fred. The parents set out for the city by road, but the breakdown of their car en route further delayed their reunion with Fred, at a time when he most needed them.

It was touch and go for Fred for a while, but he then began to pull through, and he was transferred to a general ward. Soon after his arrival there, he was inadvertently fed a formula that he was known to be allergic to, and his response to this necessitated a transfer back to the intensive care ward. From that point on, it appears that Fred began to associate illness, nausea, and trauma (which included separation from his parents) with the ingestion of food and fluids, which he began to refuse.

Over the next twelve months or so he developed into a very "finicky" eater, and his parents became increasingly concerned about his growth and development, which was clearly delayed. Further investigations were undertaken, but no untoward medical factors were identified. Subsequent to this, various behavioral programs were instituted, but to no avail. Two more years passed without any relief, and with Fred's parents becoming increasingly desperate about his meager diet and about his future. Fred was getting more and more frail.

At the first interview, the parents, Allan and Joan, tearfully filled Michael in on the history of the problem. They had little hope that further consultations would make a scrap of difference, but they did not know what else to do. They had "turned over every stone they could think of." Now they felt fatigued and shattered. They were becoming increasingly isolated from parents in their community who had healthy children and were all too ready to hand out advice. For this same reason, they had also significantly withdrawn from their families of origin. Joan and Allan's account of themselves as failed parents contributed to an acute social vulnerability. They both felt that they had nowhere left to turn. Their sense of desolation was tangible in the consulting room.

Michael speculated about the sort of conclusions they might have reached about their culpability for the problem and about their identities, not just as parents, but also as people. Joan and Allan seemed surprised to hear this. Michael then rose and excused himself, returning a minute or two later to read, and to ask them about, a list of self-accusations he had compiled in his meetings with other parents who had struggled with similar vexing circumstances. Now Allan and Joan were crying again. Michael waited, and then found a space in which to ask what was happening for them. The response took some time in the coming. Allan and Joan said that these tears felt like tears of relief, an experience that they had longed for. Suddenly they didn't feel quite so alone; others had been before where they were now.

Through further exploration of the self-accusations, it was determined that four of the list of thirteen had not occurred to Joan and Allan. This provided a point of entry to a reauthoring conversation that powerfully challenged their deficit-saturated accounts of their identities as parents and as people in a more general sense. In this conversation, both parents visibly separated from a sense of desolation and hopelessness. And they experienced an occasional flicker of pleasure as these alternative stories of their lives began to unravel.

Joan and Allan's responses to the application questions were unequivocal. They were ready to commit themselves to the bypass operation. In the externalizing conversation that followed, Fred was quick to identify his tiger strength (his tiger had swum all the way from a far-off country), although Michael had to depend on Joan and Allan's interpretations of Fred's speech to understand his responses.

"Did Fred know that sometimes when boys and girls eat they feel sick?" Fred nodded his head vigorously.

"Did Fred know that when tigers eat they never feel sick? Lots of children do know this."

In response to these questions, Fred looked at this mother, then his father, and suddenly realized that he was familiar with this fact. And yes, Fred was prepared to stand aside to let his tiger eat so that it could become big and strong and ride bicycles and go fishing.

An odd days/even days schedule was drawn up, plans for the creation of a realistic tiger suit were discussed, a tiger menu was prepared, a story about what the tiger had planned was elicited from Fred with his parents' assistance, and the "ins and the outs" of the approach were discussed. Fred and his parents entered into the discussion with excitement and a sense of fun. Michael discovered that they were actually very humorous people. The family then departed for home, via the zoo. This was to give Fred a further opportunity to become acquainted with tigers and to provide Allan and Joan with a jump-start on the album project— they could photograph some tigers and these could be pasted in the album alongside Fred's story about his own tiger's plans to grow big and strong.

The family returned for a second appointment two weeks later. Fred already looked like a different child. The black rings under his eyes had disappeared and the color had returned to his face. His parents reported that he had done what he said he would; that is, he had been standing aside to let his tiger feed. And they had all been stunned by the adventuresome nature of the tiger's eating habits. Fred had almost "gone over the top," in that on the tiger's "off days" he had been lending a hand by putting some food in his mouth and the tiger had been "coming and eating it." Fred proudly showed Michael his tiger album. It was an extraordinary work that plotted out an alternative narrative of competence and self-sustenance. Fred then donned his tiger suit. Michael got frightened, so the tiger turned into Fred again and reassured him that he wasn't at risk. Joan and Allan joined in the thickening of the alternative narrative with obvious delight and relief.

A third session was scheduled a month later. At this meeting, Michael found that the progress had been maintained despite the fact that Fred had endured a viral infection during the interval between sessions. Fred had started to ride a bicycle, one that he had been too weak to pedal just six weeks earlier. He was now playing with other children, and there was a marked improvement in his speech. Allan and Joan talked about how they now felt differently as parents. They were all getting out more, re-engaging with friends and family (who for the most part were supportive of Fred and his parents in acknowledging and reinforcing the spirit of the bypassing approach).

Michael met with this family two more times and then undertook a follow-up eighteen months later. It was a great reunion. Fred had become a healthy and adventurous young man. His tiger now rarely visited during meals. Fred had mostly taken over responsibilities for his own nutrition. Allan and Joan agreed that they were all "more into life."

Nick

Nick was six and a half when he arrived at the Leslie Centre along with his parents and three-year-old sister Olivia, to meet with Phyllis Brock and David Epston.[7] Phyllis Brock interviewed the family; David Epston was an observer and reflector.

By comparison with Olivia, Nick was wan and looked worn-out and exhausted. Despite the attractions of the playroom, he settled into his chair, resting his head on his shoulder; he was oddly immobile.

Mr. and Mrs. Foster provided David and Phyllis with an account of the problem. Up until eighteen months of age, Nick ate well, so much so, in fact, that Mrs. Foster, formerly a pediatric nurse, was reassured that he was faring well against the well-known statistical profile. Then, suddenly and for no apparent reason, Nick started refusing a balanced diet. He gradually restricted himself to white bread and jam sandwiches. This was relieved only by the occasional apple or raisin. At the time, the Fosters didn't seek help outside their family and friends, hoping that

Nick would "grow out of it." Their dismay increased over time as he grew into his stringent regime rather than out of it. Fearing that he wouldn't be able to withstand the physical and intellectual demands of primary school, the family consulted a pediatrician when Nick turned five. They were reassured that, despite his low weight, he was in no danger. He was prescribed an appetite stimulant and "something else that made him a bit sleepy."

Although Nick gained two pounds after this treatment, his diet was still restricted—he merely ate more bread and jam. The Fosters decided to discontinue his medications. Their concerns increased as Nick became more vulnerable to minor illnesses, was unable to participate in childhood games, and frequently retired to bed before 5 P.M.

By the time they arrived at the Leslie Centre, Nick's parents felt they had exhausted every avenue to the problem's solution, "from bribery to battle." In fact, David noticed a penchant for military metaphors, such as "struggle," "battle," "fight," and "warfare." Mrs. Foster felt more defeated than Mr. Foster, as she "served more in the front lines." A shift-worker, Mr. Foster was not often present at mealtimes.

Periodically, Mrs. Foster would challenge Nick and "he would go to bed with nothing to eat for three nights." "Well," she explained, "then he couldn't go to school, so back to sandwiches. He won another round." Attempts such as this would be followed by another period of appeasement, until her determination to "win a round" returned and she would try again. The Fosters had become so desperate that they took the advice of a friend and sought referral to the Leslie Centre.

The therapists explored Mr. and Mrs. Foster's susceptibility to self-accusation by reading some of the post-treatment commentaries of other families who had come to the agency with feeding problems. These commentaries focused on how other parents had freed themselves from guilt and blame. The Fosters sought to join them.

By the end of the meeting, everyone agreed that they would be unable to go any further until certain preparations had been taken. Mrs. Foster felt just enough hope to start by creating a tiger suit for Nick; that was discussed in some detail. In view of Mrs. Foster's "combat fatigue," Mr. Foster agreed to undertake coaching Nick to roar and growl like a tiger. Just as the family was leaving, something that turned out to be serendipitous and extraordinary occurred. Mrs. and Mr. Foster recommended to the therapists a book entitled *The Tiger Who Came to Tea* (Kerr, 1968).[8]

The second meeting began with Nick demonstrating his strength of purpose by "tiger growling." Phyllis Brock (the interviewing therapist) sought refuge behind a chair. Nick was surprised when the one-way screen began to vibrate. Phyllis explained, "David is behind the screen shaking with fear." When order was restored, the interviewer recovered her composure and inspected the "tigerishness" of his tiger outfit and the "ferociousness" of the screen-printed tiger on his t-shirt.

Another surprise was in order for Nick that day. Phyllis produced her own copy of *The Tiger Who Came to Tea* and invited Nick to sit by her while she told him a story. He readily agreed, saying that he knew the story only too well.

Phyllis encouraged Nick to relax and close his eyes. "When you close your eyes I wonder if you can see pictures on a TV set in your mind?" Nick nodded as she went on. "Is it a black and white TV or a color TV? Is it a big TV or a little TV?" Nick reported that he could see a "big color TV set" in his mind and started visualizing the well-known tiger story on its screen as Phyllis read.

The Tiger Who Came to Tea tells the story of an outrageous tiger who invites himself into the home of a young boy and his younger sister when their parents are absent. He has a prodigious appetite and eats absolutely everything in the house. There are many illustrations of the tiger devouring cakes, tins of Tiger Food, pots of tea, and even water directly from the faucet. His appetite seems quite insatiable. He departs only after he has eaten them out of house and home. When the parents return to their foodless home, their children tell them of the rapacious appetite of their unexpected visitor. The parents seem to take all this in their stride but that night the family has to eat out. The next day, they restock at the supermarket in anticipation of the tiger's next visit. The book ends: "The tiger never came again!"

This story was read by Phyllis almost word for word. Except that, of course, there were some calculated changes. Every time the tiger appeared in the story, alterations were made to put a boy in a tiger suit in place of the tiger, e.g., the boy with blue eyes and blond hair dressed in a tiger suit did such and such or the boy who growls like a tiger did such and such.

Also, Nick's sister Olivia was substituted for the sister in the story. Other changes were made that associated Nick with the ravenous tiger. Before the conclusion of the story, Phyllis hesitated. Nick exclaimed, "And the tiger never came again!" Phyllis took Nick's hand and gave it a light squeeze. She suggested that he return to his mental TV watching. After a moment she said, "In my story, the tiger comes every other day!"

Nick and Olivia were then asked to wait in another room while the adults talked together. Mr. and Mrs. Foster were delighted and unable to conceal their grinning. They joined the therapists in making conspiratorial arrangements for the tiger to come to tea (dinner) every other night. On the non-tiger days, Nick was to eat for himself; on the tiger days the Fosters were to play a cassette recording of Phyllis's new version of *The Tiger Who Came to Tea* while Nick was being outfitted as his tiger. Afterward Nick was to be escorted out the back door and around to the front door while Olivia ran to answer the doorbell. He was to announce himself as a tiger by the requisite growling. Then the tiger would be offered a meal of the food similar to the one illustrated in the book. If they had any difficulties with this, a tiger food lunch box would serve as a replacement.

Three weeks later the Fosters returned to the center. By then Nick's coloring had changed so that he looked normal for a boy in summer time. The family reported that "he was just eating quite happily even on the nights between the tiger visits." Everyone volunteered entries as they catalogued the wide range of meat, fruit, vegetables, and sweets he now was regularly consuming. He was even demanding seconds and had to be reproached for eating off his sister's plate!

David and Phyllis wondered if his tiger was eating so much that he might become overweight. Nick indicated that this was an unlikely prospect. His activity level was incomparable to the first meeting. He rushed around the room, exploring the toy boxes, using the chalk board, and exciting Olivia with his enthusiasm. The Fosters were somewhat baffled by what they described as "his boisterousness," although they assured David and Phyllis that this was a concern for which they would enjoy finding a solution. They stated that they were increasing the interval between tiger visits and thought they would soon discontinue them.

Six months later, when David and Phyllis had a chance to gather follow-up information from the Fosters, Nick's feeding problem seemed quite remote. But the tiger had returned five more times in the interval, which added up to ten times in total. Nick was no longer going to the doctor with minor illnesses, his hair had "life in it" compared to its being "crisp and dry" before and he was now fully engaged in the play activities of his age mates.

The following is an excerpt from the six-month follow-up interview. The interview picks up with Mrs. Foster recalling a visit to Nick's pediatrician several months before they first met with David and Phyllis.

"The pediatrician wasn't all that worried about him," Mrs. Foster began. "But were you?" asked David. "Well, we just felt it was kind of a psychosomatic thing," Mrs. Foster explained, "like there wasn't anything physically or organically wrong with him that was causing him not to be able to eat."

"Well, it was a minimally satisfactory diet, but I guess parents want more for their kids," David mused. "There's more to life than jam sandwiches—there's carrots, potatoes, and lemon meringue pies. Did you feel that he was being deprived of what was his due in terms of pleasure?"

"No," interjected Mr. Foster, clarifying further, "I just thought that he had restricted himself so much that he was in a tight little corner with the energy and things. I could see that he was restricting himself in that way."

David paused for a moment and then asked, "What is your understanding of how this situation turned around so quickly? Any ways of thinking about it that might be helpful to us?"

"Well, you sort of helped us really realize . . . " Mr. Foster started and then stopped to gather his thoughts. "You sowed the seed and gave us some ideas for a way of going about it, and then we were able to carry it out."

"Have you given yourself credit for it?" David wondered. "I worry that parents don't give themselves enough credit. Do you feel that you did it or we did it?"

"You gave us the ideas," replied Mrs. Foster. "We carried them out, but we needed the contact with you to be able to see and adopt a different approach to it."

David shared another family's outlook. "Some other people said, 'We got a different angle on the problem.' "

"Yes, yes, yes!" Mrs. Foster agreed enthusiastically. Mr. Foster concurred, "Oh yes, it was just that different approach and, as we said earlier on, you get so bound up in the thing yourselves."

Next David turned to Nick: "I remember that you listened to a story on a cassette tape—right? And what would happen in the story? Do you remember? What did the tiger do that listened to this story?" Nick responded, "Well, he would come down the pathway and come up to the house and then he'd knock at the door."

"Can you put a sample of his growling on this tape?" David requested. When Nick grinned "yes," David quipped, "Shall I stand back?" Nick laughed and let loose a mighty growl. "Wow!" exclaimed David.

"And then did Olivia open the door?"

Nick nodded.

"Then what would happen when this tiger came into the house?"

"He would go and sit at the table with my apron on."

Just then Olivia interjected, "And he would eat all that food!"

"All the food," confirmed Nick.

"He would eat all the food?" echoed David, astonished.

"Yes, and he would be the last one eating at the end because I always stopped and had two or three minutes rest."

"Why? Did you need a rest because you were so tired from all the eating you were doing?"

"Yes, and after dinner I had ice cream and I used to gobble that up and I always finished it."

"Do you think this tiger got a little bit bigger and stronger with all the food it was eating?"

"Yes," said Nick.

"And do you think this tiger that was getting bigger and stronger started having more fun? Making more noise and playing more?" David continued, building on his theme.

"Yes," repeated a smiling Nick.

"That's a pretty good tiger. Do you think this tiger is a good friend of yours?" David inquired, and when Nick nodded he asked, "What do you want to tell other boys and girls about being a tiger? Anything you want to say?"

Nick documented his comments on the tape: "Well, you start by going to Leslie Centre and they tell you a story."

"What's the story like?" asked David. Nick said into the microphone, "The tiger who came to tea and goes and eats everything and thinks he likes everything on his plate."

"You go to Leslie Centre and they tell you a story and what happens then?" David summarized.

Nick continued, "Then they tell you to make a tiger outfit and then you do your roar like this." And with that Nick let out a mighty roar. Then he paused and added thoughtfully, "Sometimes when I see it though I think, 'Oh, I hope I'm not going to be the tiger again 'cause I feel grown-up.' "

David had to wonder out loud when he heard Nick's comment: "Do you think that you don't need the tiger anymore? You've grown past it?"

Nick nodded, smiling broadly.

"Do you think some boys and girls might be helped by the tiger?" David speculated.

"Yep!" said Nick.

SUMMARY

Over the past ten years, David Epston and Michael White have used the bypass operation with a number of children between the ages of four and seven. These are children who have presented with intractable feeding and appetite problems. This approach has generally followed the guidelines presented here (it has been modified according to the circumstances of each situation), and to date it has been effective in the amelioration of the feeding problems of all of the children referred with such complaints.

Michael and David warn against shortcuts in this work. Such shortcuts are usually the outcome of conceiving of the bypass approach as simply a technique. It is essential that parents be adequately prepared prior to embarking upon this "operation". This preparation should include interventions to undermine parental self-accusations. Without such relief, the chance of success will be severely diminished. They stress the importance of the groundwork that must be laid in preparing for the this approach; this groundwork, informed by the overall orientation and the politics of the work, is a necessity.

David and Michael believe that they have by no means exhausted the possible applications of "bypassing" as a metaphor in working with a range of children's problems, especially those where the child is caught up in a mind-body impasse. They also want to emphasize that care must be taken to discern those children who are "failing to thrive" through neglect, unbelonging, or abuse, from those children and families with whom they would typically employ the bypass approach.

CHAPTER 5

• • • • • • • • • • • • • • • • • • •

Thinning the Plot, Thickening the Counterplot

It is the plot that takes a story in one direction or another, describes its intent, and shapes its meaning. Because it serves these functions one could say that the plot connects events together into a meaningful story. Brooks' aphorism that "A story is made out of events to the extent that plot makes events into a story" (1984, p. 3) aptly describes plotting as the glue that establishes a story's coherence.

Brooks describes "narrative" as one of the larger systems we use to understand our experiences within a temporal framework, while plot is the primary mode of bringing order to the meanings we glean. For Brooks, plotting is "the activity of shaping the dynamic aspect of narrative—that which makes a story 'move forward,' and makes us read forward, seeking in the unfolding of narrative a line of intention and a portent of design that hold the promise of progress toward meaning" (p. xiii). In other words, a plot organizes information from the flow of lived experience and renders certain moments into a meaningful narrative about events.

If we are to co-author a new narrative of hope in a dire situation, then the plot of the problem-saturated story has to be made available for critique and revision. This is tricky because, as Brooks points out, plotting is so ingrained in shaping the meanings we make of experience that we usually take its formative role for granted. As Brooks phrases it, "criticism has often passed over it in silence, as too obvious for discussion" (p. 3).

THE PROBLEM'S PLOT

Problematic stories have an advantage: They've been around for a while. Their plot is thick. Like a snowball, they have packed together certain incidents and episodes in the family's life, finally freezing them into a solid mass. The once innocent snowball becomes a force with which everyone has to reckon. These problem-saturated stories can be very persuasive. The trouble is that their effects are negative and discouraging. When these stories take us in, experiences that do not fit their narrow confines are overlooked and any hints of hope and possibility are obscured. They are typically informed by unexamined cultural, class, and gender assumptions; these often give them their authority and "prove" their "truths."

The problem-saturated plot has the audacity to inform a person about himself in a summary way: who he is, who he has been in the past, and who he might be. Consider the following questions for making a plot available for critique.

Let's imagine that Jack has a problem:

- What story might the problem tell Jack about who he is and how he arrived at that description of himself?
- If Jack were fundamentally faithful to the story the problem has told him, what sort of future would it predict? Who might he become according to the plot of this life story?
- How will such a problem tell Jack to experience himself, others, his nature, and his actions in such a (problem-saturated) story?
- How will the problem tell Jack to act towards himself or others?
- What story might such a problem tell Jack about the nature of his abilities, talents and personal qualities and how they are to be expressed (if, in fact, such expression is permitted)?

THE ALTERNATIVE STORY'S COUNTERPLOT

Since the problem-saturated story has mass and considerable evidence to support its momentum, a simple positive statement or reframe by the therapist is easily discounted. An alternative story must be established in which the characters, their intentions, and their circumstances are as well developed, colorful, and convincing as the problem's. Thus, Michael White (1988a/1997, p. 8) suggests a "therapy of literary merit."

A major focus of narrative therapy is the "relationship" between the child (and/or family) and the problem. If and when the problem is personified, it may be regarded as having its own traits, values, and modus operandi. One way to initiate an alternative story is to contrast the child's qualities, abilities, and knowledge with the characteristics of the problem. Therapists and family members alike find themselves protected from burnout and pessimism when they join together to analyze the pathological "values" and "intentions" of the problem instead of the pathology and pathogenic history of the young person and family.

The alternative story's counterplot is revealed by questions and comments that weave back and forth between the influence of the problem, with its effects on various aspects of family members' lives, and the influence of the young person and family on the "life" or "career" of the problem. To indicate the influence of the child on the life of the problem we highlight the special qualities, knowledges, and skills of the child, as well as any intentions, commitments, attitudes, or actions that can be construed as working against the influence of the problem. Unique qualities, such as determination, bravery, or a vivid imagination, become vital to the child's quest to free himself from the confines of the problem. The child and family become protagonists in an engaging story of overcoming the problem or of living with it in the manner that suits them best.

Going back to Jack, here are some questions for the reader to contemplate about the qualities of an alternative story:

- What kind of alternative story would be required if Jack, his family, and the "therapy" were to tell another version at odds with the problem's story?
- How might Jack, his family, and their therapist look and act in an alternative story different from how the problem's story has told them to look and act?
- Is the genre of the alternative story flexible and playful enough to point to that which is strange, anomalous, irregular, or lies outside the reach of or off the track of the problem's story?
- How might those anomalies, irregularities, and strangenesses that lie outside the predictive reach of the problem's story be considered meaningful events in the life of the child and powerful antidotes to the problem?

PLOT AND COUNTERPLOT

When the plot and the counterplot are juxtaposed, the objective is to thin the problem's plot while thickening the counterplot. The problem's thick plot can be weakened by challenging its assumptions and "facts" about a child or family. Simultaneously, the counterplot is strengthened with exciting incidents and ideas that contradict the problem-saturated story. In the following example, the problem's story was bolstered by facts like these: "Rick and his brothers fight all the time." "They can't cooperate." "The boys don't really care about each other." "They haven't gotten along in years." "The fighting was so bad last year that we had to come home from our vacation three days early." "We just can't manage our boys' behavior." "This family can just never communicate!" A tip: note that such statements are frequently spiced with "always" and "never."

Collecting a fund of exceptions to attributions like these is a good start but may not be sufficient. What is required is a collaboration between therapist and family to render exceptions into a coherent and substantial counternarrative. For example, unique outcomes to a problem-dominated story might be: "Rick and his brothers used to get along when they were younger." "They all stuck up for Jackson (Rick's youngest brother) when he got into a hassle last week." "The brothers played peacefully together twice this week instead of fighting all the time."

The therapist might propose a counterplot to the parents such as, "As you've told me, 'Rick and his brothers used to get along when they were younger,' and that 'deep down,' you believe, 'they really care about one another.' Turning to Rick and his brothers, the therapist might then say, "You've told me that you all are 'tired of Temper and Fighting turning you against each other.' You also told me that, when somebody blamed Jackson at school the other day, you all rushed in to stand together against his accuser. Does this mean that you are willing to stand together for your Brotherhood against Temper and Fighting?"

The therapist might then pose questions that invite the family's collaboration in thickening the counterplot: "I have some questions for you about these developments." To the brothers, "Do you prefer standing together or divided? What do you think Temper and Fighting would rather see you do? What do you think Temper and Fighting feel now that you are standing for each other and against them?" To the parents: "How do you think your sons were able stand together against Temper and Fighting? What does this say about your abilities as parents to communicate your values of cooperation, loyalty, and care to your sons?" To the family, "What do these developments bode for the family vacation next month? What would Temper and Fighting like to see happen? What would you like to see happen? Did reducing Fighting and Temper in your family this week help or hurt the likelihood of a fun vacation next month?"

A freshly developed counterplot often has a way of fading between meetings, perhaps being overshadowed by the old plot. To prevent this, we sometimes ask families if they would like to keep track in between sessions of highlights or sparkling events (unique outcomes) that stand apart from the problem's plot and tell us about these at the next session. At that meeting, the counterplot is immediately in the limelight.

Remember, too, that the problem is not likely to give up without a struggle—its plot supports a problem-dominated version of events, rendering evidence to the contrary either insignificant or meaningless. Some problems are quite sneaky in terms of maneuvering for a "comeback." In fact, such "comebacks" may be predictable and par for the course and should be regarded as "hiccups" rather than relapses. Acting accordingly, everyone can speculate about their likely responses if such predictions come true. For example, "Do you think Temper and Fighting might try to make a comeback and ruin your vacation?" "How would you head them off at the pass if you saw them a-comin'?"

On the other hand, if the family unreasonably expects to eliminate the problem in its entirety, they may find themselves so discouraged that they abandon any hope for any remediation whatsoever. In this predicament, the counterplot may need to offer a new attitude or way of living with the problem. "How about enough competition to spur each other on but not so much Fighting that you put each other down?"

In a "therapy of literary merit," the process of "restorying" requires painstaking work. With the ingenuity and care of birds building a nest, we create the counterplot. The therapist collaborates with the family to gather and document past events, intentions, hopes, and dreams that stand in counterpoint to the problem-dominated story. Strand by strand, actions and ideas are woven into a narrative convincing enough to serve as an alternative to this problem-saturated story.

Two case stories in this chapter illustrate the juxtaposing of antagonist and protagonist, plot and counterplot, in the development of an alternative narrative. In the following case story, the therapist, David Epston, aims to shake loose fixed and problematic descriptions of an established identity and to highlight qualities which were formerly less visible.

In Paul's story the problem of soiling is personified as "Sneaky Poo." The relationship between Sneaky Poo and Paul becomes the focus of the interview. Throughout the conversation, comparisons take place—of the character, intentions and abilities of Paul and his family versus the character, intentions, and abilities of Sneaky Poo. Paul is asked questions that reflect on the fairness of what Sneaky Poo has done to his life. Children usually agree that "it's not fair" what the problem has been doing to them. This sense of injustice incites Paul to use his skills and creativity to stand up to Sneaky Poo and to establish a very different relationship with the problem.

"You Stink and My Brother Doesn't!"

When first meeting seven-year-old Paul, his older brother, aged nine, his older sister, aged fifteen, and his mother and father, David didn't have any trouble figuring out who was most bothered by the problem. The other family members entered the room and then turned and waited for Paul, who had to be cajoled to enter. Paul grimaced as he came in and looked decidedly uneasy about what he imagined was going to happen next. No one dared to begin talking for fear of upsetting Paul and having him retreat further into silence.

Since David had already had a few words with Paul's mother, Julie, over the phone, he took a risk: "Paul, a little birdie told me that you got Sneaky Poo. By that I mean your Poo sneaks out into your pants when you're not looking." While David spoke, Paul took it upon himself to rearrange the seating. He got up and turned his chair to face away from David and his family. David kept talking: "Personally, I think it is very unfair for your Poo to be so sneaky. I guess that, like most seven-year-old boys, you would rather sneak it into the toilet, and what's more, sneak-flush it right down the toilet to the drains that run under the road outside your home to the sewage plant. Do you know they make it into compost there so flowers and vegetables will grow big and healthy? I don't know how you feel about it, but it makes me really proud to think that my poo is going to such a good cause." By then Paul had turned his head to listen more closely. "Does anyone here think it's fair that Paul's Sneaky Poo should stink him up?" There was a wholehearted condemnation of Sneaky Poo doing this to their brother and son.

David then inquired as to why Sneaky Poo should want to do this to their brother/son: Did they have any ideas about why it would want to play such tricks? Did they consider them to be dirty or clean tricks? Was Sneaky Poo getting Paul's classmates and friends to steer clear of him? Did they think it had given Paul the idea that he was younger than what his last birthday had told him and everyone else about his age?

During this discussion, a growing sense of outrage began to emerge about the effects Sneaky Poo was having on Paul's life, his self-respect, his growing up, and his participation in social and recreational activities, especially with his sister and brother.

Fortunately, Sneaky Poo had failed in its attempts to talk Paul's parents out of their self-respect and belief in their own parenting knowledges. Even so, they had to admit that they were stumped right at the moment. By now, Paul's head was twisted so far around that he appeared as if he might be at risk of injury. There was little doubt he was listening earnestly.

David then asked everyone to respond at some length to the question: "If Paul outsneaked his Poo and came clean, would you be able to get to know him better?" Everyone agreed that that would be very likely. "What would you come to know about him that you already knew about him but the poo-smell has kept you clear of? What would you guess you might come to know about him that would be new?"

Paul's father came up with the most interesting possibility: "When he makes up his mind to do something, he does it." And when he said that, he left no doubt that this was a strongly held belief.

"Say Paul lived up to his father's convictions about him," David began musing, "and put his mind to outsneaking Sneaky Poo and did a reasonable job of it. Can I ask each and every one of you what you might say to Sneaky Poo if you caught it in the toilet before Paul flushed it into sewage oblivion?"

Paul was so intrigued by this question that he almost fell out of his chair. "Paul, why don't you join us? It's your Sneaky Poo, after all," David inquired. Paul happily turned his chair around and joined in this conspiratorial discussion. Paul seemed quite delighted when his sister upbraided Sneaky Poo with, "You stink and smell; my brother doesn't!" And he laughed at his father's chastisement: "Get down into those sewers, you Sneaky Rat."

Paul now responded without hesitation when David asked the following questions:

- If you were to make up your mind to come clean, do you think Sneaky Poo could stink you up?
- What reasons do you have for coming clean?
- Why would you say that coming clean would be good for you?
- Good for your life?
- Good for your sister and brother?
- Good for your father and mother?
- Good for your family in general?
- What if Sneaky Poo had the nerve to tell you that you *should* smell and that this was good for you?
- Has Sneaky Poo ever convinced you that you did stink? Did it tell you that other people liked you that way?

David then turned to Paul's family to review the abilities that Paul could bring to bear on the problem. After all, his father had said that when Paul "made up his mind to do something he could do it." David continued to question Paul and his family about the "power to make up his mind" and gathered detailed examples about those times in his life when he had deployed his "mind power" against matters of concern to him.

David took a zealous interest in Paul's "mind power" and its potential for remedying what Paul now saw as a matter of grave injustice. He also wanted to focus on Paul's powers as preexisting and separate from the problem. It is all too easy to accept a problem-saturated description of a child and family, which can hide the child's qualities and diminish our respect for him. By getting to know Paul apart from the problem, David could maintain a view and expectation of Paul as uniquely competent, rather than troubled or developmentally compromised. David drew the distinction between who Paul was under Sneaky Poo's power and who he was under his own power. In fact, it could be said that Sneaky Poo had robbed Paul of his powers of mind, which he was now about to reclaim.

David asked Paul if he thought it was fair that Sneaky Poo had weakened his mind. Paul judged this weakening of his powers of mind to be decidedly unfair. David then learned from Paul that Sneaky Poo would typically take advantage of him when his mind was on his computer or when he was involved in play. Sneaky Poo's modus operandi was now exposed to everyone's view: it operated at a particular site (the computer) and took advantage of a particular activity (Paul's play). David ended the session by strategizing with Paul. They agreed that he would use his mind power to turn the tables on Sneaky Poo while he was playing on the computer. This would strengthen Paul's resolve and weaken Sneaky Poo's power to make him forget himself and ignore his needs to go to the toilet.

Clearly, Paul had been emboldened to turn the tables on Sneaky Poo. At the second meeting David learned that Paul had been outwitted by Sneaky Poo only a few times during the last three weeks. Everyone agreed that this was a 75 percent improvement "from the old poo days."

Thinking of Paul's powers of mind, David asked, "Did you make up your mind?" Paul was emphatic that he had. When David asked Paul why he made up his mind, Paul replied, "Because he was always bossing me around and I decided to boss him around." David then asked Paul, "What is the best advice you might give to other boys and girls struggling with Sneaky Poo?" Paul answered, "They should make up their minds."

Here is an excerpt from that second meeting:

"Had Sneaky Poo been a bit of a friend of yours when I first met you?" David inquired of Paul. "Yes it was," Paul agreed. "It was a friend of yours," repeated David. "Yet you got the better of him. How did you go about doing this?"

"When I play, I always watch out for him. If I feel him, I rush to the toilet or sometimes I hold it in."

David continued: "When we met last time, Sneaky Poo was used to making a fool of you and he would do it when you were playing with the computer. How did you out-trick him?" At first Paul wasn't sure how he had done it but after a moment's reflection it came to him: "I think how I tricked him was when I rushed to the toilet, he thought I was standing there playing!"

"Oh really!" David exclaimed, "Sneaky Poo was hanging around the computer and you had already passed him on the way to the toilet. That's a good trick! Did you leave him in the lurch? Did you leave him behind you?" "Yep," was Paul's quick reply.

David wanted to tack from Paul to the problem. He asked the next question about Sneaky Poo's point of view: "Do you think that Sneaky Poo has started to think that you are a different sort of boy?"

"I think so."

"Is he upset with you?" David asked, wishing to contrast Sneaky Poo's mood of failure with Paul's feeling of success.

"Yes."

"Why do you think he got upset with you?"

"'Cause I'm doing the right sort of thing and not what he wants me to do."

"If Sneaky Poo were your boss and you did everything he told you to do, what would he want you to do?"

"Stay and play and let him come out in my pants."

"What do you think he's thinking about you now that you are flushing him down the toilet?"

"He's upset."

"Do you mind him being upset?"

"I want him to be."

With his next question, David was interested in counterposing Paul's "mind power" with his problem, in order to strengthen a different kind of relationship with it. "Do you think that you've made up your mind to be the boss of Sneaky Poo?" he asked. "Yes!" Paul exclaimed.

"What did you used to do when Sneaky Poo was bossing you around?" David asked, seeking further contrast between how it used to be when Sneaky Poo was dominant and how it was now.

"I'd only go to the toilet sometimes—when Mom said to do it. I should have gone more but I just stayed there playing. And Mom would have to say, 'Go to the toilet!', but by then I had it in my pants."

"Now that your mom doesn't have to tell you, do you feel in any way more grown-up?" David asked, extending the contrast to matters of chronology and maturity. "Do you think that Sneaky Poo tried to talk you into being younger and not listening to your Mom?" Paul agreed that he felt more grown-up.

"What did Sneaky Poo say to you when your Mom tried to draw your attention to the fact that you might need to go to the toilet?"

"Forget about it . . . just keep playing!"

"That's a dirty trick to play on a kid, eh?" David asked, continuing to attribute to Sneaky Poo characteristics that Paul might feel were undesirable.

"Yep."

"Do you think that Sneaky Poo was keeping you young? How young do you think Sneaky Poo wanted you to be?"

David likes to ask questions like these to track the influence the problem has on a young person's self-evaluation of his age. One of the more dire effects of a problem such as this is to deprive children of some of their growing up by making them look and feel younger than they really are. Questions that clarify the problem's intent to grow them down often invoke in children a sense of purpose, providing just the sort of commitment that is needed for change. A self-evaluation of age question can also distinguish a young person's accomplishments, e.g., retrieving his growing up from the problem's sphere of influence and handing it back to himself.

"Four," was Paul's age appraisal.

"How old do you feel now?"

"Nine."

"So you grew up five years in three weeks! Do you feel different now?"

"I feel unusual."

"I know you are the same height on the outside but on the inside do you feel like a bigger person?"

"Yep."

"How many centimeters bigger do you feel you are on the inside?"

"This much," Paul said, demonstrating by holding his hands apart.

"That's nearly a meter," David estimated. "Do you think Sneaky Poo could talk you into going back and being a servant to him?"

"Nope." And that was the end of that!

ANTAGONIST AND PROTAGONIST

When the problem is made to play the role of an antagonist in the therapeutic narrative, its character, motives, and areas of influence on the life of the family can be seen more clearly by everyone involved. Then the child and family can take on the roles of protagonist, with characters, motives, and areas of influence distinct from the problem. With Sneaky

Poo as the antagonist and Paul as the protagonist, Paul and his family were able to free themselves from the demands of the problem on their lives, such as Sneaky Poo's demands that Paul's mother constantly remind him to go to the toilet and that Paul think of himself as immature.

How does such a transformation in viewpoint and outcome take place? At first glance, one might think that it was accomplished just by looking for positives in a discouraging situation. It could be said that David employed an approach in which he reframed negative incidents or told stories about the existing situation so that it could be seen in a positive light. Such pollyannism would ignore the complexities of a family and its relationships, as well as the inner world of the child.

If simply searching for and reframing difficulties as positives was enough for success, our lives would certainly be easier. However, children and adults alike sense that such an approach is phony and simplistic. If David had tried to overlay a positive perspective on this problematic situation, which had caused great distress for the family, he would not be respecting the seriousness of these problems or the painful struggles that the family members had gone through as they tried to change. Narrative interviewing enables the therapist to inquire deeply into people's painful and difficult experiences in relation to problems in a way that validates their struggles.

One could identify Paul with his diagnosis (encopresis) and its clinical implications. There is much theory attached to encopresis that would have implications for both Paul's identity and motives and those of his parents. For example, encopresis could been seen as evidence of Paul's lack of maturity. He might be seen as regressing to an earlier developmental stage. It might be interpreted as a sign of defects in Paul's early childhood mothering or some kind of abusive parenting practice. It could be regarded as a symptom of a dysfunctional marriage—perhaps a manifestation of the stress placed on Paul by marital difficulties between his parents about which they were "in denial." We choose not to let perspectives such as these dominate our thinking and tempt us toward pathological descriptions of the people we meet in the course of our work.

It is a judgment call on the part of the therapist as to whether to work directly with the child on the presenting problem. Abuse and developmental assessments need to be considered and unhappiness in the marriage should not be ignored. A therapist should be alert to the various internal and external pressures that affect the child and family, but he should not be overwhelmed by them, no matter how dire they appear to be. We have found that if more serious problems are hiding behind the presenting one, they will come to light more readily in an externalizing conversation that features the struggles, strengths, and resources of a child and his family than in a conversation that doggedly pursues pathology.

CONVINCING STORIES

According to Jerome Bruner (1986, 1990), the narrative metaphor is an apt one for understanding humans' propensity to cognitively organize experiences in story form. Conversations are social events that we rely on to build consensually based stories that explain our perceptions. Similarly, therapeutic conversations are influential in shaping the stories that organize clients' understandings of their life situations.

Therapists who are aware of this process develop practices that orient such conversations in ways that are affirming and clinically fruitful. Narratives organized by negative perceptions tend to become problem-dominated or problem-saturated, emphasizing negative experiences and negative attributions of motivation, intentions, and character. Narratives of hope and possibility are based on characteristics and incidents from a person's life that stand apart from and contradict the problem-saturated story.

These exceptions exist in the lived experience of every young person and family, regardless of the problems they face. Although families will not accept pollyannish versions of their problem situations, they are willing to acknowledge that there may be aspects of their child's knowledge and abilities that can be brought to bear on the problem. When the therapist actively inquires into this, the child's competence is reinforced and further elaborated on by the family; through this process the narrative gains substantial coherence.

While the therapist plays an active role in the co-authoring process, his effectiveness depends on the ability to listen to the family's story of pain with an "externalizing ear." In order to do this he trains himself:

- to hear the current painful relationship the family has with the problem;
- to join the family as an interested and curious observer of the way the problem operates, and the methods it uses to oppress the family;
- to hear the messages it uses to thicken its plot: the unexamined assumptions that the problem uses to gain its authority to malign family members;
- to find out what relationship the family would prefer to have with the problem.

The therapist facilitates coherent and lasting alternative narratives when he:

- is an avid reader of exceptions to the problem's influence;
- is curious and excited about the abilities of the young person and family and builds these into convincing alternative descriptions;
- takes a keen interest in new and preexisting possibilities for changing the status quo with the problem;
- serves as an editor who underlines existing exceptions and possible alternatives to the problem-saturated narrative;
- weaves a contrast between the way the problem goes about its business and the way the person works to free himself from it, thereby developing a detailed counterplot;
- ultimately becomes a co-author of a meaningful story of change within family life.

In the following story, Dean (the therapist) listens attentively with an externalizing ear to the family's story of pain. He learns how the problem has operated to undermine an atmosphere of belonging in their relationships. Together he and the family discover the sociocultural sources of the problem's authority. The young person and her family remember incidents that thicken the counterplot, which Dean contrasts with the problem's plotting of their lives. Finally, he and the family are able to nurture a coherent narrative of belonging and compassion.

Janice's Frustration

Janice's parents described their eleven-year-old daughter as "arrogant and selfish" and detailed many examples of her "negativity." They told of their disappointments, related feelings of burnout and pessimism, and assured Dean that they were not the only ones who felt this way.

Dean listened with an externalizing ear to such concerns as "Janice has always been easily frustrated and could never take turns" and rephrased them out loud first (and then into his notes) as "Frustration has gotten the better of Janice from time to time and destroyed many an opportunity for cooperation." "Janice is so demanding—maybe we spoiled her" was revised to "Frustration has invited Janice into impatience and her parents into guilt." "Janice is so negative and always ruins our family fun" became "Negativity has come between Janice and her family to the point where it is almost impossible to share fun anymore." Janice's comment that "Nobody likes me so why should I care about them?" was transformed into "Not only can't Fun be shared anymore but Caring is on the way out, too."

It is important to point out that each of these edits of a family member's statement of concern was turned over to the person concerned for approval before it was entered into Dean's notes. On post-treatment review, family members said they considered that they experienced these revisions as validating and evaluated the process as having had a significant therapeutic effect.

In order to chart the influence of the problem on the life of the family, Dean asked each member to rate the changes in Caring and Fun on a scale from 1 to 10. When had the family first noticed having less fun? When had Janice noticed less caring? There was general agreement that it dated back a year. In fact, the fun rating had slipped badly over that period of time—from 7 to 2. Caring had followed suit—from 8 to 3.

Dean began to wonder if it would be possible to rehabilitate Fun and Caring rather than somehow creating them anew. Could this provide a counterplot to oppose the problem-saturated story that everything was, and had always been, difficult with Janice? And would a reasonable counterplot be that this family had a history of Fun and Caring that the problem was spoiling?

The importance of tracking the problem and its effects, such as its suppression of fun and caring, cannot be underestimated. It serves many purposes. For example, if Dean had not accurately understood the family's experience of the problem, it would have disqualified their attempt to speak of their painful circumstances. Neglecting this task could also have deprived him of the individual members' language practices, ideas, and explanations for what was so distressing.

In order to understand the problem's plot, Dean began to formulate in his mind questions such as:

- What is the "character" of this problem?
- What values does it ground its practices in?
- What sociocultural stereotypes does it employ to persuade family members to go along with it?
- What future does it plan for Janice and her family?

Asking such seemingly odd questions allowed Dean to offer externalizing revisions that might separate Janice and her family's value systems from those of the problem. Problems are like a Trojan horse: they encapsulate unexamined gender and cultural assumptions.

Dean and Janice agreed to call the problem Frustration. They soon figured out that, in a manner of speaking, the problem didn't want other kids to like her and be her friend. In fact, Frustration told her that no one liked her. Scaring her parents with the prospect of Janice growing up to be uncooperative served the problem's purposes well. Examining the problem's values was of special interest to Dean. It was likely that, through such an exploration, they would soon identify the sociocultural constraints the problem was imposing on Janice and her family. Dean soon found out that one of the problem's primary convictions was that a young woman who was without a "best friend" among a select group of girls was not considered to be a successful person.

Dean continued to interview Janice about the Frustration that was so obviously hanging like a dark cloud over her head, along with its companions, Sullenness and Anger. In his questions Dean took the tack of framing her as the protagonist in a story of how Frustration could bring loneliness and anger into a young person's life. In order to thicken the counterplot, the methods, values, and character of the problem were contrasted with Janice's methods, values, and character.

Dean used this information to compose the following questions for Janice about her life "apart from the problem":

- Do you think Frustration likes to see you friendless?
- Does Frustration want to block your chances to get along with others?
- Has it taken your patience away?
- Is losing your patience to Frustration a good or bad thing in your eyes?
- Do you approve of Frustration's plans for you to be lonely?
- Do you like what Frustration likes?
- Do you like yourself more when Frustration has its way with you or when you have your own way with yourself?
- Do you want to see Frustration happy or you happy?
- Do you think Frustration has your best interests at heart?
- The fact that it wants you all to itself—does that suggest to you that it might be jealous of you having friends of your own?
- Do you think it's good to have jealous friends that put others off you?
- If your truth be known, what kind of friends do you prefer to have?
- Would you mind seeing Frustration frustrated?

From Janice's responses to these questions, Dean learned that she had once had a "best friend," but unfortunately Samantha had moved away a year before. With Samantha there had been a history of "having fun together" and being able "to tell each other everything." This was the start of co-authoring a counternarrative, one in which Janice had the capacity for being in an intimate, fun-loving friendship and, what's more, for being "befriendable." This description was strengthened by a series of inquiries contrasting Janice's friendship with Samantha and Janice's relationship to Frustration:

- Whom do you like hanging around more, Samantha or Frustration?
- Does Frustration want you to have a life of misery or of happiness?
- Do you want to have a life of misery or of happiness?
- Does Samantha want you to have a life of misery or of happiness?
- Was Samantha part of your happiness?
- Is that why you had so much fun together?
- Is Frustration part of your misery?
- Who knows you better—knows what kind of life you like—Frustration or Samantha?
- Who has been a better friend to you—Samantha or Frustration?
- What did Samantha want for your future?
- What did she like about you? Did she see something in you that Frustration cannot or will not see?
- Did Samantha try to keep you all to herself?
- Why wasn't she jealous like Frustration?
- How come Frustration wasn't able to get between you and Samantha and destroy your "best friendship?"
- Are you proud of those techniques for avoiding Frustration in your friendship with Samantha?

When Janice's family and friends looked at her they saw anger, hurt, and sullenness. Frustration had libeled Janice by presenting her to others as uncaring and selfish. Dean established that Janice felt resentful of Frustration. She began to protest the reputation that Frustration had rubbed off on her. The information garnered from her thoughtful responses evoked an invidious comparison—between Janice's "Frustration avoidance techniques," on the one hand, and the agenda of Frustration, on the other.

Dean wanted to outline an alternative story in collaboration with the family. Everyone seemed keen to widen the gap between Janice and Frustration and happily supplied incidents, observations, and ideas that served to foster a coherent account. Janice's parents were able to recall historical examples of Janice containing her Frustration, cooperating, and developing friendships. They understood more clearly now why friendships in her peer group were difficult to come by, and that because of the pressure to be best friends with someone in the right clique, Samantha had been hard to replace. They discussed together how such stereotypes influenced eleven-year-old peer groups. When these stereotypes held sway, the peer pressure that labeled who was befriendable and who was not could be so intense that it would invite cruelty into the relationships of its members. And this process would be hard for any young woman to get through without a "best friend" for comfort and support.

Everyone concluded that Frustration, along with Anger and Withdrawal, probably "snuck into Janice's life" when Samantha left the year before, and that Frustration provided protection from being hurt by loss and from the cruelties of peer pressure. Frustration had used exclusionary peer pressure tactics to trick her into turning against herself and her family by telling her that she was a social failure and that no one really liked or cared about her.

Everyone agreed with Dean's observations that Frustration hadn't been able to rob the family therapy session of Fun and Caring once it was exposed to the light of day. In fact, they all lamented the injury to their daughter/sister at the hands of Frustration, but said that it was good to see the Janice that they and Samantha cared about make a reappearance in their lives.

SUMMARY

Even with our best efforts to set the tone, introduce the child apart from the problem, and externalize the problem, a pathological and problem-oriented view of the young person will often dominate relationships with parents, teachers, and even therapists. When they turn to therapy, family members are often so worried, burned out, and oppressed by a problem that they will express a strong need to let the therapist know how bad things are and how much pain they have experienced. Discouragement and desperation are quite contagious, even to the most experienced of helpers; however, discouragement and desperation should not deter a helper from listening and responding to problem descriptions in an externalizing manner.

In narrative therapy, hope, possibility, and the discovery of client competence arise when the problem is set up to be the antagonist and the protagonist becomes the young person and his family. The problem assumes its power to plot events and describe personalities from within a context of taken-for-granted cultural, class, and gender assumptions. The problem's plot is undermined from within when these assumptions are exposed to discussion, critique, and revision.

This is not as difficult as it may appear at first glance, because these assumptions consistently fail to fully describe the complexity and uniqueness of a family's experience. When exceptions to the problem's storyline are gathered together, they build the nest in which family and therapist collaboratively hatch an alternative story that reflects the family's value system and defines a new and preferred relationship with the problem.

CHAPTER 6

. . . .

Building a Narrative
through Letters

Therapeutic letters are closely associated with narrative therapy (Epston, 1989a, 1994; Epston & White, 1992; White & Epston, 1990b). Epston (1994, p. 31) describes the rationale for therapeutic letters in prosaic terms:

> Conversation is, by its very nature, ephemeral. After a particularly meaningful session, a client walks out aglow with some provocative new thought, but a few blocks away, the exact words that had stuck home as so profound may already be hard to recall. . . . But the words in a letter don't fade and disappear the way conversation does; they endure through time and space, bearing witness to the work of therapy and immortalizing it.

Letters are sent home, read and re-read, told and re-told like family tales. If you imagine a letter being read privately before bed, on the toilet, or under a tree, or publicly in a family moment around the dinner table, at a party, or on the porch on a summer's evening, you're entering the literary spirit.

What distinguishes a narrative letter is that it is literary rather than diagnostic; it tells a story rather than being expository or explicatory. The letter engages the reader not so much by developing an argument to a logical conclusion as by inquiring what might happen next. Structured to tell the alternative story that is emerging along with the therapy, it documents history, current developments, and future prospects.

WHAT ARE LETTERS WORTH?

Both David Epston and Michael White have conducted informal clinical research, asking clients questions such as these:

1. In your opinion, how many sessions do you consider a letter such as the ones you have received is worth?
2. If you assigned 100 percent to whatever positive outcomes resulted from our conversations together, what percentage of that would you attribute to the letters you received?

The average response to Question 1 was that a letter had the equivalent value of 4.5 sessions. In response to Question 2 letters were rated in the range of 40 percent to 90 percent for total positive outcome of therapy. Such findings were replicated in a small-scale study performed at Kaiser Permanente HMO in Stockton, California. Nylund and Thomas (1994) reported that their respondents rated the average worth of a letter to be 3.2 face-to-face interviews (the range was 2.5–10) and 52.8 percent of the positive outcome of therapy was attributed to the letters alone. The average length of therapy was 4.5 sessions.

Soon after David first started asking young people these questions, he met Peter, aged eleven, who had had a severe soiling problem most of his life. After a meeting with Peter and his mother David wrote him a letter. This is what Peter had to say when asked to evaluate it later:

> When I got it I was surprised and happy. It went over things and I could now remember them for our next meeting. I read it quite a few times. I have my own special file for it and I put it in a special drawer. What was also good about it was that when you have something written down you can say it's wrong. I knew the letter was for me the moment I saw it. I opened it, mum read it, and then she read it out loud. Then I read it three times and put it in my file. I looked at it a couple more times over the month. What I liked about the letter was that it makes children think they know what they're talking about. I think it is a good way to communicate with children after a meeting. I would give the letter 40 percent credit for the fact that I got 75 percent over the poo problem between the first and second meeting.

LETTER WRITING TIPS

For beginners, letter writing can seem daunting and time-consuming. A useful place to begin learning "how to" is Michael White's (1995) essay entitled "Therapeutic Documents Revisited," which provides a format that "requires the investment of a bare minimum of non-contact time from therapists. And yet such therapeutic documents are highly effective" (p. 201). Although we are tempted to defer entirely to White's exposition, we here offer a few tips for the aspiring letter writer:

- Quoting verbatim from notes taken in session allows the protagonist in the letter to read her own stories in her own language and metaphors. Verbatim quotations also benefit the therapist/letter writer by assisting her to enter the world of the protagonist. This encourages a more collaborative effort, incubating new and fresh ideas. For example, if the therapist quotes Janet, "I don't want to go off on Mom anymore, just because I have a fight with my boyfriend," she will capture Janet's specific proposal to put her good intentions to work in a situation that concerns her. This contrasts with a statement such as, "Janet has been treating her mother better lately," which glosses over the particular behavior Janet wants to change (going off) and her assessment of when it is most likely to occur (after a fight with her boyfriend).
- Questions can be inserted frequently along the way in a letter, or a thought can be ended with a question. The interrogative leads forward into new and multiple avenues for reflection and speculation, as opposed to reaching a conclusion by tying up loose ends on behalf of a client. For example, let's add a question to the previous quotation: "Janet, are you saying you would prefer to get on with people instead of 'going off' on them?"
- Reflexive verbs create an agentic relationship between the subject and the object where one doesn't usually exist. They imply that you can learn and see more about yourself from yourself. Compare "Janet, did you get on with your mother by calming yourself?" with "Janet stayed calm."
- The use of gerunds (verbs that end in -ing and are used as nouns) can give a sense of progress and motion. These words are apt for externalization because they describe a relationship a person might have to herself, e.g., "Janet, has your self-calming improved your mother-daughter relationship?"
- Consider the use of the subjunctive mood. It lends itself to the wishful, the indefinite, or to a future contingency or possibility. Compare "Janet, do you think you might be developing a knack for knowing when to let something go and when to speak your mind?" with "Has Janet learned when to keep quiet and when she should stand up for herself?" The first question allows Janet

to agree or disagree with the idea altogether or to place herself anywhere on a continuum being at the beginning to the end of the process of "acquiring the knack." The second question allows only a binary answer; she has either learned or not.

- The odd pun or wry turn of phrase can add a refreshing breath of humor.

Letters often play the role in a narrative therapy of thickening the counterplot at the expense of a problem's plotting of events. When depicted in a letter, the protagonist of the alternative story becomes the reader of her own story. Her voice reverberates through the verbatim quotes, questions, and plot twists, which iterate and reiterate her heroics. Although there are a number of examples of therapeutic letters in this book, the following two case stories have been selected to show how an alternative story is developed and documented through the use of letters.

Gerald: The Boy Who Got Eleven-Year-Old Space in His Family Just Before His Twelfth Birthday

Gerald, age eleven, was the focus of concern for the Gordon family's first meeting with David. Gerald was accompanied by his sister Mimi, age six, his two brothers, Johnny, fifteen, and Barry, eighteen, his mother, Sharon, and his father, Jim. Gerald's parents and older brothers were worried that for the past two and a half years Gerald appeared to them to be pretty miserable, taking very little pleasure in his life or the activities of a fun-loving family; also, he had taken to refusing to do anything anyone asked of him. This was regrettable because the Gordons placed a high value on shared responsibility and cooperation.

Gerald did, in fact, look pretty woebegone to David, in sharp contrast to Mimi, who didn't take long to charm herself into his affection. The problem, they explained, was that Gerald was admittedly "jealous" when Mimi came along and had engaged in a fierce sibling rivalry with her ever since her birth. According to this problem plot, Gerald was competing with his sister for attention as a result of being displaced by her as the youngest in the birth order. As Gerald put it, he had been "going for the bad things." Though constantly "seeking attention," Gerald sought it in ways that were entirely negative.

Mimi and Gerald seemed to be opposites. As Barry put it, "Mimi goes to the positive and he goes to the negative." Whereas Mimi charmed, Gerald was attracting negative responses like a magnet. Meanwhile, his good qualities, such as his wildly imaginative creativity, were totally obscured.

As the family members and David searched together for a unique perspective on their situation, it occurred to them that Gerald, for "Competition's" sake, had stayed behind in the family's "six-year-old space" and so the "eleven-year-old space" was untenanted. Johnny and Barry certainly had a "secure hold" on the "young men's space." Gerald's parents and older siblings realized that they had come to think of him as about the same age as Mimi, something they were unhappy about.

Everyone was sure that, although the "eleven-year-old space was unoccupied," they would welcome having Gerald "live" in it. Gerald had to admit that such a prospective move wouldn't be against his will. Mimi offered no opposition whatsoever. Gerald and Mimi's competition immediately became passé. What then became apparent was that Gerald was already heading in that direction, as you will read below.

Piggy-backing on the enthusiasm generated by this promising discussion, Sharon came up with an ingenious proposal to usher Gerald into his rightful place, a site in his family that would dignify what was unique to him, his creative mind, and the games he made up with a very select group of friends/players. Everyone welcomed Sharon's proposal, which rapidly dissolved the way they had all been glued to the competition.

David wrote the Gordon family this letter after their first meeting. The letter follows the sequence of notes he had taken during the meeting. The commentary inserted provides information about David's thought processes as the session unfolded.

Dear Gordon family:

It was enjoyable meeting your family. If every family was like yours, this job would be a piece of cake. However, in saying this, I, in no way, wish to take away from all of your concerns that Gerald was "quite unhappy, enjoyed very little, and resisted doing things he was asked." And that all had observed this happening over a period of the last two and a half years. Barry and Johnny, you understood that Gerald appeared to have a preference for negative practices and saw how this led you, almost against your wills, to be negative toward him. We all agreed that, by contrast, Mimi has very obvious charm and was able to charm you in the same way she charmed me. As you put it, Barry, "she knows how to get people's attention" and this has contributed, we all supposed, to her remarkable "self-possession." Barry, you put your finger on it: "Mimi goes to the positive and Gerald goes to the negative." Barry and Johnny, you were clear that you would prefer to respect Gerald for his maturity rather than what you referred to as his "six-year-oldness." Gerald, you said that you, too ,would prefer being treated more like Mimi's older brother than her competitor.

Externalizing the problem's plot. In the following section of the letter, David externalizes the "negative practices" associated with Competition and contrasts them with the "positive practices" associated with Mimi's charming ways. Gerald began to sense that he was not in any way being accused. Realizing instead that he had been "fooled" into such "negative practices" by vying for the "six-year-old space," he candidly acknowledged his engagement in negative competitive practices and immediately sought a way out. The way out—his creativity—and his final destination—"eleven-year-old space" become obvious and appealing to him and his family.

In a conventional internalizing conversation, Gerald's descriptions of the ways he went about getting "negative attention" by refusing to comply with any and all requests made of him and procrastinating around his homework would likely have been experienced as shameful confessions. Within an externalizing interview, what is usually considered a "confession" becomes a summary of Gerald's expertise on how the problem "works" and its effects on and intentions for his life.

David also unearthed some important actions and incidents that were plotted into an alternative story. For example, David discovered that, over the past few months, the number of times family members had to shout at Gerald in order to gain his compliance with their requests had decreased from three to two. Lately, Gerald had got it down to one "shouting time." Counterplots are best thickened with preexisting changes such as these, no matter how insignificant they might seem.

Gerald, you thought you might have been "jealous" of Mimi when she came along. Do you think jealousy has tricked you into being her competitor? And is that a losing proposition, given that she seems to have cornered the market on "knowing how to get people's attention" by "positives"? Gerald, do you think that this only left you the option of getting people's attention by "negatives"? If so, is this working for you? Or is it working more for Mimi? What do you think?

As we got talking, Gerald, you seemed interested in the idea of being your own eleven-year-old and leaving six-year-oldness to Mimi. Obviously, she is better at it than you. Gerald, did you realize when we were speaking that "going for the bad things" isn't doing much good in your family? You certainly have found a way through to get people's attention: "I don't do any chores whatsoever until people shout at me." But why did you decide to bring the shouting times down from three to two and then to one lately? Do you guess that will win you more brotherly respect from Barry and Johnny, more parental affection, and more sisterly respect from Mimi? If you have already tried it out, is it working better than "going for bad things"? Let me know when we meet next time, as I am curious about that.

You have also found that "not doing my schoolwork and taking ages to get my pens and a book out" works. However, you thought that if you had geared your life up from six-year-oldness to, say, eight or nine you would take about a minute to get your books out and pens. And if you went so far as eleven-year-oldness, you would do it in half a minute. You also considered the idea of "older-brothering" Mimi so she might start looking up to you rather than across to you. Would you find it okay if she did start respecting you as an older brother? And Johnny, will you be disappointed if his six-year-old habit still "tells" him he is younger than he really is? I can't remember who came up with the idea of "saying it once and then one reminder" rather than "a telling off and an order."

Thickening the counterplot with maturity. David employed an age rating system to have Gerald evaluate himself in terms of how much time different "ages" would take over an activity such as "getting my pens out and a book" and commencing homework. The use of specific tasks matched up with self-defined "age levels," thereby providing a direction for him to take if he wished.

Asking Gerald "What age does the problem tell you are?" and "What age did your last birthday tell you were?", David discovered that the problem had graded him as "six-year-old-like." Not only was the problem degrading him, but it was also keeping him from being his chronological age. Could a counterplot be developed around Gerald's resistance to the problem's attempts to keep him "young"? If it could, then it would be powerfully thickened at great cost to the plot.

David guessed that Gerald wasn't living exclusively in the six-year-old space in his family. On this assumption, he asked about any aspects of Gerald's intentions, actions, thoughts, hopes, or feelings that were at odds with six-year-oldness. And when several instances were found, David asked him to age-grade these "maturities."

There were some signs of what you folks referred to as "self-regulation" on Gerald's part. For example, Gerald has self-regulated around being late. As you put it, "I stop myself being late." And even you had to admit that that was worth an 11.5. Gerald, you thought, too, that you might receive some acknowledgment from others for that. You said, "They will be positive to me." Barry and Johnny, will it be hard to replace shouting with quiet reminders?

Once everyone could appreciate that there was some eleven-year-old "stuff" around, they put their minds together to imagine what might constitute a more expanded eleven-year-old space. They then considered how they might usher him into it, should he wish to inhabit it.

We all got to talking about making an eleven-year-old space in the Gordon family to go along with Mimi's six-year-old space, Barry and Johnny's young men space, and Sharon and Jim's adult space. Sharon, you had a very interesting idea: because Gerald "has a lot of interesting things to say . . . creative games, etc.," he might need some "real interested listening." Gerald, you were of the opinion that "five or two minutes was enough of what I need." However, you were willing for everyone else to take turns interviewing you (if you needed some help discussing creative things . . . for sure, creativity is one of the hardest things to tell people about) and taking notes. I must confess myself to be exceedingly interested in eleven-year-old creativity. In fact, I am writing a book about such things at the moment. Everyone agreed that it might be a good idea to ensure Mimi goes to bed at 7 P.M. because when she doesn't, "it eats into older time." And that, Gerald, your bedtime was 8:30 P.M.

Gerald, you agreed to watch over your eleven-year-old space in the Gordon family and to let me know if there is enough space for it. I look forward to any further discussions on this matter. Do you mind bringing your notes along, Gerald?

Yours sincerely,
David

Five weeks later everyone met again to go over how many years Gerald had been able to make up in his "ageness" and if he had taken up residence in the eleven-year-old space. He had matured himself to the extent that the eleven-year-old space could barely contain him. Fortunately, he was saved by his twelfth birthday, which further expanded the "room" he could have in his family.

Dear Gordon family:

Gerald, you had your twelfth birthday and by doing so you seem to have left behind not only your six-year-old self but your eleven-year-old self. Everyone else seemed to agree with this, even Mimi. As you put it, "'I'm going to get better at getting positive attention" but you are finding that it is "hardish." Did you think, once you made up your mind to go positive, it would be really easy? Barry, you observed that Gerald was "doing things without being asked." Gerald, you considered this was a good direction for you to be heading in and that it is "okay" with you. You even went so far as to say that you "could get right out of negative attention within the next month." Gerald, who knows? You might want to go back somewhat in age and try it out again. Mimi said she was looking up to you a bit rather than across to you. And when I asked "why?" she said it was partly because "sometimes he does his homework without moaning." Gerald, does being a twelve-year-old twelve-year-old have anything to do with getting your first assembly award for hard work in math?

An alternative story grows. After reviewing these developments, David and the family agreed they had turned the corner on Gerald's reputation as a negative attention seeker. However, David was concerned about solidifying and maintaining this development. What typically occurs in therapy is that this point is often reached—but only momentarily—

until the next negative event reasserts the power of this or another problem, and the apex of attainment is lost.

The thickened counterplot develops into a coherent alternative story when the competency of a person is clearly highlighted. Then hiccups or comebacks of the problem can be met by the family and young person with heretofore unacknowledged skills and a measure of equanimity. The interviewer seeks out such skills in a reiterative and playful manner throughout the interview. The articulation and acknowledgment of extant skills and expertise are preferable to new "skill training" introduced by the therapist. Gerald's imagination had found little expression during his competition with Mimi, but now that his maturity was being exerted, his active and inventive mind began to flourish and be enjoyed by his family. David wanted to continue to highlight this.

Sharon, you had to admit that there is "an exciting world inside his head." Had you been as aware of this before everyone started interviewing him? Had anyone else been aware of such an exciting world inside Gerald's head? Barry, did you have some idea? And was it because his exciting world is something like the world you had going on when you were his age? Johnny, you put it really well, "Gerald is mind-oriented." And much of his mind, it seems, is oriented to dice roll, a game he invented with his friends. Gerald, you said that, at the moment, much of your imagination is going into dice roll, especially at the time between being awake and asleep, when the lights are out and you are falling asleep. Sharon, you were of the opinion that Gerald was now "thinking for himself" and "was pleased with himself for doing things." Gerald, do you think you were pleased with yourself? Or was it more a matter of Sharon being pleased with you?

Acknowledging the history of imagination, David turns the narrative to the history of special abilities and the suppression of those abilities in the Gordon family. Imaginative kids need space for their imaginations, and Sharon and Jim were worried that Gerald wasn't getting enough for his. They had good reason for that concern due to Jim's history.

Jim, you found yourself worried for Gerald, recalling how you had the same kind of imagination as he has. Jim, do you consider that your special abilities weren't recognized when you were young? Did they try to thrash it out of you? Are you worried something similar will happen to Gerald as happened to you when you were growing up? Jim, how is your family—the one you have co-created with Sharon—different from the one you were brought up in? On reflection, what would you have liked to have been recognized about you and your "weirdly-abledness"? Do you think there is a genealogy of "weirdly-abledness" running through your family? Jim, if so, who was before you? Were they recognized or was it drummed out of them?

The letter ends with a summary of the conversation about Gerald's relationship with his older siblings and the changes that were taking place now that he was occupying a twelve-year-old space and getting "right out of negative attention."

Barry, you thought it just doesn't work when you act as Gerald's parent. You thought that goes for Johnny as well. Johnny, you came up with a great idea: "The key is for him to do things on his own." Everyone liked the idea of Gerald regulating himself on Thursday evenings. Gerald, did you like that, too? Or would you prefer to invite others to regulate you? Which is your preference? I will look forward to reviewing this matter with you next time.

Ironically, at this point Gerald's twelve-year-old positives had absorbed so much of his attention that David was worried that he hadn't given Mimi enough positive six-year-old attention. He closed the letter by enlisting her help with this.

Mimi, I am sorry I wasn't paying enough attention to you. Be sure to remind me, next time, if I don't give you your fair share.
Yours sincerely,
     David

Don't Keep Your Secret a Secret from Yourself

In the following story, David sends a series of brief letters in succession to an fifteen-year-old girl in trouble before she gives him a letter in response, in a sealed envelope, at the end of a meeting.

By the time Yolanda was eleven, her mother, Gail, realized that she could no longer control her daughter. Gail consulted a psychiatrist who prescribed medication for Yolanda and reassured Gail that if Yolanda took them for the rest of her life all would be well. The only problem was how to get Yolanda to swallow the pills. Yolanda would go into a rage over almost anything.

In the past Gail had suffered permanent injuries at her daughter's hand. Now that Yolanda was fifteen, Gail would regularly need to call the police to restore order and protect herself and her other children. Unfortunately, this had occurred so many times that the police now refused to respond, so Gail had to flee her home, taking her other two children with her to a shelter. Besides the injuries to her family, Yolanda had done severe injury to her friendships. She was so lonely that she had even taken to feigning a broken arm at school to gain sympathy.

When David entered the picture, the situation had reached a point where Gail felt she had no other option besides making Yolanda a ward of the juvenile court if Yolanda assaulted her again. A meeting was called that David was invited to, attended by representatives of the police and the New Zealand Child and Young Person Service. When the ultimatum to make Yolanda a ward of the court was delivered, Yolanda was stunned to silence. David couldn't help but notice that for the first time that he knew of, Yolanda spent more than five minutes without tantrumming, swearing, and running from the room. Seizing on this unique event, David pointed out that something extraordinary had occurred and asked; "Does anyone know what just happened?" No one could say. He then turned to Yolanda and said, "Yolanda, you have controlled your temper for the first time in living memory. How did you do it?" Yolanda turned on him abruptly: "None of your business!" David replied with aplomb: "I don't blame you, it's too soon to unveil it. Keep it a secret, but don't keep it a secret from yourself." Yolanda's burgeoning rage turned to perplexity. "Don't unveil it for three months," David continued. "Only then will we be convinced that your secret weapon works."

David asked Yolanda if she might be willing to keep a written account of what it was like to keep the secret of her temper control for three months for the *Temper Taming Archives*. To David's surprise, Yolanda agreed. Realizing that this was going to be hazardous undertaking with many possible pitfalls for Yolanda as well as Gail, David decided to use unsolicited and randomly sent letters to keep the hope for success alive.

Here are some examples of those letters:

Dear Yolanda,

Is your secret weapon giving you force? If it is, may the force be with you! I continue to worry that you're keeping it in a safe place. If it is where I think it is, maybe you should put some mothballs with it so the moths won't eat it.

By the way, I liked your new haircut. I thought it was very friendly.

Yours sincerely,
David

P.S. I would prefer that you keep this letter to yourself for the time being as I don't want your mother or sisters to think I'm a worry wart.

Dear Yolanda,

I had this dream last night and I woke up with a fright. You had blown your top, beaten your mother up, and she charged you with assault. Then I realized it wasn't true—it was just my dream.

What happened in my dream was that you had buried your secret in a jar in the garden. A gardener came to your house and found it accidentally and took it home for his daughter for her Temper problem. And when you went to get it when you needed it to cool down, it had vanished into thin air. I hope you didn't bury your secret weapon in your garden. Please keep it in a safe place.

    Sincerely,
       David

Dear Yolanda,

    I hope you aren't finding my unsolicited letters intrusive, as that certainly not my intention. If you do, let me know.

    You know, in my last letter when I was wondering if the New Zealand Army might be interested in your secret weapon. Do you think it would be fair to offer your secret weapon to the Army before the Navy and Air Force? To do so would favor one branch of the armed services. Do you have any preferences? Or do you think you should give them all a chance? Perhaps you could sell it to the highest bidder? I wonder if there might be some money in it for you. Who knows? I've never invented a weapon so I don't know what they go for. Still, it may be worth your while to find out.

    Sincerely,
       David

Dear Yolanda,

    I was surprised at our last meeting when you told me you were making some friends and that your new friends were taking pleasure in your friendship. If that wasn't enough for one day, you told me you had advanced your maturity in the direction of a boyfriend! I wanted to go over my concern with you for him. Have you used your secret weapon on him? If you have, do you think it is fair to do so without his consent? I am worried he won't have a chance. You said that you had told him about it. But have you given him enough information for him to be fully aware of what he's up against in your secret? My advice is to not keep it a secret from him—IT'S NOT FAIR.

    On the other hand I'd advise you to keep it a secret from your family until the three months are up as we agreed. Then and only then should you consider unveiling it. I can't wait!

    Yours sincerely,
       David

These letters provided much needed encouragement and humor to Yolanda during a period when she was very close to committing an act that would have gotten her committed. Yolanda was able to avoid violence for the three months she kept her secret. She worked hard then to make amends with her mother and her sisters for her previous violence. The culmination of her reparations was planning a surprise

"Mother Appreciation Party" in cooperation with her two sisters. Such sibling cooperation was without precedent in her family.

Despite all this, Yolanda was reluctant to reveal her secret. She sought an extension for an additional three months because she considered that she was not yet quite sure about maintaining her nonviolence. After six months of keeping peace, Yolanda handed David a sealed envelope at the end of a meeting. She requested that the secret not be revealed in front of her family. Inside was this letter:

Dear David,

I am writing to tell you what I think has made me able to control my Temper. When I was placed in foster care at the end of last year, I became aware that I had lost control of my life and what I wished to do with it. My family could no longer put up with me or my Temper. At the time, I thought them very mean and unloving but now I know that they did it out of love.

I think my Temper control is caused by fear of being removed to live in an unloving, uncaring household where I would be unwanted. After the meeting with the police and the social worker when they said that I was in danger of being sent to another foster home or a psychiatric hospital I was determined to prove them wrong. I know that I belong with my family and I don't care how they treat me as long as I know they love me. I am no longer afraid of telling you my control methods because I know I can trust you. I hope they will be able to help someone who is in the same position as I was three months ago because I wouldn't wish it upon anyone. Thanks a lot for being a friend in a time of need.

Your friend,
Yolanda

CHAPTER 7

· · · · · · · · · · · · · · · · · · · ·

Publishing the News

Many a narrative practice includes the circulation of news of change and of alternative stories to concerned others. For an alternative story to take firm hold in a child and family's life, it is often helpful to catch those beyond the immediate circle of therapy up on changes. Additionally, when the views of others contribute to a given narrative, it may be important to assist in revising those views. Significant people can become an audience for notable developments and be invited to make a positive contribution to the preferred story of the child and family. Moreover, the process of gathering information to share with others invites a further "performance of meaning," thereby strengthening the narrative. Often these new meanings are documented, perhaps in a letter from the therapist which becomes a tangible and durable record for the family.

Freedman and Combs (1996, p. 237) explain the appeal of spreading preferred stories:

> Although in the dominant culture therapy tends to be a secret enterprise, in the narrative subculture the people who consult with us are usually enthusiastic about the idea of letting other people in on the process. We think that externalizing and antipathologizing practices offer people a different kind of experience in therapy. When therapy becomes a context in which people constitute preferred selves, they have nothing to hide, and much to show.

Bill O'Hanlon (1994, p. 28) notes the rewards of disclosure when the client is in the protagonist's role in her preferred story: "In this therapy, people emerge as heroes and they often want that heroism acknowledged in some social way. They are usually quite happy to communicate with others and tell their stories."

CONSULTING YOUR CONSULTANTS

The process of gathering information to share with audiences begins with the premise that a child, for example, has taken significant steps to revise his relationship with the problem and in so doing has gained knowledge and expertise that may assist others grappling with similar concerns. David Epston and Michael White (1992, 1995) have developed a practice of consulting persons in order "to document the ways in which they have resisted and surmounted the 'dominant stories' of their lives, stories organized around their problems, symptoms, and socially ascribed 'pathologies'" (Epston, White, & "Ben," 1995, p. 278).

This practice involves interviews in which a child's "alternative knowledges" are elicited and documented. For example, when a boy has achieved mastery over Temper, he may be invited to give an interview about his hard-won knowledge. Although they may occur at any stage during therapy, such interviews create an alternative model for the so-called termination process in therapy. Rather than employ a "termination as loss" metaphor for the ending of therapy, David and Michael prefer a "rite of passage" metaphor (van Gennep, 1960). They note (1992, p. 280) that according to this ritual process a person is encouraged:

> to negotiate the passage from novice to veteran, from client to consultant. Rather than instituting a dependency on the "expert knowledge" presented by the therapist and other authorities, this therapy enables persons to arrive at a point where they can take recourse to liberating alternative and "special" knowledges that they have resurrected and/or generated during therapy.

Along the way there are opportunities for confirmation and celebration of the child's new status.

When engaged as consultants, children assume an unconventional role:

- They are consulted as authorities on their own lives.
- Their preexisting and newly acquired knowledges and abilities are deemed effective and worthy of respect.

- Their ideas are considered significant enough to be documented and circulated to others.

It is hard to miss the delight that children take in the chance to "show and tell" their knowledge and skills to others. Perhaps even more important is the fact that in sharing their experiences young persons have the altruistic satisfaction of making a contribution to others.

While final meetings often consist of "consulting your consultant" interviews, such interviews are commonplace from the first meeting onward. Children can be consulted about interesting skills or knowledge that emerge throughout therapy. The interviewing process itself is validating even if the information gathered does not end up being circulated to outsiders. The major beneficiary is likely to be the therapist in terms of increasing his stock of ideas and inspiring his work.

The ideas and knowledge of a young person and his family can be circulated within a community of people who are struggling with the same problem. Madigan and Epston (1995) have coined the term "communities of concern" to describe such groups. The Anti-anorexia Anti-bulimia League (Crowley & Springen, 1995; Epston, Morris, & Maisel, 1995; Madigan & Epston, 1995) is an example of a community of concern. League members share their struggles and ideas for revising their relationships with anorexia and bulimia, including their knowledges about the social, gender, and cultural aspects of the problem. The Anti-anorexia Anti-bulimia League members have chosen to take an active role in revising the definition of the problem in the culture at large, through, for example, educational programs at high schools.

Facilitating such movements from the personal to the political is a powerful avenue for individual as well as social change and consequently a value-laden pursuit that demands high ethical standards. This requires a constant process of informed consent from clients and takes place in a context which is highly collaborative.[1]

Many of the stories in this book include "consulting your consultant" interviews, as well as the documentation that was subsequently circulated to others outside of the therapy context, including now you, the reader of this book. This chapter describes some ways we determine the focus of such interviews and circulate the information gathered in a responsible manner.

A NOSE FOR NEWS

How does the therapist gather and facilitate the flow of significant information about personal and social change in a responsible and collaborative manner? A news media metaphor is a playful way to describe how the narrative therapist engages in this pursuit. In the news media metaphor:

- The therapist has three jobs: reporter, co-editor, and co-director of circulation.
- The young person and the family members also have three jobs: newsmaker, co-editor, and co-director of circulation.
- "News" is gathered by the therapist/reporter from the client/newsmaker.
- "Readers" are identified as an audience for news of change in the life of the young person and her family.
- The news is co-edited prior to "publication" by the therapist and the interviewee.
- The news is corroborated by other sources and checked for accuracy before it is deemed newsworthy.
- The news story is prepared within a chosen media, such as letter, tape, drawings etc.
- The news is circulated to the relevant audiences.

GATHERING THE NEWS

The interview forms the basis for news-gathering. The therapist must develop a nose for newsworthy news and develop interviewing skills to engage the interviewee in discovering his discoveries and acknowledging his achievements.

Here are some sample questions (for an older child or teenager) for gathering newsworthy material to circulate to others facing asthma:

- Are you aware that there are other young people whose lives are up against Asthma?
- If I meet other kids who are facing Asthma, would you mind if I share your Asthma expertise with them in order to encourage and help them?
- Of all the things that worked for you, what are some of your favorite ideas for dealing setbacks to Asthma?
- What policies would you advise another young person to adopt if he intended to take as much of his life back from Asthma as you have?
- When Asthma had your life all to itself, how miserable did it make you? How did it go about this?

- Did Asthma try to talk you into the idea that you're a "sickly" person?
- Do you think you've been too patient a patient?
- How did Asthma hoodwink you into being so patient and long-suffering?
- What sort of future did Asthma have in mind for you? Did it try to conceal this from you or did it brag about it?
- Did you come up with any counter-tricks when you found out what it had in store for you?
- Before you reclaimed your life from Asthma, did you first have to "spy" on it to learn its means of taking your life away from you?
- Did Asthma try get you to depend on your parents because they're so dependable?
- What personal qualities and abilities have you brought to bear on Asthma that it can't stand?
- When Asthma takes your physical strength away, have you developed a moral strength to get even?
- Looking back now on how you got a fair bit of your life back from Asthma, what would you tell other kids to inspire them and give them hope?

CO-EDITING THE NEWS

Role confusion might be the trickiest element to manage when shifting back and forth from being a reporter gathering the news to a co-editor who offers suggestions on how to compose the story. Reporters have a tendency to get ahead of their interviewee when they confuse these roles. The interview process requires that any news gathered in the interview should regularly be submitted and resubmitted to the newsmaker for continued editing. Our credo is: "Don't 'run with the story'; check your facts carefully."

We have found the following guidelines to be especially helpful to the therapist for staying behind the newsmaker and maintaining his role clarity. In the following example, a boy and his father are interviewed partly for the purpose of providing a letter to the Juvenile Court on their behalf.

- Consent is always gained for any tack that the interviewer contemplates taking before he takes it. "Don, would it be okay if I asked you some questions about the changes that are taking place in your relationship with your father?"

- The ethics of news-gathering demand that the language and metaphors of the newsmaker receive preferential treatment: "You described the change as 'talking without fighting' and being 'on a better road now.'"
- Before offering a language revision, the reporter should first notify the newsmaker that he is shifting to his co-editing role: "Could I take a moment from finding out more about this to suggest that 'talking without fighting' is an example of freeing your relationship from Temper?"
- The reporter is always ready for answers that disprove any theory he might hold: "Have I got it right: You don't think that you and your Dad 'talking without fighting' was an example of getting the better of Temper; you think it was an example of what you call 'having a constructive argument'?"
- There are no trick questions. The reporter readily discloses the basis for his questions, including personal experiences or bias:"I was worried about your fighting and I wanted you to communicate without arguing at all, but maybe my idea of no arguments as the answer blinded me to the important distinction you are both making between 'constructive arguing' and destructive fighting."
- The news angle itself is always up for discussion or revision: "You said that you 'took the time to listen to Dad's point' before 'just reacting' and I notice that you are both able to describe each other's points of argument to me in quite a bit of detail. Do you think that taking the time to listen to each other's point of view makes the difference between having a 'constructive argument' instead of a destructive fight?"
- The final story is primarily a collaborative effort and is submitted to the newsmaker for final approval before circulation: "Would it be accurate to write in our letter to the Juvenile Court this? 'Don and his father have taken the first step down the road of understanding each other's point of view. They are taking the time to listen to each other before reacting and are thus communicating with what they refer to as constructive arguments instead of engaging in destructive fights'?"

IDENTIFYING AUDIENCES

Audiences range from those who are active in a person's life to hypothetical groups such as "kids your age who are dealing with the same problem." These may be variously called upon in the young person's and family's mind during reflective questioning, invited to attend sessions, put into contact with the young person through letters, reached out to through various "media," or visited elsewhere, such as at a school conference. We might name types of audiences as "known audiences," "hypothetical audiences," and "introduced audiences" (Freeman & Lobovits, 1993).

The "known audience" includes those who know and have some opinion about the young person and can be asked to witness and contribute further meaning to his life. To identify these people, we might ask the child or family if there is anyone who they feel should know about these developments or any person whose opinions have become outdated and require updating. This audience might include relatives, friends, teachers, or other professionals such as doctors and school personnel.

Some people are sympathetic and more than eager to respond and contribute to the evolving narrative in response to requests for their reflections. But others are justifiably skeptical or involved in a problem-saturated narrative. For instance, a teacher who has had a challenging time dealing with a child in a classroom will need some convincing that he is no longer a troublemaker. It is crucial that such persons be respectfully included in the restorying process. We might collaborate with a child to send a letter like this:

Dear Mr. Prothrow,

I, Burt, apologize to you and my classmates for all the trouble that Trouble has gotten me into this year. I realize now that I deserve the "Troublemaker reputation" that I've got.

When I met Dean, he asked me some questions that made me think and what I came to is that I want my "good" reputation back. I don't expect it to be given to me. I know I have to earn it. I couldn't come up with any really good ideas for getting it back, so I asked Dean. He asked my mom if I had any good reputation left at home. My mom told him I had a good reputation as a garden helper. He asked me if there were any gardening opportunities at school. I told him them there were. He asked me if I could reassure him that I know the difference between flowers and weeds.

I don't expect you to give me my good reputation back on a one-shot deal, but when you see the weedless flower bed by the entrance this just means I'm serious. Getting out of trouble won't be an overnight thing but if you don't think I'm doing good enough just tell me and I promise you I won't flip out when you do.

Signed,

Burt

P.S. Dean typed this letter and asked me the questions, but I hereby swear that the answers are all mine.
P.P.S. Dean asked my permission to put in a question of his that made me laugh. "Would you rather pull weeds out of the school yard or be weeded out of school?"

When a teacher, swayed by new information we pass along, sees past a child's bad reputation, his changed perceptions and behavior can powerfully validate the child's story of change. There is no convert so valuable as a former skeptic! When such a person's perceptions change, he may even be willing to contribute a letter that further corroborates the change.

We would like to briefly address the concern often raised by busy professionals when these practices are proposed: time, as in "I don't have time for this, especially now with managed care." We have found that the time taken to work with the family's network is a high-yield investment. The therapist's effectiveness is naturally part of what is circulated and this makes a favorable impression in the entire network surrounding the child. Additional referrals often accompany such efforts.

"Hypothetical audiences" are those called upon in imagination during reflective questioning, such as imaginary friends or significant people who are deceased but live on in a person's or family's heart.[2] Even favorite toys or pets can be called upon in a child's imagination to give supportive input. For example, an eight-year-old girl who was facing night fears was asked a series of questions that invited her to see herself in the room at night through the eyes of her beloved dog, who slept by her bed. She was asked questions like: "If your dog could talk, what would he say about what you were able to do last night when you stroked him and calmed yourself down instead of being taken over by the Fears? Knowing you as well as he does, would he be surprised at your bravery? Did you learn any of your bravery from him?"

CLUBS, NETWORKS, LEAGUES, AND PROJECTS

Finally, there are "introduced audiences," such as reflecting team members who may be present in the consulting room. Although we will not attempt to cover this topic here, reflecting teams can be powerfully supportive in the development of therapeutic narratives.[3] Members of a therapy group are, of course, another potentially valuable audience for change.

Communities of concern may be introduced via letters, newsletters, or other media. These communities have "the power to appreciate alternative stories in the making, and to offer locally based knowledge and techniques for changing dominant, problem-saturated stories that equate a person with a problem" (Freeman & Lobovits, 1993, p. 222).

White and Epston (1990b) were the first to form clubs, such as the Temper Tamers Club, for children facing the same problem. Epston pioneered the first actively networked communities of concern, such as the Anti-anorexia League. Since then several networks and leagues have sprung up that link young persons and their families for support, knowledge, and information, as well as social action. A few of these are The Fear Facers and Worry Stoppers Club, The Peace Family Project, and The Freedom from Ferpection (Perfection) Network.

Activities such as these can shift the work of therapy from an individual family-based effort to a more public and social endeavor, in terms of learning about and dealing with specific problems and their sociocultural aspects. When children and families are invited to join or create clubs they become audiences for others, and when they serve as experts and consultants to other kids their own stories are also validated.

CORROBORATING THE NEWS

One of the main benefits of circulating news is that it provides an opportunity to corroborate the newsmaker's story. The corroboration process itself enriches the meaning and validity of new discoveries and understandings. Corroboration can be provided by someone who has been directly in contact with the child and seen the change, someone who was adversely affected by the problem, or by someone who was skeptical about the possibility of change. These parties are often close at hand—in the family, at school (e.g., a teacher, vice-principal), or in the community (e.g., a probation officer).[4]

Corroboration and verification can be obtained in various ways and from different people; they might be written to or interviewed. For example, when child applies to the Temper Tamers Club of America the application process might include a letter of reference from a corroborative source (Figure 7.1).

NEWS MEDIA

The media for communicating the story are many: essays, letters, lists, taped interviews, certificates,[5] proclamations (Figure 7.2), art, poetry, and transcripts. These range from the personal, such as a "Document of Identity" (White, 1995, p. 144), to the public, such as REVIVE: The Magazine of the Vancouver Anti-anorexia Anti-bulimia League.[6]

For younger children, lists and charts are useful media for keeping

---

TEMPER TAMERS CLUB OF AMERICA.
LETTER OF REFERENCE

Name of Applicant:_____

Name of Referee:_____

- In what capacity are you aware of the applicant's prior relationship with Temper? (tantrum, argument, fight, etc.)

- In your opinion, what sort of person did Temper make the applicant in those circumstances?

- Can you provide one or more examples in which the applicant showed her or his temper taming ability?

- During those times what strengths or competencies did the applicant reveal?

- Can you recommend the applicant to be admitted to the Temper Tamers Club of America, where she or he will have the authorization to share her or his temper taming skills with other young people who are similarly beset by Temper?

Figure 7.1 Letter of Reference Form: Temper Tamers Club of America.

track of developments. A particular project, such as Virginia Simons and "Carrie's" "Bravery Project" (Freedman & Combs, 1996, pp. 232–236), can be kept in the form of a list. Another use of a list is to compile a child's accomplishments apart from the problem. For instance, a young child can be asked, "Have you done something that you're proud of as a

---

THE SIMONS FAMILY PEACE PROCLAMATION

Whereas quarreling has corroded the Simons family communication up until recently, leeched love and respect out of it, and replaced them with bitterness.

Whereas the Simons family has declared itself a Peace Family and has proven through its quarreling free mealtimes that it has the will to head off quarreling when it is nipped in the bud.

Whereas each family member has sworn an oath to do everything in their power and knowledge to sound a warning if they consider that quarreling has made its way into their communication in any shape or form.

Be it resolved that this proclamation will be lodged in a prominent and accessible place, e.g., refrigerator, mantel, answering machine.

Be it further resolved that upon the occasions that a warning is necessary, any member may cause said proclamation to be read to the entire the family aloud.

Be it finally resolved that each family member has sworn to lend an ear to the reading in order to hear and reaffirm the end of quarreling and hostility and herald the return of cooperation and peace to their family.

Signed and witnessed on the tenth day of June, 1996, in Berkeley California, County of Alameda.

Figure 7.2 The Simons Family Peace Proclamation.

six-year-old lately? What things can you do that you think that I couldn't guess by just looking at you?" The family is usually happy to give examples of the child's growing skills and abilities. The list can provide reference points for the story of the child's competency with the problem. Subsequently, another list may be started that compiles specific successes in relation to the problem. For example, "Can we add to your six-going-on-seven list of things you're proud of, your new skill in calming yourself down?"

Members of a community of concern may be connected to each other through various media (Freedman & Combs, 1996; Lobovits, Maisel, & Freeman, 1995; Madigan & Epston, 1995). These include personal letters, poetry, art, or taped interviews that are shared by two or more particular members of community of concern who are linked by the therapist. To hear and perhaps respond to the letter of someone else struggling with habits (obsessive-compulsive disorder), for example, can be a very moving experience. Such letters may be reviewed and read by everyone in that community. *REVIVE*, which began as a letter exchange, provides a particularly sterling example of this.

HANDBOOKS: THERE ARE MANY PATHS

A few years ago Jenny asked herself, "What if therapists kept files on problems rather than on patients?" This inspired her to develop handbooks on children's knowledges and successes associated with specific problems. In these, children and families either make an entry for themselves or offer their own stories of success and advice to future readers. They have the option of reading about how others before them approached the selfsame problem.

An invitation to write in a handbook can be seen as a form of "consulting your consultants." A child could make his contribution simply as a way to document his knowledge on a topic. Or, if it is appropriate, a potential audience for the entry might be introduced to the child as "other kids I [the therapist] might meet in the future who are facing the same problem and who would benefit from your discoveries."

This project has several aims:

- to empower and respect children by inviting them to consult for the benefit of other children facing a similar problem;
- to validate their accounts of struggle and success;
- to provide a way to have fun in showing off success and reaching beyond themselves;
- to keep these accounts for inspiration and reference in case they themselves experience a setback.

Children are invited either to write or dictate in unlined notebooks their story or statement, question, or poem and to illustrate their contributions with pictures, cartoons, maps, or graphs. The handbooks include colorful pictures and cartoons added by Jenny. They have been circulated to other therapists working with children, who in turn have added their own entries. Some examples of handbooks are: *Kids' Temper Tamer Handbook: How to Cool Off and Be Cool; The Fear Facer's and Worry Stopper's Handbook; Making Friends with Your Imagination; Sleeping Soundly; The Freedom from Habits Handbook;* and *The Different School Book.* Figures 7.3 and 7.4 show examples of two handbooks with their collage covers.

It is important to note that a handbook is not intended to be a record of those who are successful and experienced to be presented to those who are new and less competent. Neither is it intended to be used as a manual or guide. This is not in the spirit of the handbook. Nevertheless, children entering therapy can sometimes be offered the stories of those who have traveled the road they are on. Children who are ready for such input from other children will show their readiness by their high interest level. However, we consider the main value of the handbooks

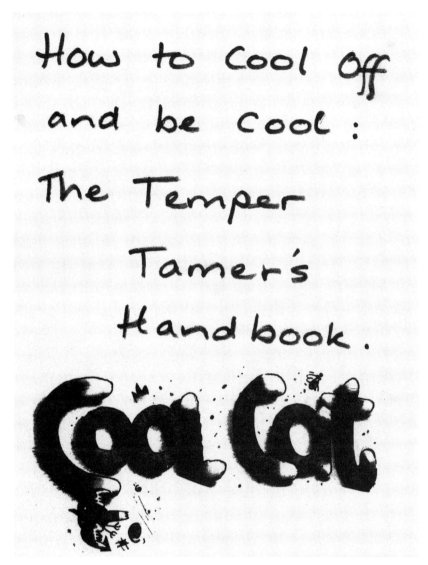

Figure 7.3 Kids Temper Tamer Book: How to cool off and be cool!

to be the child's participation as he makes his own entry. Many children are so interested in being contributors that they don't even take the time to read the previous entries. When a child does read the entries of his predecessors, he is typically inspired to make his own contribution.

The handbook is like a "summit log," the book placed in a watertight container on the top of a mountain. Having reached the summit, the climber takes in the vista, feels the thrill of his "peak experience," then perhaps reads the log and makes his entry about the journey up. A large part of the pleasure of a summit log lies in making one's own record.

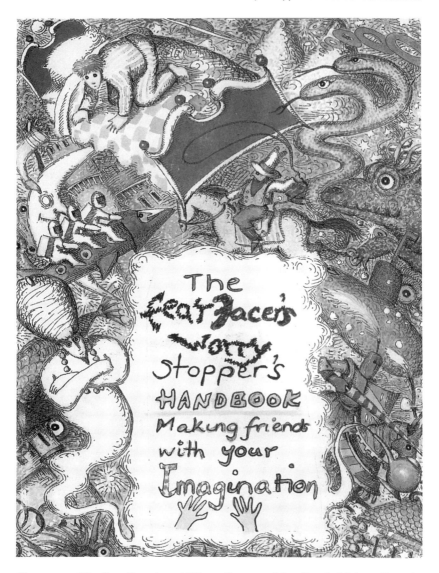

Figure 7.4 The Fear Facer's and Worry Stoppers Handbook: Making Friends with Your Imagination.

Some entries are made as a culminative statement, but others serve as a record of milestones along the way. Each journey up the mountain is different because of the various routes, weather, and other conditions the climber faces; each experience of the summit and of the view is also unique. Handbooks are the summit log of young person's journey of knowledge while changing their lives in relation to a problem.

A therapist who can co-author a narrative of change with a young person is qualified by this skill to develop new contributions to the handbook. If the therapist uses the handbook in place of his or her own guiding skills, it can be intimidating or off-putting to the child. Children are generally invited to make an entry following a unique outcome, in order to develop and confirm a story of change.

Here is an entry from the *Sleeping Soundly Handbook* dictated by Rachel, five years old:

> *I wanted someone to stay with me 'cause I was scared of monsters under the bed. I went into Mom's bed and she sent me grumpily back because she didn't want to get up. So I had the idea to turn on the radio and fell asleep and woke up at 4:44 and fell back asleep after listening to the radio. Then I got into Mom's bed at 6 A.M. when we agreed. Mom and I were happier and we liked being in bed at 6 A.M. I also felt happy and proud of myself. It helps to have a Teddy light on too!*

Another five-year-old child dictated to her therapist, Suzanne Pregerson, some comments to accompany a drawing of herself getting out of bed in the morning (Figure 7.5):

> *I went to bed by myself because my grandma helped me. It's 6 o'clock and it's time for me to get up. I am getting out of bed and going to check my dogs because my sister isn't up yet. I am learing how to sleep by myself. Me and my slippers are smiling because I slept by myself.*

A seven-year-old contributed some advice from her own experiences dealing with night fears:

> *I found out some ways to like my bed. Make a cosy nest with pillows and stuffed animals and pretend gossamer stuff. You can change your scary dreams when you're in them. Get a relaxing music tape to play if you wake up.*

Here are a couple of sample entries from a *Temper Tamer's Handbook*:

> *I think it's better to play instead of staying mad. If your temper comes up when you're playing, just go away and do something else until it goes away and calms down (Risa, age six).*

> *I figured some ways to get rid of the temper. I can do it all the time now! I spied on it. It used to creep up behind in a straight line, but since I spied on it, it creeps up in a spiral. I wait till it's close, 'cause I like to trick it, then I blow the whistle and it jumps up and runs in the air. Then it goes away and falls down. Or, sometimes, I call it names: "Stop you big bag of clattering screwdrivers, you poophead!" Then it stops and goes away. Like Mommy and Daddy were going out at night but Mommy mixed up the schedule.*

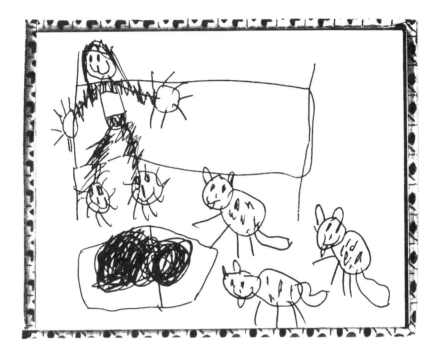

Figure 7.5 "Me and my slippers are smiling because I slept by myself."

We were going to have a different baby-sitter than I thought, and I could have been really upset, but I used my ideas and calmed down. Daddy and Mommy didn't even know about this, I was so calm (Maria, age eight).

Maria also made an entry in the *Fear Facer's and Worry Stopper's Handbook* describing a chart she drew of the race between the Fear, Anger, and Fun in her life (Figure 7.6).

GRADUATION, CONFIRMATION, AND CELEBRATION

Doesn't termination sound like something needed for a household pest? Graduations and confirmations are examples of rituals that take place when significant transitions occur in the lives of young persons. The rite of passage provides a metaphor for sharing the fruits of a young person's transformation with his community. Families and children enjoy such rituals at the end of therapy. Summaries of their accomplishments in the form of consulting your consultant interviews or contributing to an archive bring the meetings to an affirmative conclusion. However, some of us just like to plan a plain old-fashioned party where changes are reviewed, a certificate is given, a letter or poem is read, or a celebration sandtray is made along with food and festivities.

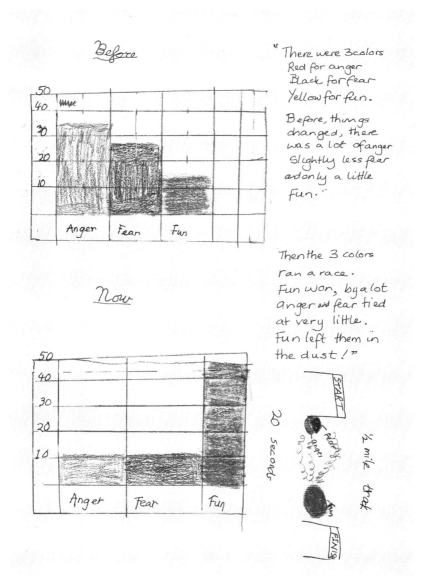

Figure 7.6 Maria's chart showing the race between anger, fear, and fun in her life

Jimmy's Honesty Speech

David's last meeting with twelve-year-old Jimmy took the form of an honesty party (Seymour & Epston 1992). In preparation, David asked Jimmy, aged twelve, about his party's guest list: "Who do you think would be keen to celebrate your return to honesty? Who do you guess has been concerned about what dishonesty was doing to your life and the life of your family? Are there any victims of your dishonesty whom you would like to invite to see if you can make it up with them?"

Jimmy suggested that his grandparents be special guests. Unfortunately they couldn't attend the party, so David proposed an idea: "Since they can't reach the party, what if the party were to reach them?" The highlight of an honesty party is, of course, the "honesty speech." Jimmy asked his parents to audiotape his honesty speech so that his grandparents could have a copy. Here is a transcript of the speech that was delivered at Jimmy's honesty party and circulated to his special guests:

> *You are all aware of what I did earlier on this year. I now realize that what I did was not only stupid but selfish. And I am sorry for that. Since the incident occurred, my mum, dad, John, and I went to see Mr. Epston, a family therapist who suggested I go on a program of honesty testing which you all know about. I did this to prove to myself and my family that I could withstand the temptation of taking things that did not belong to me. I have now successfully completed the tests which have led to this gathering. I'd like to thank you all for your support which has certainly made me realize what I did was wrong. And in the future, I will be earning money and not taking it.*

SUMMARY

Interviewing for news and circulating it to appropriate audiences is a special feature of the narrative approach to child therapy. In doing so narrative therapists are challenged to:

- develop an ear for discerning the expertise and hard-won knowledge of a child struggling with a problem;
- develop unique questions that evoke rich and detailed accounts of such expertise;
- edit and amplify alternative narratives about the young person;
- consistently check their theories for accuracy with the young person, family, and others;
- identify appropriate audiences, real and virtual, for circulation both within and outside of the family;
- devise means of publication that are apt to engage the audience (letters, archives, handbooks, certificates, artwork, etc.);
- co-develop and support communities of concern (clubs, leagues, networks, projects etc.);
- co-create rituals of confirmation, graduation, and celebration.

11

PLAYFUL MEANS

CHAPTER 8

· ·

Therapies of Aesthetic as well as Literary Merit

Drawn in by the adventure of overcoming an externalized problem, many young people open up and engage actively in verbal conversation. But, as we all know well, children prefer to express themselves in more ways than just sitting and talking! Much has been written in the field of child therapy about the limits of verbal interaction in therapy with children and the need for other forms of communication (Axline, 1987; Brems, 1993; Case & Dalley, 1990; Combrinck-Graham, 1989; Gil, 1994; Moustakas, 1973; Oaklander, 1978). Many alternative and playful ways to communicate can easily be integrated into narrative therapy (Barragar Dunne, 1992; Freeman & Lobovits, 1993).

In this chapter we offer some ideas on the importance of paying attention to nonverbal cues and of making expressive arts and play therapy available to children. The integration of expressive arts with narrative therapy is illustrated by a longer case story. We then elaborate on various ways of expanding narrative conversations with the arts.

Parents seek art or play therapy for their children, knowing that this will be fun as well as effective in helping them to communicate. Most kids jump at the chance to communicate in different ways; even those who are quite comfortable with verbal conversation usually appreciate being offered various forms of expression, such as painting or puppets. If they are not provided with alternative means of expression, the unique "voices" of certain young persons may be excluded from a family therapy conversation.

It is worth considering play and expressive arts therapy with:

- children who are not very verbal in therapy, including those who experience verbal shyness, speak another language as their first, have language-based difficulties, or are just too young to talk;
- children for whom art, sandtray, or dance are preferred means of expression, considering that they may be primarily visual or kinesthetic processors;
- those who have experienced a constriction of verbal expression at certain times, for example, due to threats made during abuse, and who may be uncomfortable with "talk therapy" (Barragar Dunne, 1992);
- with families where differences exist between therapist and child in terms of family style or cultural expression and where parents have expectations about appropriate ways for children to communicate.[1]

We may notice, for instance, that a child is expected by parents to communicate with any adult in authority (including the therapist) with displays of deference, e.g., limited eye contact, or polite abbreviated answers. The therapist may then inquire about such manners and how best to observe them, or about the possibilities for altering them in therapy without being disrespectful. We might, for example, compliment the child on her polite behavior and ask her parents if it might be a good idea for their child to communicate with drawings or a journal.

Children caught up in an emotional experience of the problem may have great difficulty expressing themselves in words, yet they may be communicating nonverbally, broadcasting their experience with facial expressions, posture, and movement. To what extent should we keep persevering in the attempt to verbally engage young people who are immersed in such an experience?

Information about problems may be lodged at a somatic level even when it is barely within conscious awareness. Approaches are then needed to bring such experience into focus. Elsewhere we have referred to these as "somatic conversations" (Freeman & Lobovits, 1993, p. 198).[2]

In the above situations, nonverbal encounters offer alternative means of communication while demonstrating acceptance of the child.

MIND-BODY UNITY AND EXPRESSIVE ARTS

For some time learning and communicating unfold for babies in the social context without words. As Mills and Crowley (1986, p. 92) put it, "Although the baby has no language capacities during this period of time, a vast array of qualities, feelings, and needs are communicated."

As young children become verbal, more and more sensory input is organized by the brain into narrative form.

Implications for our work arise when we consider the complexities of perceiving and making sense of the world. If we limit our conception of a person's life to what is "storied" in words, ignoring the functional biological whole of mind and body, we may slip into the dualism of Descartian philosophy. The map of verbal description does not fully represent the territory of lived experience, including the richness of visual symbolic processes, feelings, emotions, and sensations. Expressive arts therapies directly engage auditory, visual, and kinesthetic senses, as well as emotions. When we pay attention to nonverbal cues and facilitate expression through a variety of arts that evoke different senses, new dimensions of experience arise that are aesthetically rewarding as well as effective in our conversations with children.

EXPRESSIVE ARTS

Children and whole families can be invited to develop a narrative conversation using the expressive arts with media such as drawing or painting, cartoons, poetry or journal writing, sculpture, guided fantasy, charts or maps, sandtray, dramatic play with puppets, dress-ups and role-play and drama therapy, movement, mime, or mask-making (Barragar Dunne, 1992; Freeman & Lobovits, 1993; Smith & Barragar Dunne, 1992).

Although many of the approaches in this chapter describe working directly with a child or children, they are also applicable to facilitating alternative forms of communication among family members who are interested in trying, for example, a family drawing, puppet play, or sandtray.

One does not have to be an artist or be specially trained to use the expressive arts in combination with narrative therapy. There are straightforward ways to broaden expression. For example, many children can be invited to show problem or counter-problem ideas in graphic form in a drawing or cartoon. It is not necessary to be an expert in expressive arts or play therapy, since the child is already an expert at play and, given a simple invitation, will go a long way; the adult merely has to be willing to tag along and take up the meanings that emerge.

The field of expressive arts therapy has some things in common with narrative therapy. While the theories behind these approaches may differ, the "expression" of problems in art form is inherently akin to the practice of externalization. The very process of drawing, sculpting, or dramatizing the relationship with a problem naturally evokes a visceral sense of the problem as located for reflection outside of the self. The act of expression, in this sense, is often reported as beneficial in itself—it can be a relief for children to literally "express" the externalized problem in a symbolic yet physically experienced way. This allows them to "see" the problem and ponder it more easily. Just as they do when left alone to play, children often like to work and rework stories in oblique forms, such as puppet theater, rather than talking about things directly.

In some expressive arts therapies, the client creates and dialogues with figuratively expressed problems conceptualized theoretically as "parts" of the self. For example, "the critic" within a person is personified, drawn, and brought into a more agreeable relationship with the person (McMurray, 1988). We have found that similar benefits result from the artistic expression of a problem in expressive arts therapy as from the practice of externalization.

Rather than being employed for objective diagnostic and interpretive purposes, both expressive arts therapy (Weller, 1993) and narrative therapy invite clients to make meaning of their own expressions. The therapist takes a stance of curiosity and facilitates the expansion of preferred meanings for the client, rather than offering an expert opinion on her artistic productions.

THE PERFORMANCE OF MEANING

Narrative therapists are interested in the "performance of new meanings" (Bruner, 1986; White & Epston, 1990a/1997), which leads to the co-authoring of alternative stories. Our use of language actively shapes meaning and, therefore, experience, rather than just representing or describing it. As Michael White (in White & Epston, 1990b, p. 12) puts it:

> If we accept that persons organize and give meaning to their experience through the storying of experience, and that in the performance of these stories they express selected aspects of their lived experience, then it follows that these stories are constitutive—shaping lives and relationships.

This idea takes on new dimensions in the context of expressive arts therapy. The "performance" of a new meaning or story that includes other realms of expression helps solidify the new experience. To literally see in a picture a different vision adds a sensory dimension to the performance of meaning. For example, a child may draw herself as the problem would see her and then as she would prefer to be seen, thereby gaining a problem-free version of herself to match the emerging alternative story.

Children revel in performing new stories about their relationship with the problem via drama or puppet play. Imagine a special project for the performance of meaning: a videotaped "documentary" of a child or family's preferred story, which includes interviews, testimonials, poems, and meaningful images in drawings or sandtrays.

When integrated with verbal commentary and questions, the performance of meaning in any of these art forms becomes multidimensional and is thus enriched.

AESTHETIC MERIT

Expression in art may be experienced as inherently rewarding and healing. In expressive arts therapy, the process of creation is regarded as being of value, instead of the main focus being on the technical viruosity or artistic merit of the product. When expressive arts are combined with co-authoring narratives, we invite a child into alternative forms of expression, respectfully inquire into the nuances of her meanings, and allow our own imagination to overlap with hers, rather than using stories to interpret or evaluate the product.

Paolo Knill, Helen Nienhaus Barba, and Margo Fuchs (1995, p. 71) have noted the value of an aesthetically satisfying expression:

> An *aesthetic response*, as we will use the term here, refers to a distinct response, with a bodily origin, to an occurrence in the imagination, to an artistic act, or to the perception of an art work. When the response is profound and soul-stirring, we describe it as "moving" or "breathtaking (Atem-beraubend)." Our language suggests a sensory effect associated with the image, what Hillman describes as revealing itself in the quick in-breath (or inspiration) we might experience when in the presence of beauty (1994).

Multimodal or intermodal expressive therapies invite a person to move flexibly among media, following her creative instincts and interests (Knill, Barba, & Fuchs, 1995; Robbins, 1994; Rogers, 1993). Satisfaction is afforded as different senses are employed and a deepening effect takes place. This model can be loosely applied in the context of narrative therapy. For example, a sandtray is reflected on by writing a poem or short story. Its meaning could be further developed in movement, which then leads to a painting or sculpture.

Knowing that various media are available, a child or other members of the family may choose to express themselves in different ways at any time during therapy. Sometimes important meanings for a child emerge in concert with this aesthetic experience. Eleven-year-old Arianna had been in individual play, art, and bibliotherapy for several years, freeing herself from the effects of severe physical and sexual abuse. One day she entered the playroom and, after saying a quiet hello, walked over to the sandtray.

Starting with her finger in the center, she carefully drew a spiral in the sand, covering the whole sandtray. Arianna invited Jenny to look at the sandtray, but did not choose to say anything about it right then. There was a gentle silence. Jenny inquired as to whether she might like to express herself in any other way, perhaps with a poem or drawing about her sandtray. She sat down on the floor and wrote the poem in Figure 8.1.

After Arianna read the poem, Jenny asked if and how she might like to continue expressing herself. Arianna thought she might want to do some journal writing or share something of her knowledge in a handbook. Aware that her writing might be shared with others in the future, she wrote this commentary to accompany the poem.

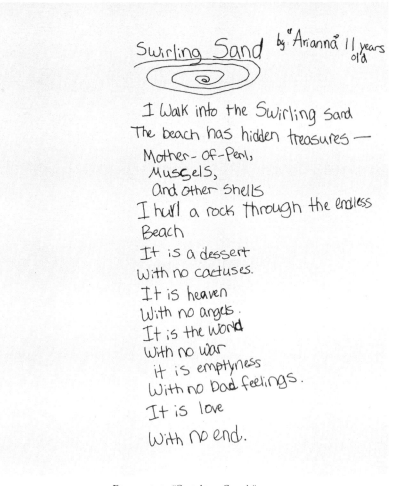

Figure 8.1. "Swirling Sand."

Changing Fear

This story-poem is about one girl, walking through an endless desert, which seemed like an endless desert of fear, but really the girl finds that it is a beautiful place. She finds that really she is not alone and that every grain of sand is as precious as a pearl. The mussels and shells were not only dead animals but live treasures.

I have learned to use my sensitivity positively instead of negatively. Instead of crying when someone calls me a bad name, now I think "that's just your problem" and I can laugh about it. The fear is like sensitivity, you have to change it. Fear is actually hidden bravery. Fear is an arrow—it points to things—it can be your friend. There are two kinds of Fear: (1) Stupidness Fear, when you're afraid of your feelings, then you have hurt feelings. (2) Fear for a Reason. How to tell the difference? You just listen to your feelings, what your heart is telling you, not what fear is telling you. You have to listen with your heart, through your heart.

Considering that up until this point in their work together dissociation had seemed the main option for Arianna when anything having to do with fears or abuse was raised, Jenny was moved by the vividness and eloquence of her expression.

Jenna and the Temple of Life

Now we offer a longer illustrated case story so that the reader may read and view the creative journey of a child who used several art media to express herself. Jenna and her mother Rachel met with Jenny in individual and conjoint family sessions intermittently over a period of two years.

Jenna, age eight and of mixed African American and Jewish descent, and her mother, Rachel, came to see Jenny, because, as Rachel put it, "she seems ready to deal with some issues around her dad's death from cancer a year ago." Rachel related that Jenna had been very close to her father, Gene, who had been her primary caretaker, but his lengthy illness meant that he had been tired and grumpy a lot of the time. Their family had faced a double crisis: Gene had been diagnosed with cancer while Rachel was finishing treatment for cancer herself. Fortunately, she was now in remission. Rachel went on to describe her daughter as "a vibrant, intense, charismatic, artistic tomboy."

Jenna was facing a lot of fear and grief. And one thing was certain—she was also angry and volatile. She wet her bed regularly and often spent most of the night screaming as an aftermath to "bad dreams." Jenna never slept through the night and was quite demanding in general. This was a serious problem for Rachel, who was extremely fatigued and required sleep for her health and well-being. She felt that everything had become a battle and found it hard to decide "where to draw the line between her needs and mine."

Jenna was now so controlled by Fear that she was having trouble attending school, as well as reading or watching anything "scary" on video or TV. When Jenny asked Jenna about the effects of Fear on her life and her relationships, she complained that it "stops me from reading books and hanging out with my girlfriends." Rachel and Jenna both wished to get through this time following the loss of Gene, without Fear taking over Jenna's life. They had already come up with some practices that Jenna used to calm herself down, such as playing a music tape at night.

Rachel sought art therapy for Jenna, knowing this was a favorite way for her daughter to express herself. Jenny made a loose plan with Rachel and Jenna to divide therapy between conjoint meetings and individual art/play/talk sessions. Many of the narrative conversations took place with Rachel and Jenna together and much of the expressive arts with Jenna alone, although her productions and thoughts were usually shared later with her mother.

Jenna's late father, Gene, was included in the therapy from the start. At Jenny's suggestion, Rachel and Jenna brought in photos of the family's times together, along with stories of his life and death.[3] The family performed simple rituals for Gene's inclusion in their lives, such as lighting candles and remembering him at times he typically would have participated in events in family life. Jenny would ask questions about what Gene would want for Jenna. What advice might he give on Jenna's struggle with Fear or any other problem? What would he say about her successes and how would he celebrate them? Jenna would exclaim that she wanted her father to know about her accomplishments or steps she had taken.

For a while Jenna was satisfied with simply externalizing her fear as "Fears." The anger and demanding behavior she engaged in became known either as "Fear " or "Frustration." Later Jenna also came up with the term "the Trickster" for when the Fear was being particularly intrusive. In order to overcome the frustration and fighting that was coming between mother and daughter, Jenny suggested they stand together to view these problems, in the form of two large puppets, from across the room. From this united perspective, they decided to form an Anti-Frustration Team so as to spot Frustration building up and to stand together to rebuke it. This conceptual shift changed their relationship at home.

Jenna's grief was something she was unable to talk about for some time, until Jenny invited her to draw a picture of her experience. Jenna drew a picture (Figure 8.2) showing water pouring over a girl "like a bucket of tears" from an overhead shower. She said quietly that these were partly her mother's tears. This opened the way for her to say she was overwhelmed and scared by her mother's grief and had trouble crying herself.

"When I talk about my dad and she cries and it's noisy and scary, it's like a shower," she explained. "It makes me mad to see her so upset." By the next conjoint session, Jenna was prepared to show this picture to

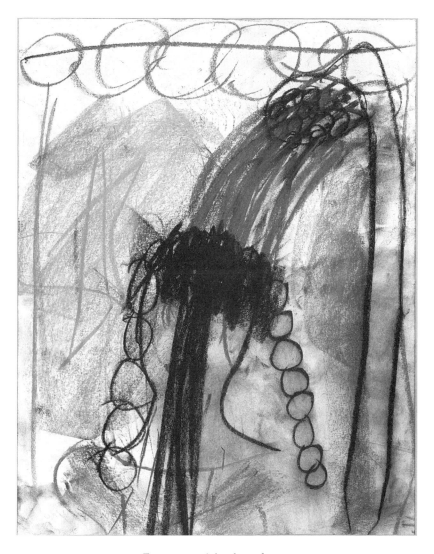

Figure 8.2 A bucket of tears.

her mother. The picture spoke a thousand words to Rachel about Jenna's feelings and inspired a conversation about how Rachel might express her grief in ways and places that were "unscary" for Jenna. Jenna asked her mother if she could help make sadness and crying less overwhelming for her.

Several months later, Jenna made a picture of a rainbow and took up Jenny's suggestion to write a poem to go with it.

> *Stormy Day Rainbow*
>
> I am a stormy day
> I have a little lightning and black streaks
> and all kinds of colors in my sky:
> Peach and Green,
> Magenta, Pink and a little Lavender,
> through it all you can see a rainbow on me.
>
> I'm a storm,
> I go rumble, rumble
> I feel very neat,
> It feels good to be a storm.
> Clatter, crash, bang and bam,
> that's the lightning in Alabam
> Pink, Yellow, Purple, Brown,
> Put it all together and you get a storm.

It seemed easier for Rachel and Jenna to discuss Jenna's relationship to Fear and Worry and to consider how damaging Fear was to their sleep. They realized that Worry, which was not at all surprising in their circumstances, had turned into an "overgrowth" of Fear. Jenna particularly resented that this stopped her from feeling able to read books or stay with friends for fear something scary would be on TV or in the book. "It's a Trickster that gets you thinking you can't handle things and tells you you're dumb," she said. In response to Jenny's inquiries, Jenna decided it was unfair that much of her life had been taken over by the Trickster Fear; now she was ready to stop it in its tracks. They decided that as a first step Jenna needed to be able to tell the difference between Worry and Fear and to draw the line between the two.

Jenny suggested that Jenna draw pictures (Figures 3.3 and 3.4, pp. 66 and 67) showing how it was when Worry had the better of her and when Jenna bested Worry. Jenny recorded her comments about the pictures:

Worry good, Worry bad

First the worry succeeds. Then Jenna beats worry. You know how? Instead of getting teased herself, she teases him. Then she's not as worried anymore. She likes that better. Worry should stay in jail in solitary confinement so you can get him when you need him, like when you cross the street. You should also worry when you're throwing up. If you didn't and went to school, you could get someone else sick, or get much sicker yourself, dangerously.

This distinction was encouraged by Rachel, who reviewed with Jenna her "realistic worries" and what she could do about them along with times that Worry turned into the Trickster Fear. Since they knew by this time that the Trickster thrived on physical tension, one project was to identify and foster "Friends of Relaxation," such as music, deep breathing and affirmations, as well as Jenna's own courage and strength. When she needed them, she could call on these Friends to help her relax and get past Fear instead of rousing her mother during the night. One of Jenna's original new ideas was to invent "an imaginary brain transmitter that you can use to switch your brain back on and free it from Fear's tricks that shut it down."

For her part, Rachel decided she needed to define some limits. She employed the time-honored chart system, marking early bedtimes and sleeping through the night with star stickers and a weekly reward for success.

Rachel and Jenny helped elaborate the story of Jenna's ability to be in command of the Trickster Fear. The next time they met, Jenna announced with excitement that she had started watching "scary funny movies like the *Return of the Killer Tomatoes*." Rachel added that she had also noticed with delight that Jenna was comfortable saying what she didn't want to watch. Jenna had been invited to watch *Psycho* at a friend's party and did not hesitate to take a book into another room.

Jenny likes to thicken the counterplot or enrich the picture of alternative stories through means that include other senses, such as the tactile and visual. As Jenna's confidence in dealing with Fears grew, Jenny invited her to make "a Fear mask and a Freedom mask." She made three masks; each was played with, tried on, given a voice and story. Jenny interviewed each mask, asking questions like: "What is your name? What do you do? What is your purpose in life? How do you bother kids like Jenna? How do you help kids like Jenna? What would you like us to know about you? How can Jenna make peace with you?" Jenna recorded the following stories about her masks:

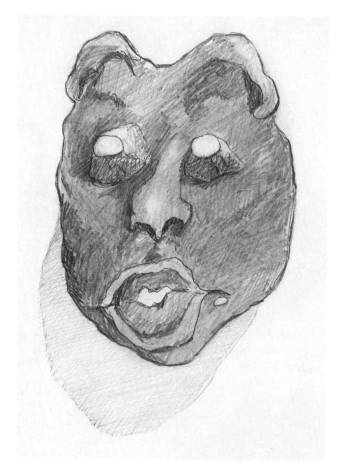

Figure 8.3 The Trickster Fear, Ricky.

Fear Mask (Figure 8.3)

"My fear mask's name is Ricky. He's the empty face of fear . . . surrounded by happiness. He has empty eyes and he's sad, because the happiness has surrounded him. He has been named Fear now. I say to the mask: 'You're no longer nothing . . . being nothing made it hard to know you. Once you're named, you can be known and conquered!'"

Freedom Mask (Figure 8.4)

"I'm me when I'm twenty years old. I have short curly hair. I'm a family doctor. I like my work. I live with my roommate. I'm funny, happy, sad, and love to play games. Mom is at home. I could be called Sarah Lee, a girl who knows what she's doing, she's taking the right track, she's in control of her life. She's not worried, she's lucky. She won't be scared on dates and at her wedding."

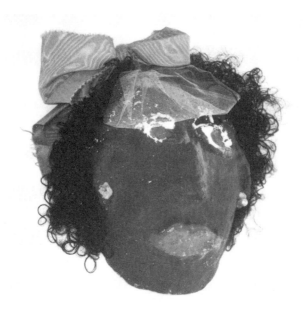

Figure 8.4 Freedom Mask, Sarah Lee, "a girl who know what she's doing."

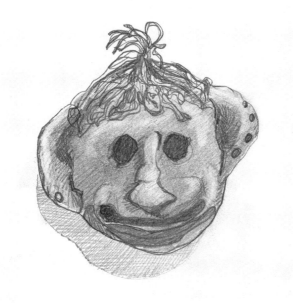

Figure 8.5 Another Future Mask, "It would be a bright life."

Another Future Mask (Figure 8.5)
"He's a rocker, he loves rap, he has red and blue hair. He's leader of a band. He's twenty, he wants to have a different career when he gets a bit older. That's what I've dreamed of 'cause it sounds fun. It would be a bright life."

Several months later, Jenna's grasp on Fear and Worry was put to the test. She came home from school to find her mother absent. It turned out that Rachel had been caught in traffic. Instead of panicking, Jenna collected herself and called her mother's friend, who came over to be with her. Jenny hoped to weave this breakthrough into Jenna's new story of courage, humor, and freedom from Fear. She asked if Jenna wanted to find a way to celebrate in an art form. Jenna was in the mood to create a sandtray, one of her favorite media (Figure 8.6). Afterwards, she wrote a poem to reflect on her sandtray. While Jenna was writing her poem, Jenny wrote a letter.

Here is Jenna's poem:

The Temple of Life

Gods and Goddesses watching the things of life,
Venus, Buddhas and more, standing watching,
The Tiger is the sign of bravery against danger in life,
the jeweled frog the sign of passion and beauty in life.
Venus and Buddhas with the other gods and goddesses
   watch over the things of life.
Food for health, cones for money, flowers for love,
A jeweled frog for beauty,
A tiger for bravery and for life,
That's what the gods guard!

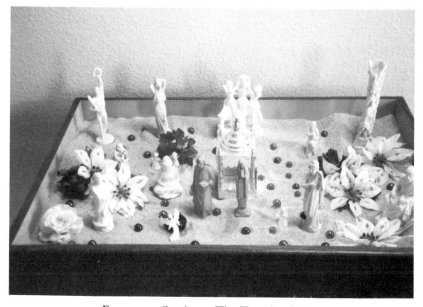

Figure 8.6 Sandtray: The Temple of Life.

Here is Jenny's letter, which was reviewed by Jenna and completed after their next meeting together.

Dear Jenna,

As we said when we talked about writing the latest installments in your story, Jenna: "This is the story of a girl who is challenged in her life to deal with fears. She finds again her bravery and trust, realizing that she can take care of herself and get taken care of in life."

You have dealt with fears before. You said you found out recently that you had been worried about taking care of yourself, in case you had to deal with something when your mom wasn't there. A very important thing happened recently that showed us— and you—how you were able to take care of yourself. This gave you confidence to let go of these fears, knowing that you are now learning to take care of yourself.

You told me about the time that you came home from Hebrew School and nobody was there. You could have been scared, but instead you stayed calm, used your head and thought about what you could do to solve the problem. You decided to call your mom's best friend. This told you that "I knew how to handle myself in emergencies, and that if something ever happened to mom I could take care of myself." You said, "I learned I could think clearly, and think ahead, face the unknown and make it fun instead of scary . . . this made me know I was brave and could take care of myself and I knew that now I didn't need the fears."

Jenna, what other times have you been in touch with this freedom before? What other signs are there that you don't need fears anymore? Perhaps your mom or others might have some stories of trust and bravery to add to this one? You thought that Anna wouldn't be surprised to know that you had these abilities, knowing you as she does.

When I asked you how these realizations were affecting your relationship with the fears, you said: "Now I'm sleeping better at night, and once again I don't have to have my life run by fears, but can run my own life instead."

Jenna, as we have talked about before, it is natural that you would have to recover your trust and bravery after your dad died. You said that you thought your dad would be proud of you! Perhaps you or your mom could also remember some earlier stories of trust and bravery, ones that your dad knew about or was part of? I think, too, that he would love to know that you are learning this trust in yourself and can go on and be free from the fears . . . and that you can feel confident to enjoy and celebrate life.

After we talked about these things you made a very special sandtray about the Temple of Life. This can remind you about your own special story of trust in life, and about your confidence and bravery.

Yours for trust in your freedom,
    Jenny Freeman

FOLLOW-UP

Jenny met with Rachel and Jenna during the preparation of the story for this book. Thankfully, Rachel is still in good health. Jenna is now fourteen, and by both of their accounts is thriving at school and in her home and social life. Jenna offered the poem on pp. 295–296, written when she was thirteen.

The rest of the chapter is devoted to forming a collage of ideas about the mixture of expressive arts and narrative therapy. We start with thinking about how children may be invited into making use of expressive arts and then offer maps for some of the many possible ways that expressive arts media may be combined with narrative therapy.

INVITING CHILDREN INTO PLAY AND EXPRESSIVE ARTS THERAPY[4]

From the time the child walks into the room, nonverbal clues may suggest to the therapist a move into other realms of communication. If a therapist notices that a young person seems uncomfortable talking, is shy or antsy, is not responding to questions, is overwhelmed with emotion, struggling for words, or that her attention is glued to the art materials, it is worth considering offering other choices of expression. The therapist can initiate a shift with a question like, "Sometimes things are hard to talk about in words; could we find another way?" Alternatively, she might say: "There are lots of ways we can communicate. What ways do you like?"

Jenny sometimes picks up a puppet who makes friends with the child or children in a family; she offers the child and other family members puppets so that they might establish a different way of talking together.

When making the shift from conversation to expressive arts activities it can be helpful to offer warm-up exercises such as guided relaxation, imagination games, or physical games (Barragar Dunne, 1992; de Mille, 1976; Oaklander, 1978).

To invite conversation using specific media, we might ask the individual child or family members:

- What does the problem look/seem/feel/sound like to you?
- Can you show it in a cartoon or drawing, or make a mask?
- Does it look like one of these puppets to you? Would you rather use puppets to talk?
- Could you show me what you mean by making a scene or map in the sandtray?
- Could you dance or move and show how it feels when the problem takes over?

Emma's Decision

Jenny and twelve-year-old Emma were having a hard time talking in an individual session about whether Emma wanted to visit her mother, from whose home and custody she had been removed because of abuse. Emma could not decide if she was ready for a visit, although she and her caretakers had agreed that it was time for her to involve herself in this decision. For several weeks she had been unable to resolve her dilemma.

Emma was literally squirming. It was obviously easier to change the subject or to play a board game. Knowing that there were risks on either side of her decision, Jenny wondered about the "Bind" that Emma was in. "Does the Bind make it difficult for you to sort your feelings out?" she asked. "Does the Bind make it so that you're damned if you do visit and damned if you don't?" Emma nodded vigorously. "It's stopping me from making decisions," she said. "But it's too hard to talk about," she added, grimacing. There was a pregnant, rather awkward pause.

Jenny invited Emma to wonder if there might be a more interesting way of looking at the Bind and exploring the two sides of the decision, without talking. "How would you like to check out the Bind and get in touch with what you want to do? Do you want to do some art or use puppets?" she asked. Emma jumped up, ran across the room and grabbed two puppets, a dragon and a butterfly. She returned to her place and said expectantly, "Now what?" There was a lengthy silence before Emma suggested: "Hey, they could argue the different sides!" Jenny thought this idea had great potential and proposed that they make a colorful chart with two sides that the puppets could fill in to explore the pros and cons of her decision. The puppets drew pictures and wrote phrases on each side of the chart, revealing thoughts and feelings that Emma had not previously been able to put into words. She was also able to articulate the Bind she was in and to make plans to share her concerns with her family. By the next morning, Emma had reached her decision.

PLAYFUL WAYS TO EXPLORE THE RELATIVE INFLUENCE OF PERSON AND PROBLEM

Children can interact directly with the "personified problem" to dramatize their relationship with it. For example, a puppet, mask, or drawing can be put on or propped up, given a voice, and interviewed as to its plans and intentions. When a young person is invited to create a "problem mask," she is also invited to create a solution or "personal agency mask" (Barragar Dunne, 1992) to develop the alternative story.

The masks can be brought into dialogue with each other to explore and advocate for a preferred relationship. Nine-year-old Jeremy, for example, made a Fear mask and a Bravery mask. When he was playing the part of Fear, Jenny asked him, "So, Fear, how are you stopping Jeremy from enjoying his life?" Jeremy gave the Fear mask a voice and responded, "I like to whisper to him that the night is full of ghosts and robbers." Jeremy then switched roles by donning his Bravery Mask, and was asked, "Bravery, what do you want to tell Fear about you that it doesn't know, that might scare it away?" Jeremy responded, "That's baloney, Fear—you just like to make things up to scare me. You're still using that scary show on TV, but those kinds of shows are meant to make you scared. I don't need to listen to you! We've got a security system, right Mom? . . . And anyway, I'm getting braver every day!"

In another example, Mickey, who was dealing with a lot of trouble at school, was drawing a cartoon. He depicted in graphic form answers to questions, such as: "Tell me, what does the Troublemeister say to you about yourself? If the problem were drawing you in a cartoon, how would it make you appear?" Mickey drew the Troublemeister with a caption saying, "Why bother about school? You're just a deadbeat anyway!"

In order to further expose such "motives" of the problem, questions could be asked, such as:

- What does the Troublemeister want you to do?
- How does it try to get you to go along with it at school?
- What are its plans for your future? Is that fair to you?

Then, to clarify the preferred relationship with the problem, Mickey was invited to draw an alternative picture. He was playing at recess and the Troublemeister was in detention:

- Do you like this picture of yourself? Does it suit you?
- How did you get Trouble out of the picture (of your life)?
- Was it fun to "draw back" and show "the untroubled you"?

Problem plots and alternative story counterplots can also be depicted with topographic maps. A tangible map is created using sandtray or drawing. This appeals to a child's love of adventure stories and magic. The map can represent territories, chart paths to freedom, and so on; the possibilities are endless. For example, a child in a magical quest for bravery or peace creates Lake Fear, a Brave Team on the Trail of Happiness, the Peace Meadow, and the Lair of the Worry Wart-Hog. Games can also be made up to map out a family's relationship with problems (Davida Cohen, personal communication, 1995).[5]

Below we elaborate on several specific expressive arts approaches[6] and give case story examples of their narrative application.

SANDPLAY

Anyone who remembers the magical appeal of miniature figures and creating an imaginary world with figures is likely to be intrigued by sandplay. A young person, dyads such as a mother and daughter, or even a whole family can be invited to play in a therapeutic sandtray (Kalff, 1971). Children are usually attracted to the array of miniature figures on the shelf, which stand ready to be chosen and arranged in the sandtray. For those who do not consider themselves artists, the sandtray is an accessible and satisfying form of symbolic communication.[7]

There are several ways to approach sandplay in a narrative context. A child or family can be asked to create a problem-saturated sandtray: "What does the world of the problem look like?" "Is there a figure that reminds you of the problem?" "How does it live?" "Who are its cronies? What supports it?"

A sandplay world can be used to map the influence of the problem: "Would you like to show me how the problem takes over?" "Could you make a picture of it or map it out with symbols in the sand?" Having laid the problem out visually, the child may find it easier to describe its effects.

The therapist offers the option of leaving the problem-saturated sandtray as it is or creating a "transition tray" by introducing elements of change:

- Would you like to leave the tray as it is, or change it, or make another tray?

If the child chooses to change the tray, objects can be removed, added, or moved around. The therapist can ask questions, such as:

- Would you like to put some other figures in the tray or change things around in some way?
- What would you add to or take away from this tray so that it feels better?
- What would free things up?

Working with unique outcomes, we might ask:

- What are you doing in your life that changes the way the problem works in this scene?
- Could you show how you are taking back your life?
- Can you show what happens when you're the boss of the problem?

As the conversation progresses, the child or family can be invited to create an alternative story sandtray or series of trays to symbolically map how the child or family is relating differently to the problem. The sandtray may show a scene of battle, a triumph over the problem, or a vision of life as it will be without the problem. The child's experience shifts as she make the various sandtrays and as she performs new meanings in this tangible form.

An alternative story sandtray can also be created if a child is ready to envision a new story without first portraying the problem. Something akin to the "miracle question" (de Shazer, 1991) can also be posed for consideration in a sandtray: "How would it look if things were already the way you want them to be?"

From session to session, sandtrays can be used to signify progress or to explore setbacks. Sometimes children are more comfortable representing the problem-saturated sandtray when they have moved safely past the problem. Jason's story in Chapter 15 illustrates this.

Polaroid photographs and slides serve to archive the sandtray. These may be used to "depict" narrative change over time. Children often pick a figure to represent themselves or their team, and these take on a magical quality. The symbols and story of the tray are often referred to and woven into future conversations or art forms, rather like the contents of a narrative letter.

Children and families can take up a simple invitation to "make a map of how it works" or "show it in the sand." Before making a tray individually, children are informed of possible ways to approach it: While they make the tray, some choose to tell a running story; others prefer to complete the sandtray in silence and then have the family and therapist gather around to listen to the story. Sandtray pictures should receive the profound respect given to any artistic production. They should not be touched unless the child invites participation and they should not be disassembled in front of the child.

Zoe Dumps the Worrier

During a therapy whose main interest was to help release seven-year-old Zoe from her fears about being away from her parents, Jenny mentioned that a kid she had met before used a pouch to store notes about good ideas for getting over Worries. It turned out that Zoe and her parents had previously invented the practice of sending her to school with a "pocketful of kisses." However, the Worries still tried to convince her that her parents would not return at the end of the school day. Together the family and Jenny then came up with the idea of "a remembering pouch" with a touchstone for bravery and charms for recalling her parents' caring. This was intended to back up the discovery made through unique account questioning, that such "remembering" was already occurring in her life. Although an actual pouch was not made, the next week Zoe was keen on reporting about the days she remembered, thus fortifying the new story that was developing about her preexisting bravery and trust.

A running story sandtray (Figure 8.7) was created over the final three meetings (out of a total of six). Zoe was asked to show in the sand how she was taking back her life back from the problem or, as she had put it, the Worrier. First she chose a large blue dragon as the Worrier, putting it in the middle of the sandtray. She talked about how it had been affecting her life. When asked if she wanted to leave the tray as is for now or change it, she picked a symbol for herself and assembled a team of various animals and magical characters who helped her back the Worrier into a corner with taunts and threats. In the next session some of the team buried the dragon and sat on its head.

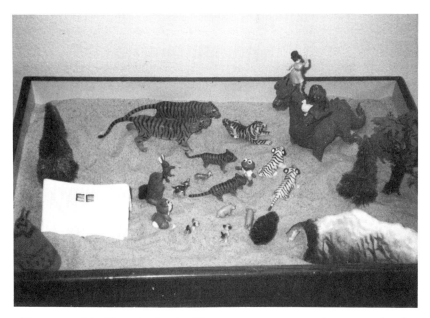

Figure 8.7 The Team backs the Worrier into a corner and sits on its head.

The large team established a clubhouse with a meeting space where they could come up with ideas for getting free of the Worrier. It was here that they had the great idea of having "happy good-byes" instead of "sad good-byes." It turned out that Zoe had been experimenting with this idea over the past week and that "happy good-byes" had already changed the experience of parting from her parents in the morning. By the end of the story in the final tray, the magic team had taken over so much space that they set up a "game house" just to enjoy the fun they could have now that they weren't so busy worrying about the Worrier. More of them, including a chicken and an owl, enjoyed sitting on its head.

Parents, when they witness a tale like this, are often inspired to perform meanings of their own. As Zoe finished telling the tray's story, her father, Robert, joked that since the Worrier was in such a boring position, buried in the corner, he must be considering a long vacation, if not retirement! At this point, Zoe, Marina (her mother), Robert, and Jenny each took up puppets, who had a conversation among themselves about all these developments.

The following letter was written by Susan Andrea Weiner in response to the sandtray. As part of her training, Susan had joined the family meeting as a one-person reflecting team.

Dear Zoe, Marina, and Robert,

It was very nice to meet you several weeks ago in Jenny's office. Thank you for "catching me up" on the wonderful and very smart tricks that Zoe and her team have been using to keep the Worrier from bothering Zoe. Having been introduced to you, Zoe, Marina and Robert, and the rest of Zoe's team, I can see that the Worrier, despite his three heads, does not have the brain power to keep Zoe from growing up and having a good time in the process.

Zoe, among your many ideas, I especially like the idea of the Flying Unicorn sprinkling sleeping powder over the Worrier, to "keep him snoozing in his cage," and the use of sweet roses to "make him sneeze and keep him confused so he forgets" to bother you as you make plans to visit with your friends. Zoe, you recruited such helpful and creative members to your team!

Marina and Robert, your very obvious love and support and your commitment to working with Zoe to discover creative ways to tame and let go of fear seem to have helped keep the Worrier in his cage, guarded by the loyal and protective tigers. What have you noticed lately about Zoe's growing ability to relax around partings, and find a way to experience happy good-byes? Which of your clever ideas, like putting hugs and kisses in Zoe's pockets, has Zoe been using? Have the Fears made any attempt to re-trick her? What other ideas have you all come up with to outsmart the Worrier?

With the Worrier backed into a corner, has there been more room for happy good-

byes? Am I right to guess that your good-byes before drop-off at school are continuing to get happier, as Zoe shakes off the mean tricks the Worrier played on her and skips off to join her friends? Which of her many ideas has she been using to help grow her confidence into believing that she can relax and know that she will be picked up after school?

Zoe, is the Worrier still asleep or sneezing in his cage, or have you let him slink away? Hopefully, he won't bother other kids, but would it be okay for me to share the tricks I've learned from you about not letting fears ruin fun and friendships? Have you noticed, like I have, that after "goodbye" comes "hello" . . . hello to a fun day at school with your friends, hello to new experiences, hello to hugs and kisses giggling in your pockets, and hello to your mom or dad when they pick you up after school? How much easier is it getting to say hello to school? Are your parents pleased, knowing you are filling your days with hellos?

Zoe, are you reminding yourself that these are "silly tricks" and that you have a strong and supportive team on your side? If you ever want to fill me in on any of the smart tricks you and your parents have been using to keep fear from spoiling the fun, all you have to do is call me up and say—you guessed it—"Hello!"

Thank you again for sharing your clever ideas and powerful strengths with me.
Warmly,
    Susan

In a follow-up conversation eight months later, Marina said that Zoe was still living with some fears but she felt that Zoe and the family had more tools to deal with them. For her part, Zoe said she was enjoying going to school. When the subject of the Worrier came up, she giggled and said she was imagining putting two fingers for ears behind the Worrier's head—"to make more fun of him."

MOVEMENT AND BODY AWARENESS

In the kinesthetic realm, we pay attention to the embodiment of the problem and of its resolution. A person can have a visceral experience of being "overtaken by the problem" and with finding a way out of it in dance, movement, or posture. Through movement, one can journey toward freedom in relationship to the problem (Smith & Barragar Dunne, 1992).

The therapist can invite young persons to notice what holding a problem story about themselves does to their body—to their posture, breathing, and movement. A child might try to "walk in the shoes of the problem and see things from its perspective" (Clover Catskill, personal communication, April, 1991) A child and family can play, use dance or body sculpture to explore the influence of the problem on the body.

For example, a girl battling "Self-doubt" might be asked:

- Where does Self-doubt live in your body?
- When it has a grip on you, how does it get you to walk, stand, breathe and move?
- What does it want your face to do?
- What stance/posture does it have you take in the world?
- How does it color your senses?
- Can you show what happens in your body when Self-doubt shows up in class?
- How does that feel to you?
- What do you prefer to feel instead?
- How do you sit or walk when you're feeling relaxed and confident?
- What happens when you buck Self-doubt's messages about girls and walk your own walk and talk your own talk?

The therapist may then invite her to explore, in a transitional movement or body sculpture, a way out of the problem's influence, gradually developing a movement of agency and freedom. These liberatory movements or gestures may become easily recalled signatures, serving to remind a person of an alternative stance in relationship to a problem story. In pantomime, family members might try peeling off the mask of the problem, shaking it out of their bodies, or otherwise removing it in a visceral manner from a person or relationship.

Younger children love the intrigue of "spying" on how the problem tricks them in their body or how it gets them to walk or act. The way in which a problematic story influences the body can be noticed in between as well as during meetings. We suggest that the child record her findings, as any good spy would do, and bring her inside information to the next session. When the problem's tricks are deciphered, the child can play counter-tricks on the problem, outwit it, by changing her posture, facial expression, breathing it out, or deciding to let it go.

Dan, Julia, and the "Weight of a Problem"

Here is an example of using somatically-based awareness and communication with an eight-year-old boy who was not exactly the type to leap at the idea of doing some "dance or movement therapy." At Jenny's first meeting with Dan and his mother Julia, Dan sat with his jaw set and his arms tightly crossed over his chest, while Julia described the frequency of his fighting, along with eruptions of swearing. Attempts to externalize the anger or fighting kept getting derailed as Dan rolled his eyes or protested angrily and scuffed his tennis shoes against the edge of the carpet. "He started it" or "It wasn't my fault" Dan repeated insistently in his defense and concern for fairness. This concern seemed to preclude Dan's taking any responsibility for his anger or his part in the fighting.

Jenny felt it was important for her to examine the operations of fighting and blame in the family, including assessing for possible abuse. Her persistent attempts to initiate an externalizing conversation to accomplish this were going nowhere. Finally, she asked, "Would it be okay with you two to talk about things in a way that would take Dan out of the hot seat of blame and put the anger and fighting problem there instead?" Julia consented, but Dan continued to look uninvolved yet wary. Jenny pondered momentarily and then asked Dan if he knew what she meant. If not, could she show him?

She stood up and walked slowly over to him. She asked him if it would be okay for her to hold a book near to his chest. He agreed, so Jenny approached Dan, who was still sitting, and then held a book a few inches away from his body, saying, "Let's pretend this book is the fighting problem and that it's pressing on your chest. You know how it keeps getting you in trouble, putting you on the spot, and making it look like you're to blame—does it feel like there's a pressure on you? Do you feel like the blame falls heavily on you?" Dan nodded.

"What would happen if we were to take it off your chest and put it over here on the floor where we could all take a look at it?" Jenny asked, as she began to lift the book away from Dan's chest. "Would that be a good idea?" Dan nodded again. Jenny lifted the book, dramatizing the sense of its heaviness, and tossed it down on the floor, where it landed with a thud. Dan emitted an audible sigh of relief. Pointing at the "externalized" problem on the floor, Jenny asked again whether it was fair of the fighting problem to be weighing him down and getting him into trouble all the time. "No, it's not," Dan said emphatically, shaking his foot menacingly at the book.

The physical sense of having the problem lifted from his body seemed to help Dan relax. He stretched, sat back in his chair, and turned slightly towards his mother as she began to speak in a sympathetic way about the effects of so much fighting on his life. This opened the way for a lively discussion, in which Dan and Julia began to look at how Fighting and Temper worked in the family and what they could do about it.

Attention to somatic dimensions in a safe and relaxed atmosphere opens the way for emotionally charged information to become part of the conversation. When a child like Dan is more relaxed and less defensive, it is more likely that difficult topics such as abuse will emerge.

Along these lines, Griffith and Griffith (1994, p. 66) write about how "emotional postures can either open or close possibilities for therapeutic dialogue." They differentiate between ethologically based postures of tranquillity and those of mobilization. Postures of mobilization may be expressed without language as "exploring, investigating, showing alarm, mobilizing, readying to attack or defend, stalking, fleeing." In language, postures of mobilization show up as "justifying, scorning, shaming, controlling, distancing, protesting, defending." Postures of tranquillity manifest in behaviors such as resting, gazing, and playing, and in language, as "reflecting, listening, wondering, creating, musing, fantasizing, day-dreaming."

These ideas provide useful guidance in therapy with families and children. If we pay attention to the postures people arrive with or that are evoked in conversation and use our skills to facilitate tranquillity in the room, tension dissolves into a readiness to relax and to converse openly in an atmosphere of safety.

WHEN ANY FORM OF COMMUNICATION SEEMS NEXT TO IMPOSSIBLE

What happens when all your most playful and creative questions, as well as invitations to respond in verbal or nonverbal ways, fall flat? It is tempting to keep trying to get children to express themselves one way or another, but by doing so we may create unnecessary pressure.

If alternative forms of communication are not terribly successful, there are other ways of moving forward. David has a way of carrying on the conversation even when there is a lack of direct communication with the child. Rather than trying hard to elicit a response, he may choose to interview the other participants in the room about the young person and her situation. This might draw forth a fresh response from the child or she might just listen and absorb the conversation. For example, he might address Jill's mother like this: "If you were Jill, how would you answer this question?" Then, turning back to Jill, he would ask, "How close was your mother's Jill to your own Jill? As she tries to get her understanding of Jill closer to your Jill, would you nod your head 'yes' if she is getting warmer? Or shake your head 'no' if she is getting cooler?"

Jenny has experimented with codes for communication. For example, one boy was so emotional about the problem that he did not feel like talking. Jenny noticed that, although he refused to speak aloud, he was making movements with his head in response to questions. She suggested they invent a code so that he could answer her questions without having to talk. He grunted and nodded slightly in response to this suggestion, and she asked if this meant yes. He grunted again, and proceeding thus, they continued. The system of signals they came up with included a grunt for "yes," a head wag for "no," a wave for "I don't know," and a look down for "I pass on answering." This allowed him to continue the conversation merely by responding to her questions and guesses. Having established this code, Jenny then asked him to draw or communicate in other ways his experience of the problem's effects and his influence over the problem. This turned out to be much easier for him than talking.

A child might also crawl under a blanket, stick her hand out, and give us thumbs up or thumbs down in response to our musings. Some children choose to speak through a puppet, even if it just nods or wags its head in response as the adults question and guess.

On the other side of things, sometimes the challenge with children is that they are so keen on talking that we cannot focus on the conversation we need to be having with others in the room. When children are having trouble speaking in turn in a family meeting, an "interrupting card" can be used (Jeffrey Kerr, personal communication, August 1996). Index cards in different colors can be handed to the child to make "interrupting notes" on, notes that can help remind her of the important things she wants to say when her turn comes to speak. We can also suggest drawing, poetry, or other media as a way for the child to keep expressing herself while the adults are talking in a family meeting.

· ·

CHAPTER 9

Unlicensed Co-therapists

In many children's stories, children are befriended and helped by their nonhuman companions: dogs, birds, dolphins, guinea pigs, their own pets, stuffed animals, and imaginary friends. Where would Calvin be without Hobbes, Christopher Robin without Winnie the Pooh, Timmy without Lassie, or Max without the Wild Things?

Child and family therapists have written of the value of puppets and toys in facilitating communication with children in therapy (Barragar Dunne, 1992; Brems, 1993; Gil, 1994; Oaklander, 1978). Talking about things in a one-step-removed fashion is usually freeing for the child. As Oaklander (1978, p. 104) puts it,

> It is often easier for a child to talk through a puppet than it is to say directly what he finds difficult to express. The puppet provides distance, and the child feels safer to reveal some of his innermost thoughts this way.

As for the therapist, who among us has not wished for a little help, relief, or fresh insight? Enter the imaginary or nonhuman co-therapist! Co-therapists in the form of puppets and other toys or even imaginary or mythic entities can be called upon to support the therapist and enliven the conversation. Among the first published experimenters in narrative therapy were Wayne McLeod (1985), who was assisted by his "stuffed" therapy team members and Andrew Wood (1985), whose imaginary friend and colleague King Tiger lived in a cave and liked to correspond with children.

Some of us dream about having co-therapists around all the time! Although the use of reflecting teams has increased, it is rarely practical to have human co-therapists on board for most of our sessions. Instead, we may invite members of the family or anyone else present at the session to pick up a puppet and form a reflecting team with it. Puppet reflecting teams can bring a range of voices into the room. Imagine a team consisting of a Wise Owl, a Snail, and a Wizard, or a King and Queen, a Dragon, and a Frog!

Child therapists each have their own favorite cast of characters to use as co-therapists, as well as their own ways of playing. Jenny's office has an array of puppets large and small, as well as other toys, waiting patiently but eagerly to be called upon. Sometimes either Jenny or a child will notice that one puppet in particular seems to be squirming about, asking to jump into the action. A disproportionate amount of the time, this character is Rascal, a young brown dog who sits up on his hind legs, with an intelligent, alert, and perhaps even mischievous expression on his face. Rascal knows a lot about mischief and trouble and can sympathize with kids who are caught up in it. However, he has become something of an expert on getting free of trouble and is very curious to ask children about their own ways of doing this.

With children who are feeling shy, sometimes it is Snail who peeks her antennae slowly out to make friends. Other times it's Juno, a friendly mop of an English sheep dog, whose eyes are hidden behind his shag. He is a bit of a pest as he rolls on his tummy, asking to be scratched a lot, but he is a patient listener to stories of pain and hope. Harpo the Hippo has a great sense of humor; he has a talent for making big muddy fun of problems and loosening up serious dilemmas. As these co-therapists accumulate years of experience interacting with children's stories, they become better questioners and reflectors. They serve as an audience, as archivists, and as circulators of children's knowledges and accomplishments, offering to share some of the tips and stories of other children they have played with in the past.

It is also a good idea to have some puppets that are rather plain (such as a simple ragdoll puppet or a rabbit with a non-descript expression) and whose "personalities" have not been well developed by the therapist, giving the child a chance to use his imagination and make a "friend" for himself (Sallyann Roth, personal communication, August, 1996).

The Listening Rabbit

Sometimes even an experienced co-therapist doesn't seem to be of much use. In Dana's case, not one of the puppets was able to talk to her or listen adequately to her pain. Even the charm of Rascal had no impact. You see, Dana, who was seven years old, was not only sad and conflicted about her parents' divorce and her grandmother's recent death, but frequently taken over by desperate screaming fits, during which she shouted that no one was listening and no one understood her. This perception was so powerful that whenever any topic with the slightest emotional charge came up in a conversation she would fall apart, putting her hands over her ears and screaming, "You're not listening to me!" Dana's obvious pain and the isolation that she suffered due to these outbreaks would often bring her mother's heart to the breaking point. She hated having to give Dana "time-outs" until she could calm down enough to be with others again. Both parents were keen to help her gain control over the fits and to find a bearable way to communicate. Different attempts, both gentle or firm, to externalize the temper and isolation and to inquire into her experience of not being heard soon deteriorated under the pressure of this intense sensitivity. As soon as anything problematic was mentioned, Dana's hands would fly up to cover her ears and the screaming fit would take over the room.

Dana's parents looked at the pervasive influence on all family members of the blame, shame, and criticism that had escalated during and after the divorce. Over time, work progressed on a family anti-fighting project, but this was of more interest to the adults than to Dana. They worked hard on setting their own limits on the temper and screaming, limits that had been previously impeded by their fear of piling more shame on Dana. This inadvertent cooperation with shame and blame had strengthened the idea that Dana was terribly injured by the divorce, that she could not deal with her father's new relationship, and that she needed to be treated with kid gloves. Her reactions to the mention of any difficult issue provided ongoing proof of Dana's injured vulnerability.

As this story lost some of its ability to make her parents guilty or to define her as overly vulnerable, Dana began to develop and demonstrate her ability to calm herself down. This was a step in the right direction, but still, when an adult wanted to communicate anything that was uncomfortable to Dana, the conversation might easily grind to a halt as desperate screaming took over.

One day, as Jenny was struggling to find a way to talk with Dana, an idea popped into her head. She suddenly cupped her hand to her ear and softly told Dana she had just heard a whispered idea that she should make a magic listening rabbit. Dana smiled. Rabbit's head was soon sculpted from white Sculpey.[1] He had large ears and a gentle smile and during the intervening week a little furry body and tail was added.

The next time Dana started to tense up and scream "You're not listening to me," the magic rabbit finger puppet stuck its head out of Jenny's pocket and introduced itself as Listening Rabbit. Listening Rabbit said to Dana, "Temper and shame have unfairly got your tongue and convinced you that you can't be understood or heard. I have appeared to help you work a little magic to take talking and listening back from shame and make them your own again. Listen. To start with, whenever you need me I will do some magic listening to what you have to say and I can help you remember about listening and talking. Look at my ears. Do you think they are good listening ears?" Dana smiled shyly. "Do you like to just be listened to? Do you think I could listen and understand?" Dana smiled again and nodded. This was a first.

Her new co-therapist solved Jenny's dilemma: How could a narrative therapy proceed without any conversation? Previous attempts to communicate any of these ideas had been immediately cut off. But who could resist the appeal and surprise of a tiny magic Listening Rabbit? Coming from Listening Rabbit, the message started to get through. Dana became a little curious and started to relax. Whenever things became tense again in the conversation, Jenny called on Listening Rabbit to help sort things out.

Soon after Listening Rabbit's appearance, Dana said that she wanted to make a Listening Rabbit of her own. Her rabbit could become "friends with the first one, and they could listen to each other." Indeed they did; they found they could listen very softly and safely to each other, to keep the shame and temper out of their talks. This new relationship between the listening rabbits began to open the door to a gentle change. It might best be described by a quote by Lynnea Washburn found on a postcard:

> We sat there in the quiet stillness that happens just as the day
>   meets the night.
> "Listen," he said, "Did you hear that?"
> "I didn't hear a thing," I replied.
> "Sometimes everything being right makes a kind of sound."
> "I wish I'd heard it," I said softly.
> Then it seemed, just as I stopped trying so hard to listen, I could
>   actually hear it too.

Kevin's First Job

It took some time before Kevin the temper-tantrumming monkey had his first serious out-of-office employment. From his performance on his first job, however, David was quite sure that he had a brilliant career ahead of him.[2] David met Jackie and her three children, Brad, who was about to turn nine, Jerry, seven, and Suzie, five, about a year after he had been given Kevin by his American friends Dian Barkan and Lucia Gattone. Kevin had the ability, when his hand was pressed, to shake and make strange noises. He also had a large red heart on his other hand reading, "YOU MAKE ME WILD."

Jackie had been in an abusive relationship with her then husband for many years and, as she put it, had just "gone numb." Finally, she had ended that relationship because, assisted by her mother and her doctor, she came to the justifiable conclusion that it was "a matter of life and death."

Not surprisingly, in order to make up for the terrible things that had happened to her children through the abuse, Jackie went about her parenting by "satisfying everyone's whim." This didn't help matters, as she hoped it might. She began to realize that having no discipline won't make up for or replace abusive discipline. Jackie felt pretty helpless in the face of her children's continual fighting, aggravation, and signs of distress. Brad temper-tantrummed at the slightest provocation. Now, sometimes children's tantrums sound the alarm of abuse in a family. This was once the case for Brad. His tantrums had served such a purpose and the alarm had been heeded by Jackie, her mother, and her doctor. Brad's younger brother Jerry had been in a similarly stressful situation, but instead of tantrumming Jerry was letting Sneaky Poo have its way with him—his pants were soiled four or five times a day.

David decided to introduce the whole family to Kevin the stuffed monkey, who was given a co-therapist's chair beside him. David showed off Kevin's screeching, panting, and hooting by pushing the PRESS HERE button on his left palm. Everyone was wildly amused at Kevin's tantrumming and marveled at how he looked just like a real monkey.

This brought to mind a few questions David wanted to put to Brad. "Have you ever seen a monkey?" David asked. Brad had and he described the antics of monkeys he witnessed at the local zoo and on a visit to Bali, Indonesia. "Do you think your temper has you looking like a monkey to your family, classmates, and friends?" David asked. Brad thought this was probably right. "Do you think it's right and proper for a monkey to act like a monkey?" Brad agreed it was. David posed a final monkey question: "How do you feel about your temper making a monkey of you?"

Everyone knew it was Brad's birthday the next day. David asked him if he thought it was unfair that this was happening to a boy about to turn nine. Brad turned his face to one side, seemingly deep in reflection.

He agreed that it was indeed unfair—in fact, something of an outrage—for a boy only one day away from his ninth birthday to be made a monkey out of in this way. "Will you give yourself the present of maturity tomorrow?" David wondered. Brad looked uncertain but said he thought it was a possibility.

While Brad was thinking, David engaged in conversation with his new co-therapist: "Kevin, how do you feel about a day-away-from-nine-year-old boy being made a monkey by his temper?" Kevin was shy and was only willing to whisper in David's ear, so David was required to translate for him. "What Kevin told me was that if you are upset by this, he will take the Temper back from you. He says he doesn't mind Temper making a monkey out of him because he is used to being a monkey. Matter of fact, he really likes being one because you can climb right up in tall palm trees and screech and generally scream your head off. Other monkeys don't mind because that is the way of monkeys." David then turned to Brad: "Do you want Kevin to take it back? Or do you want to keep it for yourself, your family, your friends?" Brad exclaimed that he didn't want it anymore and that Kevin could have it. Hearing his assent, David proceeded, "Would you like me to ask Kevin how to go about the pass-over? You know what I mean? You pass over your temper to him when you really don't want it for yourself."

Brad beseeched David to ask Kevin about it right away. David directed the request to Kevin, who indicated that he wanted to whisper in David's ear. He did so at some length. David was quite delighted by Kevin's proposal and couldn't help expostulating while Kevin was whispering in his ear: "You don't say! Well, that is quite an interesting idea! Are all monkeys as clever as you are?" Finally, David understood Kevin's plan and translated the proposal to a very interested young man: "Brad, this is what Kevin said to do. He will lend himself to go home with you today. Whenever you feel a temper tantrum coming on (or anyone else sees it before you do), go to Kevin and pass it over to him by squeezing his hand and stand back so you won't get hurt. And please don't laugh at him when this causes him to demonstrate his monkey antics." David winked at Kevin as he left with Brad that day.

After this meeting David was not able to catch up with Jackie and her family for another seven weeks because of a move by the family to her parents' place. By then, Brad had well and truly turned nine. He had had only two tantrums in all that time. Tantrumming already seemed like history for Brad and his family, but he was willing to "remember a little bit" about what had happened when he had passed over a tantrum to Kevin the monkey. Here is his account of that first pass-over: "I went into mum's room and I pressed Kevin's hand. The temper went into Kevin.

Then I went and put Kevin in the cupboard." Brad continued, "I felt okay afterwards and more grown-up. I got the badness away from me. He (Kevin) gave goodness to me." David could not have predicted Brad's answer to his next question: "How much goodness has Kevin given you?" "A whole room size of goodness," replied Brad.

Jackie supported Brad's claims, acknowledging that "he has improved a heck of a lot." She admitted that she and her parents were surprised. "Are you ready to part company with Kevin or do you think you will still need him around in his special cupboard place?" asked David. Brad seemed very confident that he could go it alone. David then informed Brad that this was Kevin's first job and asked if he thought that Kevin had a good future ahead of him helping young boys and girls whose lives were being bossed around by their temper. Brad said he could certainly give Kevin a good job reference.

To complete the day, David found out that Jerry had only had two "sneak-outs" with Sneaky Poo in the seven weeks since they had met. At their first meeting, David had informed Jerry that Kevin was also an expert in general all-round sneakiness and could help him to outwit Sneaky Poo. David told Jerry that if he wanted to out-sneak Sneaky Poo, all he had to do was put Kevin close to his ear and ask him how to be sneakier. To David's surprise, Jerry had not had cause to consult Kevin. According to Jerry, he just "started going poos" and he was not very interested in making much of a fuss about it!

After the successful completion of his first job, Kevin has returned to the corner of David's office, where he patiently awaits his next assignment.

CHAPTER 10

. . . .

Weird and Special Abilities

Emily,[1] aged ten, came to catch David up with exciting developments about the recent actions she had taken to resist her thumb-sucking habit at night. They had met several times before when she was eight. At that time, her habit had been ruling her both by day and by night. In fact, no one could recall ever having seen her without her thumb in her mouth. She acknowledged that it was very distressing for her. She worried that she would have a misshapen jaw and teeth, and there certainly was visible evidence of that at the time.

After the second meeting, Emily intervened in the "life" of her thumb when she took umbrage at the effects that thumb-sucking was having on her. Everyone was so pleased that Emily was having a life of her own by day that thumb-sucking by night was set to one side. Now, two and a half years later, Emily was clearly excited about something or other. It didn't take David long to find out what it was. Emily reported that she had gone five nights in a row not sucking her thumb.

Naturally enough, David was extremely curious about this and asked her to let him in on the secret of her success. She informed him that it all had to do with her imaginary family: Jim Harritt, Jim's mother and father, and John and Lisa, aged fifteen and sixteen. David was not surprised Emily had been granted older imaginary friends, as she seemed somewhat beyond her years. Since David is always keen to talk with young people about their imaginary friends and family, he was excited to find out that Jim Harritt's father had the franchise for assigning imaginary friends to weirdly abled kids in New Zealand.

Who or what are the weirdly abled? Well, they are kids who are so abled that other kids and adults think their abilities are weirdnesses. This means, as Emily told David, that you may "get teased and pushed around" and be greatly misunderstood by kids and adults less abled than you are. The "weirdly abled" have special abilities that allow them, in Emily's view, to "see things that aren't there" or "see things in a different way from others . . . at times, they can think that the real world doesn't matter too much."

David decided to take the opportunity to learn more about imaginary friends[2] and what part they might play in the lives of the weirdly abled. He asked Emily lots of questions and she was very gracious and kind in telling him who they are and who needs them. In return for her favor, David said he would tell any weirdly abled kids he met in the future about Mr. Harritt and how they might apply to him.

"How do you apply to Mr. Harritt for an imaginary friend?" David asked. Emily told him that in your imagination or in secret writing you let him know your age according to your birthday and then, more importantly, the age of the person with whom you feel at home. You also tell him what kind of person you are. For example, Emily said in her application that she was a "kind person, a helping and strong person." You then tell Mr. Harritt what your interests are and what special abilities you have that you have found it best to keep secret from most people your own age and certainly from adults. You also tell him your favorite things, such as music, books, food, or clothes, and any spare time activities you particularly enjoy. It is also a very good idea to get a photograph of yourself, so Mr. Harritt can get a good idea of your appearance. Emily thought that other kids should know that Mr. Harritt's head office is under the sea somewhere between Tasmania and the Cook Straits.

David asked Emily, "If there were only so many imaginary friends to go around and too many applications to be filled right away, who would go first?" She answered immediately, "The most lonely, weirdly abled kids."

David started wondering to himself first and then out loud so Emily could hear, "How have your imaginary friends helped you in your life so far?" He was very surprised to find out how large a part they had played and continued to play in Emily's life. "First of all," Emily said, "they help me when I'm feeling lonely or when I'm in trouble at home or at school." David realized he could have guessed that if he had really tried. But there was more. Most of what Emily then told him, he could never have guessed, no matter how hard he tried.

Emily continued, "They help me with homework that I can't work out. They give me helpful hints but never do it for me and they also give kids personal strength to overcome habits that they don't want or like, for example, thumb-sucking or crying all the time."

David hadn't been aware that Emily had been crying all the time since she was always so bright and happy when they talked together. Maybe the reason for her good mood was that she knew that David knew she was weirdly abled.

David asked, "What would make you cry?"

"A little hit or word would set me off crying, but now I am turning crying into laughter."

"Have your imaginary friends helped you with teasing?"

"With teasing, you can almost automatically see the funny side and show it . . . the teasers can no longer get you that worked up!"

"Quite apart from what has been bothering you, have your imaginary friends done anything to make your life a better life than it was before you knew them?"

"They have helped me to be more adventurous. I am no longer scared of heights. I used to be scared of thunder but now I look forward to a storm, hoping there will be some thunder. I am not scared of spiders anymore either."

"Hold on now, spider fears are hard ones to overcome. How did they encourage your bravery there?"

Emily told of the nature of her imaginary friend John's assistance. "John told me that this anti-fear approach had worked for him within a day. He told me and asked me if I wanted to try it. Even though it was weird, I liked the sound of it. What he did was have a spider in one cupped hand and some lollies in the other cupped hand and refuse to tell me which was which. Then he told me to hold my hand out. Well, I did and it only took five times before I wasn't scared of spiders anymore. I did have to throw a few spiders away but they really didn't hurt when I think about it."

David asked if there were any more weirdly abled ideas like this. Sure enough there were. It seems that once Emily was afraid of crabs in rockpools. John showed her how to first use a long stick and then keep getting shorter sticks until she could pick a crab up with her hands without getting nipped by its claws. This meant that Emily could enjoy herself a lot more walking over the rocks from Palm Beach to Boatshed Bay when the tide was out.

David supposed he could have expected that Emily would save the best for last. "What's really good about imaginary friends is that they're good practice for when true friends come along, as they will . . . imaginary friends treat you like you would like to be treated."

David had one last question for Emily, "If you could thank your imaginary friends for one thing and one thing alone, what would you thank them for?" Emily replied, "I've come to understand the ways of myself and my shortcomings like spelling and in physical education when balls come at me. But I'm even starting to overcome that."

Emily recommends imaginary friends to lonely young people who have to wait a while to find true friends. Unfortunately, people like Emily may be thought to be weird, despite the fact that really they are just weirdly abled.

After talking to Emily, David considered a way that imaginary friends might be better than real ones—imaginary friends always know that you are really wonderful and weirdly abled. If you have imaginary friends who try to convince you that you are bad or try to get you into trouble, fire them and get in touch with Mr. Harritt for imaginary friends like Emily's.

RESPECTING WEIRD ABILITIES

Sometimes a young person's abilities may be assessed as weird. With Emily, however, playfully engaging in a conspiratorial discussion of weird abilities honored her imaginary friends; when that happened she was only too willing to fully appreciate them and herself. When David took an interest in the "special abilities" of children, he noticed not only that many adults categorized them as strange or weird but also that the children themselves often believed this to be the case.

Musing about children who had condemned themselves or were accused of being "weird," a "nerd," "spacey," a "day-dreamer," a "liar," or "living in a fantasy world," David became more and more curious about their closeted experiences. He wondered about the oppressive effects on these children of being misunderstood, put down, ignored, or otherwise undervalued. He thought it prudent to discuss special abilities in a way that respected their very contradictory nature: They simultaneously afforded the young person marvelous delights and pleasures and were deemed weird by important adults in the child's life. After all, parents and teachers usually have the monopoly on what constitutes knowledge and what constitutes nonsense and evaluate children accordingly. However, not all children are silent about their abilities due to suppression. It just hadn't crossed their minds to disclose their abilities to adults since they had never considered such activities to be abilities.

Once David began asking children questions about their special abilities, he was flooded by disclosures and revelations. Children reported that some adults in their lives seemed to fear what they didn't understand. Others seemed impatient with "weirdly abledness," which they took to be signs of childishness. Children said that adults (presumably thinking to help their children with this "immaturity") had often tried to convince them to "grow out it"—the sooner the better.

Children recalled being made fun of or teased over their abilities. They soon learned to suppress such abilities or to reveal them to only very trusted adults or friends. When young adults were asked by David at what age such suppressions had occurred, they told of incidents in the age range of ten to thirteen.

While the revelations of children surprised David, they left parents incredulous. Parents learned for the first time about amazing aspects of their children's lives. The parents who witnessed these revelations soon began to remember and discern "traces" of weird abilities in their own taken-for-granted but unnamed special talents. Some parents were even interested in rehabilitating special abilities that they had either renounced or spurned.

Those children whose special abilities now attained a featured role in their lives soon joined David in playing around with ideas such as t-shirts inscribed "I am a nerd and proud of it." Some proud "nerds" considered forming groups they called "nerd-doms."

We have found that the detection of special and weird abilities expands our horizons and challenges us to substantiate children's ways of making meaning and dealing with problems. When we assume that a young person is not resistant or "out of it" but may be concealing her resources, some questions may arise: "What is she into?" (Rather than, Why is she out of it?) "What realm is her mind inhabiting at this moment? Is she busy fantasizing, involved with an imaginary friend, or engaged in a one-handed game?" Such questions lend weight to what is usually considered flighty or count what is often discounted. If we do not ask, we may never find out about these children's inner experience and expertise. This is our own loss as well as theirs.

Special abilities exist in the realms of intuition, imagination, or wizardry. They may also lie in the child's specific talents, such as playing music, practicing magic tricks, or juggling. If you trace these talents back to their source, you turn up weird abilities: for example, reading hearts; turning oneself into an imaginary animal; using telepathy to know things in dreams; hearing harmony in a discordant argument; or calming oneself down by using juggling skills.

In general, while family therapy includes children it excludes their "special abilities." For example, some family therapy schools have viewed children as "acting out" to call attention to difficulties in the parental relationship. The couple relationship then becomes the center of the therapeutic attention and the "worlds" of children become marginalia, quaint but decidedly irrelevant.

Imaginary foes can also take up residence in a child's imagination and wreak havoc in both her inner and outer worlds. The child is in a relationship with these inhabitants, whether benevolent or malevolent. Some relationships bless the young person with unfailing support and nurturance; they furnish wise counsel or constant companionship. Others curse the young person by humiliating, shaming, tormenting, and persecuting him. We take up the latter case in the next chapter.

REALITY-TESTING

Adults sometimes express concerns when they enter the child's worlds of play and learn of imaginary friends or weird abilities. They may ask: "Isn't it confusing or scary for the child, whose reality-testing is still developing, to have an adult confound reality by joining the child in the fantasy world?" To the contrary, children often express considerable relief when they feel safe to disclose such friends and abilities to significant adults. If they are sure that their inner world is accepted, they can put aside their fears of censure and allow adults full access to their imaginations. Then they can either call upon their imaginations to serve their purposes or take back the imaginings that are serving the problem.

In an externalizing conversation, adults and children can espy not just the mere existence of such experiences but also the kind of relationship children have with such friends and abilities. Satisfying aspects of the relationships are noted and cherished, while the ways that the young person is being misused, maltreated, or hoodwinked in the relationship are exposed and called into question.

Clinicians may also have concerns about confounding the child's reality by supporting these friends and abilities. This may be due to the fact that at one time phenomena such as imaginary friends were believed to be the private fantasies of disturbed children. Yet research since 1973 has consistently shown that the capacity to create imaginary worlds and friends is quite separate from the capacity to distinguish between fantasy and reality (Taylor, Cartwright, & Carlson, 1993). In our own practices we have observed that even very young children develop an accurate ability to tell what's make-believe and what's not. Children with active imaginations fare no worse than other children with reality-testing and may fare better than other children in terms of their capacity to imagine and play happily.

THE GENEALOGY OF THE IDEA OF WEIRD ABILITIES

While reflecting on weird abilities, David began to reevaluate his own childhood experiences and think about those who had acted to foster his own abilities. He was obliged to reconsider his long-standing conviction that his father was an endearing fool. David's father was known in the small Canadian town where he grew up as "Benny the Peanut Man." Benny derived from Benjamin and "the Peanut Man" from his occupation running a small lunch bar that sold the peanuts he roasted daily. Here is one of the stories David recalls about Benny the Peanut Man (1991/1997) that exemplifies his reconsideration of his father:

When I was fifteen, I informed my parents that I had engaged in underage drinking along with my somewhat older friends. My parents, as I expected, took it pretty well but my father, unexpectedly, did not leave it at that. Since he was a man who only drank on very rare occasions and kept little or no liquor or beer on hand, I was surprised when he arrived home soon after my disclosure with a very large bag from the liquor store. On reflection, I suppose he chose an opportune time to start unpacking this bag. I observed him putting away bottles of rum, rye, scotch, vodka, and gin. In all my life, I had never seen so many different kinds of hard liquor in one place.

I couldn't help inquiring what was up. My father told me that he had been thinking about hard liquor ever since I had told him about my drinking and he had got to wondering if hard liquor was as "hard" these days as it was when he was my age. I arrogantly replied, "So what's that got to do with all these bottles you've got here?" He told me, "The only way to find out for sure is to try each kind out." I must admit to having been somewhat bemused. He invited me join him in testing the "hardness" of hard liquor. "How do you do that?" I innocently asked. "Well, it's pretty easy, really. What you do is drink it. That's the only way to find out."

Now I knew I was on to a really good thing—free drinking at my father's expense. I had to laugh at my father's naiveté, considering the risks my friends were taking in diluting their parents' liquor supplies with water to ensure their own supply. I had always considered my father something of a fool so this was nothing new to me.

Every so often, my father would convene tests in which we would drink together, comparing the hardness of, say, rye whiskey, when he was my age to its current proof. He would engage me in considering how "hard" whiskey was for me as we talked and drank together. We both got the odd headache, but that just went to prove how hard whiskey could be. My friends marveled at how I was duping my father and I seemed to gain a lot of respect from them for what I took to be my guile.

It was many years later that I realized that Benny's idea of "hardness" had a strong resemblance to the familiar concept of "knowing your limits." He had persisted with our experiments until he had gained sufficient evidence that I truly knew my limits. Because

I had demonstrated my more carefully-considered drinking habits to him, my father rested more easily on nights he knew I was "out with my friends."

With his father's example in mind, David gained new appreciation of weirdly abled perspectives. He began to stand alongside young persons as a comrade in exploring and rehabilitating weird abilities. With respectful curiosity, he started experimenting with lines of questioning that highlighted and confirmed these abilities. Here are some examples:

- Do you find adults boring in the way they can only see things through adult eyes?
- Can you see things more than one way?
- Do you suspect you know more about some things in your life than anyone else does?
- Have adults (or your friends) tried to talk you out of imagining things the way you do? Has your imagination gone underground? Are you keeping it just to yourself?
- Would you be willing to let me in on your secrets?
- Do you have magic (imaginary) ways of doing things? If you were to tell me, do you think I would make fun of your magic (imagination)?
- Do some people think you are weird when, in fact, if they really knew you inside and out, they would know you are weirdly abled?
- Do you find it hard to believe that your parents were once children with wonderful imaginations of their own?

INFORMAL RESEARCH ON SPECIAL AND WEIRD ABILITIES

Perhaps this chapter has sparked memories of abilities that you had as a child or were aware of others having. Is it possible that these abilities were surrendered on growing up or are they still part of your life? David has developed the following questions for use in workshops for therapists working with children; you can explore them on your own or with a friend or group.

- Do you remember what special and now seemingly weird abilities you had as a child? What delights and satisfactions did these abilities afford you? Did you ever use them to make things better?

- Did you share these delights and satisfactions with anyone else or did you keep them pretty much to yourself?
- Can you recall any adult—say a parent, uncle, aunt, grandparent, schoolteacher, coach, or even the person who sold you candy at the corner store—who fully appreciated your special abilities?

If you have recalled someone (or even more than one person), ask yourself these questions:

- In what ways did that adult indicate to you that she knew you were "weirdly abled" and that your abilities were not "'weirdnesses'"? Was it the way she spoke to you? Was it the twinkle in her eye? What else about her conveyed an interest in and respect for your inner world?
- Did you surrender or deny these abilities, say between the ages of ten and thirteen, perhaps in response to a critical comment from a teacher, parent, or friend, or to misunderstandings and subsequent fears about these abilities? Or did you conclude at some point that these abilities were childish and leave them behind you?
- When you became an adult, did you consider acknowledging or rehabilitating any of your seemingly weird abilities? Under what circumstances?
- If you maintained these abilities, how do they play a part in your life? How do you foster them?
- Do any of these special abilities now play a feature role in your work with children or adults?

If you cannot recall anyone who knew of and acknowledged your special abilities, ask yourself these questions:

- If you had been available to your child self as the person you are now, how might you have shown an interest in and appreciation of your special abilities? How might you have acted toward your child self so that your appreciation was in no doubt?

While for many respondents, special abilities had gone unnoticed or were suppressed by others, others recalled significant people in their pasts who recognized and encouraged such abilities. When David interviewed adult therapists who recalled such people, he asked, "Can you recall the questions such acknowledging people asked you? Or, if not, can you guess what questions they would very likely have asked you?" They recalled questions that commonly followed these formats:[3]

- What have you been thinking about?
- What big ideas have you been working on in your mind?
- What is going on in your imagination?
- Tell me what you see when . . . ?
- What do you think might/would/could have happened if . . . ?
- What could/would you do about . . . ?
- When was it fun? What made you laugh?
- What do you guess will happen next?
- What do you see up/out there?
- What surprised you/shocked you?

According to the adult therapists David interviewed, these questions would not have been experienced as an interrogation of any kind. They were in no way evaluative of the young person's intelligence quotient. They described the stance of the questioner as "one who is truly curious about what another knows." In other words, these questions share the premise that what the young person "knows" is unique to her, important and interesting to the adult, and potentially amazing.

Robert's Heart-Reading

Robert, age fifteen, was referred to David because he had just experienced debilitating flashbacks on watching an Oprah Winfrey program about child sexual abuse. Robert confided to David that he had been tortured for five long years between the ages of three to eight at the hands of members of his foster family at that time. Because of this Robert had found it necessary to scrupulously gauge the motives of anyone who promised to care for him. When this came to light David and Robert were able to redescribe what others might refer to as "distrust" as a legitimate survival ability. Suffice to say, Robert was by now a very astute judge of people.

A new description of Robert's ability began to take shape when he told David, "I can read people." David was curious about this skill. "Do you think that you can see inside people?" Robert assured him that he could. At the same time, however, he downplayed his ability as commonplace. David pursued his line of inquiry, "What can you see inside to?" Robert nonchalantly acknowledged that he could tell if a person was good or bad. "Can you read hearts?" David wondered. For the first time since their meeting began Robert grinned with bemused self-acknowledgment and responded enthusiastically, "Yeah, I can read hearts!"

David introduced Robert to the notion of "weirdly abledness" as a desirable personal description with the question: "Do you think that reading hearts qualifies you to be considered by me as 'weirdly abled' or not?" Robert agreed that it would. David then asked, "Do you consider reading hearts to be a weird ability that you can add to your collection of less weird abilities?" With his confident "Yes!" Robert qualified himself as weirdly abled. This allowed Robert to establish a separate domain of "knowledge" that stood apart from adult knowledges and which could not be subordinated by them.

Over the next few months Robert extended the range of his heart-reading to find classmates and teachers who had "happiness, joy, and good humor in their hearts." He did such a good job locating "hearts" like these that he became surrounded by a loyal group of friends. He also earned respect throughout his school as a person who was willing to stand up for anyone who was bullied and to look after those who had suffered injuries or had a disability.

More Imaginary Friends—Martin and Dirk

In the following interview with David, Martin, aged sixteen, explores the qualities of his relationship with his imaginary friend, Dirk. Martin had been expelled from his high school because of his persistent and reckless drug use and drug dealing and was now pursuing his studies by correspondence. Relations with his father had become so vexed that his father had notified the Child Protection Services. The expedient they all agreed on was that Martin should go into foster care for the time being.

David met with Martin around this time, as it was thought prudent for him to have some counseling as a prelude to family reconciliation. Martin, a very tall young man, looked older than his years and acknowledged that his father had "lost all belief and trust in me and we couldn't talk to each other but already we are beginning to making amends."

As David and Martin were exploring the nature of his "special abilities" near the end of the first meeting, Martin introduced his imaginary friend, Dirk, and by doing so broke the secret. David was honored to be the first to get to know Dirk.

At the beginning of their second meeting, David began by summarizing: "You felt very comfortable with the idea of being a weirdly abled person. Let me go back to some of your comments. You have always felt 'pretty weird,' but some people, like Peter, have made you feel that you are unique, weirdly abled. You told me that it had been good to know this. And that these abilities of yours have grown on you over time."

David wondered how long Dirk had been an imaginary friend of Martin's. Martin explained to David that Dirk had been around "for about a year" and that he "dresses in World War I clothes with a leather hat and goggles, and a cigarette in his mouth."

"Did Dirk just show up or did you sort of invite him into your life?" asked David.

"Half-and-half, sort of," replied Martin, "I formed him in my mind and then he just sort of appeared in my hand—if I cup it, he sits in it."

David was curious as to whether Dirk was a help in Martin's life: "Can I ask you if Dirk has played any part in assisting you to get free of problems with drug dealing and drug taking? Could you have done it without him?"

"No, he played a major part in it," Martin said.

"Is it okay to tell me how he featured in all this?"

"He was sort of like my counselor really."

"Did you turn to him often?"

"I could call on him but sometimes I would be sitting in my room and he would just appear."

"Can you remember any counseling sessions with Dirk that stand out in your mind as turning points in taking your life back from drugs and dealing?" David asked.

Martin replied, "He just told me: Look into the future and see what you are going to be and so I pictured myself with lung cancer and damaged brain cells."

"Is Dirk pleased with your therapy so far?"

"Yeah, he's pleased I made a change, and he's pleased I'm seeing you."

"Oh good. Why is he pleased?"

"You're someone different with a different point of view."

David felt happy to have a good working relationship with his colleague. "You know," Martin continued, "I used to think I was sort of a freak, going nuts. I was really scared there for a while."

David now pondered with Martin the possibility of an imaginary friend being part of the solution rather than part of the problem. David helped Martin consider what was "nuts" and what wasn't "nuts." This relieved Martin's fear and allowed him to feel more comfortable revealing Dirk. Hiding Dirk could have had negative ramifications for Martin, stigmatizing an important part of his inner experience and depriving him of a valuable resource in his fight against drugs and dealing.

David offered some criteria for evaluating whether Martin's relationship with Dirk had been a destructive, confusing, or oppressive force in

his life: "If your imaginary friend were more like an enemy and perse-
cuted you or called you names, I would be asking you if that is the kind
of friend you wanted to keep. After all, some enemies can dress up as
friends like wolves in sheep's clothing. Are there any grounds to suspect
that Dirk hasn't been a good friend?"

"No, he has always been a great friend."

"Has Dirk ever found you wanting?"

"There was one instance when a guy came in drunk and I told him to
stick his finger down his throat and spew up. So he did that and ended
up in the hospital. He choked. Dirk told me I should have sent him
home to bed."

"Can Dirk be severe at times?" asked David.

"Yeah, my dad walked in and I was yelling at the palm of my hand."
Martin laughed uproariously when he recalled this incident.

"It's funny," Martin mused, "because I can see him in full color. He's
got a mustache and the lines on his face are all there. That's what used
to freak me out, because imaginary friends are not here, they are in your
mind."

"Does embodying your imaginary friend make him friendlier?" wondered David.

"I see him in my dreams, too, and my subconscious talks to him. I
suppose I programmed him, for want of a better word. I put what I wanted
in him."

This piqued David's curiosity: "When you were making up Dirk, what
ingredients did you use?"

Martin replied readily, "Friendship, kindness, respect, just a helping
hand, laughter, funniness. I made him a place to live in the back of my
head. I can close my eyes and see a lounge suite for him. It's funny how
he came to me. I was sitting there one day and I drew him. I just drew
this guy."

Reassured that Martin and Dirk's relationship embodied liberating
qualities, David asked, "When you are withdrawing from drugs, how do
you turn to him?"

Martin pondered this for a moment. "His advice to me was go and
get ten packets of chewing gum. Every time you feel like smoking something, shove a piece of gum in your mouth. He gave me good advice
about staying away from rolling cigarettes because it reminds me of
rolling up some dope. You know, once I thought I was 'schizophrenic'
because I was hearing this voice. I have accepted him now; he's mine
really," Martin reflected.

David sought his advice: "Would you recommend such a friend to
other people?"

Martin responded thoughtfully, "You just put all the goodness you can find into him. He cautions me about hazards and dangers."

David had one last question: "Can I ask you, without Dirk where would you be today?"

Martin replied immediately, "In a drug treatment program or dead!"

. . . .

CHAPTER 11

Family Politics in Action

Many family and child problems are not entirely of our individual making or under our individual control. Rather, they reside in the imbalances in our society—which value the individual over community, the secular over the sacred, the masculine over the feminine, money over time, the affluent over the poor, etc. These imbalances press on families, threatening to "divide and conquer" them. Fear, frustration, or desperation can take over, leading to hostility and resignation. Everyday family interactions can become tinged with bitterness, sarcasm, and accusation.

Families in the midst of such experiences need to be listened to very attentively and respected in the context of their individual and social circumstances. This chapter is about how the perspective of family therapy can change its focus to those points at which the personal and political intersect. This is a requisite to revising personal and family relationships to such problems.

OF WAR AND PEACE IN THE FAMILY

Family tensions can run high when there is fear of rupturing the fabric of the family, for example, when there are threats of a stepparent leaving due to conflicts with stepchildren, of an impending divorce, or an adolescent running away. Abusive fighting or excessive punishments may accompany these threats.

When a family is in crisis a young person who is asked his opinion may be co-opted by family politics. If he has had the experience of being deployed in a power struggle, he knows that any statement he makes is likely to be taken as being on someone's "side." This situation may silence him or provoke his angry protestation but neither response is likely to serve his purposes. If he opts for silence he may be victimized by siblings or ignored by adults. If he chooses provocation he is likely to be understood as seeking attention in a negative way, being disrespectful, or just plain behaving badly.

A child (or woman) under physical or emotional threat of being co-opted or put at risk might also choose to communicate her distress covertly, fearing that any assertion will increase family volatility. The child will be inhibited from commenting directly on the tension and intimidation in the family. A vicious cycle of concealment and persecution may ensue. For example, a child under stress might conceal that she is having trouble with homework to avoid a family uproar. When she conceals her difficulties there is ever-present danger that they will be discovered by the abuser and the child will be blamed as the source of family tension. Eventually, the fact that her grades are suffering will surface. When the discovery occurs, the child's concealing, rather than the intimidating atmosphere, will be the focus of fights.

Typically, her mother is likely to be blamed as well "for not being on top of things." When this kind of uproar occurs, the abuses of power by those that are contributing to a threatening atmosphere will go unnoticed or be condoned.

Even in non-abusive circumstances, covert tactics to equalize power imbalances on the part of women and children may compromise rapport with the therapist. For example, a boy is identified as having psychological problems by his school counselor and referred to therapy. His father constantly accuses his wife of making poor choices "for the family." He states, "My son needs her" and "there's enough money for her to leave that damn job she cares more about than us. She gives them too many hours for no promotions or raises." He says they could "get by on my pay if she would take care of our children so we could use less daycare, do more house cleaning so we can let the house cleaner go, and do more cooking so we can spend less money eating out."

He does not take into account that his greater pay and rapid pace of promotion are supported by differential advancement for men in the workplace or that his wife is battling both a glass ceiling and a negative attribution in the culture at large that working mothers are neglecting their children. He complains that his wife "is always forgetting things that are important to me and the kids." He then vociferously encourages the therapist to attend to and correct his wife's "forgetfulness and poor priorities," so that his son's problems will improve. He claims that his standards for guiding her choices are "normal" and "what anyone would expect of a good mother and wife."

The mother states that since her son began to have problems she has "felt confused, overwhelmed, and neglectful." She continues, "I have been forgetting a lot lately and I really haven't been there for our son." The therapist can easily get caught between the husband's demands and the wife's acquiescence and exclude the child's voice. Also, if the therapist doesn't help the wife behave "normally" he will be seen as ignoring the "discovery of her neglectful parenting." If he calls into question the husband's prerogative to set the standards that she must measure up to as a wife and mother, he runs a great risk of being seen by the husband as "taking sides" against him and by the wife as not "understanding my family problems." The therapist walks a tightrope in trying to name and externalize the effects of such power differences in a way that includes and supports each spouse and includes the child's voice as well.

In the event that the husband prevails on his wife to acquiesce, it is unlikely that the son's problems will remit. The patterns of overt and covert behavior described here are likely to escalate to the point where a pall of fear, hostility, and resentment descends on the life of the family. Seriousness seems to be the appropriate response when such emotions are so thick that they can be cut with a knife. A complete discussion of how to take up this couple's power struggle is not in the purview of this chapter, but so as to not leave the reader hanging we have included a little food for thought.

When a therapist finds himself in one of these untenable positions, he can, along with including the child's voice, explore the relationship between the family and various societal pressures. For example, he can externalize the "divide and conquer strategy" of gender inequities: Gender-based inequities such as differential pay and promotion in the workplace support and prescribe rigid roles for men and women. These roles place inordinate pressures on the man to be a "super" provider and the woman to be a "super" carer. Neither can live up to these expectations, so they are divided against each other if something goes wrong in either domain. If their problem is financial—he's failed; if their child or marriage has a problem—she's failed. Articulating the negative influence of the problem on family communications can provide an incentive for change and a source of hope and possibility.

The family members can band together and launch a playful conspiracy or project that undermines the divide and conquer tactics of gender inequities. They can rediscover ancestors who burst out of the constraints of restrictive gender stereotypes. They can identify heroes in their current lives who have actively resisted gender role limitations. They can speculate about the virtuous effects that new roles for each of them might have on their family communications. They can choose roles that suit the unique economic and relational needs of their family and join together with other families who share their spirit and concerns.

In the case stories below we offer some reflections about situations in which the therapist's attention is drawn away from the children and toward the power struggles that shape family communications. It is hard to imagine engaging in a playful approach in an atmosphere like this, but it is important that we do so. Otherwise the power struggles that accompany societal imbalances will eclipse the concerns and the contributions of children, reinforce inequity, and the family will lose a valuable source of creativity and change.

Evan Stands Up for Noncompetition

Evan, aged eight, and his sister Brianna, aged ten, were caught in the crossfire of an impending divorce. Both their parents wanted to separate, but each insisted that the other go first. Not surprisingly, they were stalemated. The father had been laid off due to downsizing and had to take a job with a reduced income. Despite both parents' working long hours, the family lived under economic duress. Financial changes such as these have real effects on a family (such as shifting gender roles and fracturing marital bonds). While these should be addressed in the therapy, it is important that they not be allowed to limit the child's participation and influence.

Evan had been caught stealing small sums of money from both his mother and his sister. There were also concerns that he had no interests except TV-watching; he had few friends and was doing poorly in school. Although both parents believed their continual conflict was detrimental to their children, they felt hopeless about reconciling their differences and were unable to initiate their separation.

Evan's response to any query from either his parents or Dean was "I don't know" or "I guess so." Whenever he stepped outside his position of being noncommittal, he immediately found himself on one side of a dispute or the other. For example, when he commented that he had fun on a recent weekend boating trip, he was accused of taking his father's side (boating) against his mother's side (other kinds of weekend recreations). When he talked of enjoying a school activity, his sister accused him of being "a goody two shoes" and condemned him as an ally of her parents against her. His mother accused his father of being a "Disneyland Dad" and currying the kids' favor by spoiling them, while his father looked at the therapist as if to say "See, with her I can't do anything right." Conflict swirled around everyone in the family like a dense fog and no one knew where to put a foot down without stepping on someone else's toes.

Dean decided to meet Evan on his own, as there seemed no possibility of his being able to speak for himself in the family meetings. However, he was no less noncommittal on his own. Dean thought of another option. Why not have a family therapy session where the problem might be played around with despite its seriousness?

Dean suggested this and they all agreed to try it. They made up a game that everyone could play. Each family member was to write down something for other family members to guess, e.g., a favorite movie, gripe, restaurant, accomplishment or vacation plan. Then each member would write down his/her guess of the other persons' replies. Dean proposed two ways in which they could approach the game: competitively or collaboratively. If they chose the competitive alternative, they would try to stump everyone else. The person who made the least correct guesses in a round would be eliminated; the winner would be the last person to survive. The collaborative alternative would mean that they would think of things that other members would be very likely to guess. The family would play as a team and accumulate the highest total of correct guesses they could in a single round. The object would be to set a family "personal best."

Evan had a strong preference for the rules and outcome that were noncompetitive. Dean asked him if he would back down on his preference for compromise over conflict if his sister said that the game would "be no fun if nobody won." Evan said he would keep his position and refuse to back down. Dean then asked Evan if he would back down because he might be seen to be "on your father's side." After all, "your father has said he would rather switch than fight." Evan was still adamant. Dean asked him another question in the same vein: "Would you back down because you may be seen to be on your mother's side because she believes you don't have strong opinions like your father and here you are having a strong opinion?" Evan remained steadfast.

Dean then proceeded to interview each family member about why he or she thought Evan would not back down. There was agreement that he was truly committed to family collaboration. After this discussion the family decided to try the game both ways. It turned out their family spirit was more important than how the game was played. When it was high-spirited, infectious humor broke out and took the bite right out of the competition. By acknowledging Evan's firm stand, his family was able to move towards more humor, harmony, and cooperation.

Their first initiative at home involved deciding on a specific arena of family life and freeing it from contention and conflict. Dinnertime was declared the first conflict-free zone. They agreed that all arguments between Evan and his sister had to be delayed until after the meal and before dessert. The parents served as referees to guarantee the fighting was "fair" and "above the belt." They consulted with Dean to develop their "refereeing skills." They even made a special ring for bouts and foam bats for their children to use.

Strangely enough, when the time came for the "bout," everyone preferred to have dessert instead of a fight. To celebrate within their means they decided to "feast on peace" rather than have an expensive meal ending with a "just dessert." Humor started to creep in and they created a new favorite dessert—the "peace-o'-cake." Soon Evan and his sister asked their parents to declare dinner a "work-and-money-discussion-free zone." The parents were pleased to comply.

It did not take much encouragement on Dean's part for Evan's parents to decide that, whether they stayed together or not, "conflict-free" events were vital for their children's well-being, as well as theirs.

Simon, the Transformer

When parents bring their children or themselves to therapy, they are often in disagreement about child-rearing practices. They turn to the therapist to arbitrate their disputes. One familiar example of this is the "you're too hard . . . you're too soft" debate.

Sarah opens the discussion by telling Dean that eleven-year-old Simon has become increasingly shy and sensitive. She is worried that he cannot express what is causing him to withdraw. His withdrawal has meant that he has few friends and is disinterested in school. She hopes that Dean can "draw him out of his shell." She is concerned, too, that her husband, Jeffrey, is "too hard and intimidating."

On the other hand, Jeffrey is of the opinion that Sarah is too soft and "rewards Simon with sympathy and concern even when he is just a little bit upset." He believes Sarah undermines his attempts to establish consequences for Simon's underachievement at school. In fact, he argues further that "she's undermined her own authority over him" by alternately rewarding his misbehavior with sympathy or entering into interminable arguments with Simon.

When Dean queries Simon about this, he replies that he does not know why he acts the way he does. He says that school is boring, that he does have friends, and he likes TV and Nintendo. Sarah interjects that "none of his friends are his own age," while Jeffrey interrupts to add that "he'd rather play Nintendo and watch TV than do his homework."

Dean is caught in a bind. If he offers Simon a sympathetic ear, Jeffrey could construe this as letting Simon off the hook and taking Sarah's side. If Dean helps with the limit-setting, he may alienate Simon and be viewed by Sarah as on Jeffrey's side. If he identifies the parents' dispute as the problem, he may very likely diminish Simon's viewpoint in his considerations.

Jeffrey believes that Simon is guided by the maxim "negative attention is better than no attention at all." According to this "theory of negative attention," children will behave problematically to be rewarded with attention. Should parents subscribe to this, they will ignore or distance themselves from the child when he is behaving in an undesirable way, hoping that the unrewarded behavior will disappear. The option of rewarding desirable behavior is ruled out because it can be seen as part of "being too soft." "Why should I reward him for doing what any kid his age is supposed to do?" Such a parenting tack can place a family in a bind. If parents pay attention to the problem they are rewarding negative behavior, but if they ignore the problem they may be ignoring a "cry for help"—which is Sarah's concern. You might say that problems "attract" attention, but it may not be as useful to say that young persons behave in problematic ways in order to attract attention.

According to the "cry for help theory," the child would not behave in a problematic fashion that upsets everyone around him if there were not some underlying pain that needed attention. Accordingly, a parent would look for a way for the child to open up and express the "true" meaning underneath the symptom, so that the cry could be answered. We have found more often than not that men are proponents of the negative attention theory, while women tend to support the cry for help theory. Parents often find themselves divided between theories and the solutions implied by them.

A family therapist may be requested to arbitrate. If his ideas are at odds with one or both parents, he may be become a disputant. For example, he might believe the child does need more sympathy, or consistent limit-setting, or that the parental dispute itself is the source of the problem.

Within a child-focused family therapy, it is not up to the therapist to judge between competing claims. The therapist's task is to encourage everyone involved to consider how the problem operates in the life and relationships of each family member. An externalizing conversation enables family members to develop some appreciation of the problem's effects. Here the opposing approaches can have their virtues as diverse perspectives on the operations of the problem, as long as everyone is included.

Jeffrey pointed out that some problems receive altogether too much attention from family members and deserve a good dose of ignoring,

while Sarah's experience showed her that problems can silence and dis-
qualify a child's cry for help. Simon's theory and approach to understanding or changing the problem may seem fantastical, simplistic, or
even irrelevant next to the competing theories promulgated by the adults.

In such a disputatious atmosphere the expression of Simon's view is
limited to I-don't-know's or does not even make an appearance. Although
it is tempting to describe Simon's lack of response as "unmotivated" or
"withdrawn," this would be more than short-sighted. Simon may have
the resources of an imaginary friend, a weird or hidden ability, a mental
practice, or a hero or a story that may be drawn upon or enacted with
puppets or miniature figures in a sandtray. He may, in fact have evolved
an approach of his own at odds with adult logic. It is important that
Simon's vision be included in the conversation.

In the course of play, Simon's vision emerged. He said that he was
bored and disinterested in school. He also felt that he was uninteresting
and that it was no wonder that no one sought him out. He said he preferred the play of younger children, since he could entertain them with
his imaginary games.

Simon's play with Transformers (miniature action figures that change
from people-like robots into weapons and back again using the same
parts) gave him the means to represent both his concerns and the means
to remedy them. In the course of his play with the Transformers Simon
revealed his ability to use his imagination to transform himself through
mime. When Dean wondered if he had used this body ability to transform himself in ways that he might not have noticed, Simon was intrigued. When Dean asked him if he had transformed his quietness into
a talent for miming, and if he thought his miming skills might be engaging of his friends' interest, Simon's image of himself as boring to his
agemates was called into question.

Dean asked Simon if he thought his school life might be less boring
if his reputation as an disinterested student was transformed in the eyes
of his teacher. Simon thought it might, so he readily took up Dean's
invitation to co-write a letter to his teacher about his interest in movies
and video games. In response to this letter his teacher allowed him to
run the audiovisual equipment in the classroom. This activity engaged
Simon's interest in movies and his physical dexterity in school.

It was almost as if Simon was waiting for the parental debate to be
decided one way or the other before he could take any initiative. Simon's
parents' debate had inadvertently supported his apparent disinterest and
inactivity. When playful communication upstaged the highly charged
debate, Simon's enterprise became the focus of the therapy. As a conse-
quence the debate soon became hypothetical: Simon's father was pleased

to see that Simon "finally took the initiative" and Simon's mother was satisfied that once Simon began to speak "we really got to the bottom of it." Simon's opinion was that he liked having "a cool thing to do at school" that the other kids admired.

THE PEACE FAMILY PROJECT

Dean and Jenny have been recruiting families that are beset by Tempers, Fighting, Bickering, and other forms of contention to join others in becoming a "Peace Family." Dean came upon this idea while interviewing various family members about their preferences for "peace" in their family life. Many spoke against hostility and violence in their own histories, their current lives, in the media, and in the culture at large. They wanted to draw the line at permitting such ways of relating into their own homes and lives. They were willing to band together to protest the effects of a culture that condones violence within families. For example, they went to such measures as turning off TV at times, not buying violence-supporting products, signing "non-proliferation treaties," or circulating peace proclamations announcing their peaceful intentions.

Andrew, Temper-Teacher

The story of how Andrew became a Temper Tamer has been told in Chapter 2; this is the story of how Andrew inspired change in those around him.

Brian and Jean, Andrew's parents, had something of their own to say about Temper and Aggression. Brian acknowledged that he found himself caught up in power struggles with his son or becoming impatient and snapping at Andrew when he was "in a bad mood." Jean told of growing up in a family addicted to "rageaholism." They were intent on developing different ways to parent their son.

When Jenny asked how Brian and Jean might like to approach this, they responded that they wished to explore what growing up in their own families had taught them about anger and communication. The conversation soon expanded to considering what messages they received from the media and the culture at large about these matters. Jenny, pleased to join them in this endeavor, took the opportunity to inform them about the "Peace Family Project." Jenny asked them if the peace family idea fit their concerns: "Would you like to join me to research your own ideas and practices as a prospective peace family? And perhaps even share this with other families in the future?" They liked the idea so much that from then on each meeting included time spent reviewing their Peace Family Project.

Although Andrew's parents had begun by encouraging Andrew's tem-per-taming, now it was he who became their temper-teacher. He took to reminding them to tame their own tempers when he heard anger rising in their voices. Brian and Jean were beguiled by this at first, but over time they came to consider it a milestone on their road to becom-ing a peace family.

This is but one of many temper-teaching anecdotes that became part of their peace family lore: One day while driving in heavy traffic, Jean was unaware that she was muttering imprecations until Andrew piped up from the backseat: "Mom, watch out, the Temper's getting you!" Her amusement dissolved the Temper before it could take her over. Instead of becoming further "stressed out," she found herself thanking Andrew for "making me aware of it sneaking up on me."

The following is a letter Jenny wrote to the family about their work together:

Dear Andrew, Brian, and Jean,

I thought it might be useful to write to you and ask each of you more about your Peace Family Project.

Andrew, it has been fun to see you getting over the worst part of the Temper. It used to get you to do things that made you unhappy, like hit your head, have tantrums, and not like yourself. Remember when your parents said that you are "liked oodles" by the important people in your life? We figured the Temper must be tricking you by getting you to say you don't like yourself. You said that Temper "gets me to kick a rock," and that "an Anger makes you yell and scream and makes you scared."

At our first meeting you declared "I don't like it, and I'm sick of it." I could tell that you were ready to take over and make peace with the Temper, too. Some signs that you were ready were: (1) You wanted to be a big boy and decide for yourself how to be instead of losing control to the Temper. (2) You felt "old enough, like I can stop the Temper." (3) You're having good ideas that solve problems. (4) You decided to use the bathroom like a big person. (5) You have been going to bed and going to sleep more easily like a big person—which helps the whole family to get their rest and be more peaceful. I am very impressed by how ready you were and by how quickly you got a handle on your Temper. Would you mind if I tell your story to some other kids who want to tame their Tempers? It could give them hope and courage.

Now I'd like to ask your parents about the Peace Family Project: Jean and Brian, you both came from families where Temper was rife and where people succumbed to "rageaholism." That's a difficult way to grow up—a way that you didn't want for yourselves or Andrew. Did you worry that an out-of-control Temper would infect your young family? These infections do seem to get passed down through generations. The Temper was bothering your family with "yelling and tension" and "getting An-

drew afraid." You said you were "sick of this pattern." How did you decide that it would stop in this generation?

I am moved and impressed when I meet young families like yours who have the interest and courage to peacefully resolve conflicts. What gives you the strength to not accept the legacy of rageaholism? How did you come to your decision? How are you supporting each other? What "peace family practices" have you discovered? What were you already doing that you will keep doing? What effects do you think that this project will have on your family's future and on your son's growing up?

Brian, you are currently tackling the issue of power struggles between fathers and sons. Is this part of your overall peace project? You said you were tipped into a power struggle when you found yourself thinking like your dad did: "I don't want to be controlled; I don't want to be a puppet." Do these thoughts trick to you into forgetting that you have so much more power than your four-year-old? What forces do you think come into play that encourage domination and aggression between fathers and sons? Since dominance issues are part of our social existence, I am very interested in how people make conscious choices to reduce their effects. I would like to keep track of what you discover about this in your relationship.

Jean, I am struck by your determination to overcome the after-effects of growing up with "rageaholism." What is the effect of your sharing more limit-setting with Brian? Is this supported by his work on dominance reduction? Is this reducing overall family tension? I agree with you that there is "love and good communication" in your family. Andrew feels respected and trusts you and his dad. Does this provide a foundation that will make the full development of a peace family in your generation a less formidable task? You are well on the way. Can you see how I might say this? What do you think is your next step?

I am looking forward to hearing about how your Peace Family Project is evolving when we next meet,

Jenny Freeman

SUMMARY

When social pressures threaten to divide and conquer a family, it is tempting to partition them off from the world they live in—by pulling a "professional" curtain around them. Therapists can be very comfortable in that "room." There is always much to talk about with a family about themselves, their parents, and the families from which they came. If we ourselves are myopic, how can our conversations with families reach to vewing their predicament as beyond themselves? Families fracturing under social pressures should not be further burdened by the likes of us (Boyd-Franklin, 1989; Pinderhughes, 1989; Tamasese & Waldegrave, 1993). We need to think about, talk about, and act where the personal and the political intersect. This we refer to as *family politics in action.*

CHAPTER 12

• • • • • • • • • • • • • • • • • • •

An Imagination of One's Own

Many of the young people we have met who are struggling with fears or other problems also have rich imaginations. While the topic of imagination is a thread running throughout this book, in this chapter we discuss some children's changing relationships with their imaginations. A young person's relationship with her imagination may be a wonderful resource that can bring her much delight. But it can also terrorize. Captured and driven by fear, a rich imagination can spin out of control. As a comedian Jenny heard on the radio quipped, "Fear is a darkroom where negatives are developed."

Most of us remember from our own childhoods some version of imaginary monsters or witches under the bed or in the closet. A fear-possessed imagination may convince a child that burglars are prowling outside the house, a ghost is slinking along the bedroom wall, or every dog is a monster ready to bite her. Nightmares may be so vivid that they are experienced as almost real and can have a devastating emotional effect. A child can come to be tyrannized by one of her greatest potential resources. Under such circumstances, is it any wonder that a child sees little prospect of bringing this ability back under control?[1]

We need to be aware that some fears arise from real and frightening life circumstances, such as trauma and abuse, and it is up to us to ascertain whether the child has been traumatized and whether she is currently safe. Sometimes it is our job to reveal such circumstances and to address them. However, once the child is safe she can be encouraged to reclaim her feelings and imagination from the abuse—to reserve her fears for present dangers, and to employ her imagination to serve her own purposes.

Ginger and the Dream Screen

Eight-year-old Ginger was beset by nightmares in which she was terrorized by fearsome beasts of tooth and claw who chased after her until she awoke over and over, breathless and sweating. Jenny, after determining to her satisfaction that Ginger was safe, concluded that this was a matter of her vivid imagination having been taken over by Fear.

Ginger's most recent "scary dream" involved a huge and terrible lion pursuing her. At a lake, she set out in a boat with a friend to the other side, seeking safety. They came to the far shore, landing at the mouth of a cave. The cave seemed dark and foreboding. As they peered into it, they saw, to their horror, a huge, hideous crocodile. It stirred and started moving toward them. There seemed nowhere to turn, no safe haven. At this point in the dream, she awoke. She didn't know how it turned out. Even in her daytime retelling, Ginger's voice had a nervous tremolo and shadows of fear played across her face.

Jenny broke the spell of the dream by inviting Ginger to make a puppet play. Ginger leapt up and created a delightful play on a matter of her own choosing. Her improvisational skills and her rich imagination were very impressive. Her family witnessed this and confirmed her "wonderful imagination." They told of Ginger's ability to visualize and her love of pretend play.

Jenny questioned her parents about when Ginger enjoyed her imagination freely in contrast to the times when Fear ran away with her. She asked Ginger, "Would you prefer to be even more in charge of this talent of yours? Or would you rather have Fear run the show as often as it does?" She chose the former. Jenny asked Ginger if she might be interested in some imagination games where she could practice using her imagination for herself instead of letting Fear use it. In a warm-up,[2] Jenny initiated a game in which she asked Ginger if she could close her eyes and imagine a video screen in the room; if so, could she see a picture on it in her mind's eye? Could she project an imaginary puppet play onto the screen? She agreed she could. Once her play was projected on her inner screen, Ginger was invited to improvise. Ginger both created and watched several versions on her imaginary screen, chuckling all the while. The exuberant freedom of Ginger's imagination was entrancing.

After a while Jenny asked Ginger if she would be interested in playing with some scary dream images in her imagination. Although nervous, she said she would like to give it a try. She projected a monster from "an old dream." They experimented, much to Ginger's delight, with some comic variations. She found she could make the monster run around in red spotted undershorts, sing opera, and turn around in circles. Ginger laughed along with everyone else. Jenny asked if she had previously realized how capable she was at bringing her sense of humor into her imagination. Had she realized how playful an imagination she really had? What would happen if Fear realized this, too? Would it run away in red undershorts? Ginger's "Yes" got caught up in her giggling.

Jenny asked Ginger if she might be ready to play with her recent nightmare. She said she was ready and willing. Ginger put it on her inner screen and then "rewound" for a while. She began to play it through, but this time, when it came to the really scary part, Jenny asked Ginger if she was ready to let the dream continue to see what else might happen.[3]

Ginger took a breath and imagined the dream movie playing on. The cave and the threatening crocodile loomed up. But this time, as Ginger watched, she saw a prison fence rise up from the lake and close off the entrance to the cave. She looked inside and the crocodile appeared, wearing purple spots and looking a bit sad. Just then she heard the lion roaring from the far shore and tensed up for a moment. She checked in with her dad, who encouraged her to relax and see what would happen if she kept playing the dream. Now she saw a lovely fairy fly down over the lake. She pointed in the direction of the lion, and the fairy flew over and sprinkled shimmering dust over it. It turned into a purring kitten, and she smiled. Before long it turned back into a lion, but with the fairy around Ginger wasn't so worried anymore. In fact, Ginger and her friend sat in the boat in the middle of the lake and appreciated the great animal's awesome nature from a distance.

Ginger's excitement at being able to play with her dream was palpable. Later, Jenny questioned her about the implications of these abilities of hers now that she was more in charge of them. At a follow-up session Ginger surprised Jenny by telling her that she remembered a time several years earlier when she had discovered she could actually become aware that she was dreaming during a dream and decide to wake up or change it. It had happened again during the last week. Ginger, Jenny, and her family mused about how fascinating dreams can be when they're not so frightening.

It's Blueberry Pancakes or Nothing!

Jenny has noticed that certain children who are prone to Bad Moods, Upsets, and Tempers, as well as Fears, also possess the particular ability to visualize future events, thereby creating expectations of how things will go. When reality fails to live up to these expectations, a child can be sorely disappointed. For example, Jenny was trying to find out in a first meeting with a family exactly how Misery took over eight-year-old Phoebe's life. Although it took some time to draw out the details, she was told of an event that was pretty typical of Misery. They told of a "miserable day" on Saturday when Phoebe seemed mad and unhappy about a family outing for no apparent reason. Following her hunch that Phoebe just might be a child with an imagination that creates elaborate expectations, Jenny asked for details about the actual event that the family members described, as well as what Phoebe had imagined would happen.

It turned out that when her family planned the night before to go out for breakfast, Phoebe had visualized going to her favorite restaurant and having blueberry pancakes with real maple syrup. She could almost smell and taste those delicious pancakes. Next she imagined stopping at the playground on the way back and could see her father pushing her on the swings while she lay back as far as she could so she could see all the blue sky and clouds "upside down."

On Saturday, the family set off. By the time they arrived at the restaurant of their choice rather than the one Phoebe expected, she was feeling very hurt. She was unable to speak of her imagined breakfast; all she could say was a grouchy, "I don't like this place." By the time they ordered, she had been swept up into an inexplicable and embarrassing tantrum about her seating. This cast a shadow over the rest of the day, in which everything seemed to go wrong for Phoebe and they could do nothing to put anything right. Jenny's interview of Phoebe's "disappointed imagination" revealed her sense of attachment to her vivid but inflexible imaginings about the future.

The family eagerly embarked on a quest to help Phoebe release her imagination from Misery and Disappointment. They soon found that it was important for them to "tune in" to her expectations in advance and prepare her if those expectations could not be realized. They took to apprising her of what was going to happen in the near future. Phoebe came to a fuller appreciation of her imagination and learned to use it more flexibly. Soon she was starting to use words instead of tantrums to express her wishes and expectations. Phoebe's summing up at the last meeting was "My imagination's my friend, but it's gotta be open." To this day, Phoebe's imagination conjures up visions of future events and she has to struggle to adjust, but her family reported on follow-up that at least they have ways to talk about it now.

Timmy and the Great Silver Monster

In this next story, David Epston weaves the imagination of seven-year-old Timmy together with his own to write a story of transformation for Timmy and his family.

The first phone call. Alice, Timmy's mother, phoned David seeking an appointment. Alice wanted to come in alone because she felt that there must be something wrong with her as a mother. She ruefully informed David that her feelings about Timmy had become very negative. She expressed herself in a tone of such sorrowful self-abasement that David felt he had to make a request. He told her that, although he had fully taken in what she said, he wanted to meet her together with Timmy and anyone else she would like to have present. He wondered if there might just be some alternative way to comprehend her concerns.

First meeting. David welcomed Timmy and Alice into the room. When they sat down, David was hard-pressed to say who looked the gloomier. Despite the despondent atmosphere, David asked if he might "get to know Timmy without the problems. I want to know what resources we've all got to put together against the problems, whatever they be," David elaborated. Alice was quick to tell David that Timmy "has an amazing imagination, lots of enthusiasm for certain things, and that he is very strong-minded."

"How does he show his amazing imagination?" David wondered. "He's good at writing," Alice said. Turning to Timmy, David inquired, "What is your favorite thing to write about?" The enthusiasm that Alice had referred to broke out all over Timmy's face as he told David, "The Great Golden Monster!" Timmy expounded on the Monster and all the ways he was able to delight both himself and others with his amazing imagination.

As Timmy spoke, Alice looked happy and sad at the same time. She went on to tell David that, although Timmy's imagination was wonderful sometimes, his mind could "turn the world black" and darken his moods. The other problem was that he would often soil his pants. Timmy explained the trouble by complaining, "I get told off all the time for not doing what I am told."

"At times does your mind run away with you?" David asked Timmy. He agreed that it did. "When it takes hold of your mind, can imagination play tricks on it?" According to Timmy, this was certainly so. "Why do you think the Problems would want your mind to themselves?"

Timmy thought for a moment about this unusual question. He wasn't sure how to answer it, but he replied, "I would like to talk to my mind so that I can have the kind of days I want."

"What kind of days do you have in mind for yourself, Timmy?"

"A good day in which I don't get told off."

"Why would the Problems want to run away with your mind and its imagination?"

"It makes me get into trouble and I think of bad things that could happen. At the amusement park it told me I wouldn't have a good time on the roller coaster."

"What did you say back when it tried to take your fun away from you?"

"I fought back and I decided to shake it off."

"How did you go about that?"

"I said in my mind to my imagination, 'I don't want you.' Then I played a trick on my imagination. I tricked it into being good. In my mind I made the park into a jungle. And I had a paint brush in my mind, and wherever my imagination was walking, I drew a crocodile underneath it. I scared it back!" After describing this amazing sleight of mind, Timmy affirmed to David and his mother that he was proud of himself for tricking his imagination rather than being tricked by it.

While interviewing Timmy and his mother about this incident and his abilities and interests in general, David was impressed by a number of things about Timmy, which he wrote down in his notes. Since some of the most impressive things were Timmy's imagination and his writing ability, David felt inspired to ghostwrite a story about Timmy and his family. David asked Alice and Timmy for permission to take notes for such a story right then and there in the session. They agreed. He told them he would make a rough draft and show it to Timmy and get his help. He planned to finish it off after the meeting and send it to them in the mail.

In order to write the story, David looked at the list of impressive things he'd written about Timmy. Then he looked at the list of ways that problems such as excessive anger and fear had been depriving Timmy of enjoying his imagination. When he put these together he could see how they could fit into a story. After he made up the story, he consulted Timmy about ideas and details, which Timmy provided readily.

The Great Silver Monster Story

There was a boy I met who had an amazing imagination. His imagination made him really good at writing and painting and thinking and telling stories. Everyone agreed also that he has a really strong mind. Everyone thought he was so lucky. This made him feel like a very special person. And you know, he was a very special person. His stories, pictures and clever expressions gave him great joy and gave many people who knew him much joy, too. It looked like this boy was going to have a great life.

He was an only child until two years later when a sister came into the life of his family. And two years later another followed her. Now there were three. His parents were very lucky indeed because each of their children was amazing in his or her own way. No mother or father could have hoped for more.

David recalled Timmy's familiar antagonist the Great Golden Monster. He changed the metal to Silver so as to not plagiarize. This allowed Timmy to have his "amazing imagination" champion his own interests.

It looked like they were going to live happily ever after until the Great Silver Monster figured out what was going on. You see, the Great Silver Monster hates amazing children and happy families. The more he spied on this family, the more sour he became. He thought to himself, "Hey, why am I so sour? Why don't I sour the life of this family instead?" He wondered who he would start with and figured it was right and proper to pick on the oldest child. He thought to himself, "This kid thinks he is so smart, so strong-minded, and with such an amazing imagination! I'll show him. I will take his strong mind and imagination away from him and use them to turn him sour. And when he goes sour, everyone in his family will go sour, too." So the Great Silver Monster decided to sneak into this amazing boy's mind through Anger and Fear. But first he had to find a way to turn his insides sour.

David was aware that one of the worst things that was happening to Timmy was that Sneaky Poo had tricked "your poo into staying inside of you rather than coming out and going where it belongs—the sewage works." Alice and Timmy agreed that this trick was even "sneakier" than the one where it "puts it in your pants when you aren't looking or thinking about it." David guessed that Sneaky Poo could very well be an agent of the Great Silver Monster, so naturally it would be an important character in the story.

The Great Silver Monster had a friend called "Sneaky Poo." I suppose you all would like to know how it got its name. It's pretty obvious, really. He is so darned SNEAKY. He has lots of tricks up his sleeve, like getting kids' poo to sneak out in their pants when they aren't thinking about it. Or worse, telling them to keep it inside of themselves, which turns them sour. Everyone knows that the best place for poo is to be flushed right down the toilet with a great big flushing noise.

David then worked out how the Great Silver Monster was in league with Sneaky Poo to turn Timmy sour both on his insides and the outside. It scared Timmy and made him grumpy and cranky, too, and worst of all it did this using Timmy's own imagination so it could hide what it was doing from him. Timmy would just think it was his own fault, or someone else's in the family.

As the Poo started turning this boy sour from the inside out, the Great Silver Monster said to himself, "It is now time to take over his imagination and make him mad." And he did. The boy's world turned black and he became grumpy and cranky. Like so many grumpy people, he stopped doing what his mother and father asked of him, even though he had a really nice mum and a really nice dad. He didn't seem to be able to help himself. He couldn't understand it. His mind seemed to have a mind of its own. But you see, the Great Silver Monster never let on what he was up to. He had the boy think his mind was his own. So this boy found himself angry all the time, not knowing quite why.

This was not enough for such a monster, so he then decided to start scaring this young boy. He knew it was really easy to scare amazing kids with amazing imaginations. All you had to do is get their imagination and run away with it. The Great Silver Monster started playing fear tricks on him. Some of these were dirty tricks. When they worked, they took the fun away from the boy by talking him out of things. For example, once at the Rainbow's End, it told him that he wouldn't have a good time on the roller coaster. Now, don't you think that is a pretty dirty trick to play on an amazing kid?

A hero often sees the light when the hour is darkest. David laid out clearly how the Great Silver Monster had been having its way with Timmy's imagination. Together they surveyed all the havoc the monster caused in his life and his relationship with his parents. David suggested that Timmy use his mind's eye to see who was making the trouble in his life and how his antagonists were going about it. Timmy was mad at the monster and determined to make it stop. David wrote into the story that Timmy planned to do this, but he did not investigate how. This he left up to Timmy.

Finally, it dawned on this amazing boy with an amazing imagination that his life was really getting sour. And his nice mum and nice dad were getting pretty sour, too. So, he thought and he thought and he thought about it. Finally he said to himself, "Hey, I know who is behind this. It's that miserable Great Silver Monster. Hey mate, I know what you are up to." With that, he decided to take his imagination back. After all, it really is his property and not the Great Silver Monster's. So he planned to take it back in a rather amazing way. But he decided not to tell anyone how until he met with David

Epston and his mum and dad and sisters at The Family Therapy Centre. They couldn't wait to learn his amazing way.

How would Timmy seize the initiative and take his imagination back from the monster? Well, that was the mystery that ended the first chapter of the story and made anyone who read it look forward to the next installment!

Second meeting. Timmy's father, Robert, and Timmy's younger sisters, ages three and five, joined David, Timmy, and Alice at the next session a month and a half later. David checked in with Timmy to find out what had happened in the next chapter of their story: "Do you remember we met about five or six weeks ago and I wrote you that story? I want to know what has been happening to that Monster of yours." Timmy told David that he had been good. David was curious about how he had accomplished this: "How have you been good? Did you have to do something to the Monster to get your life back and be good?" Timmy replied that he had. "What did you do?" David asked, dying with curiosity, "This is exciting!"

"I drew things with a paint brush," Timmy replied.

"You drew things with a paint brush? What did you draw?"

"A trap," Timmy replied, "A Monster trap!"

David had come across traps while helping other kids deal with monsters, so he immediately asked, "How did you trick the Monster into it?" He looked at Timmy for an answer but he couldn't resist guessing first, "Did you put some special food he liked in the trap so the Monster would go in it?"

David had guessed wrong but Timmy was merciful and didn't make him guess again: "People, fake, dummy people."

"Really," replied David, wanting to hear all about this, "and how big was the trap? As big as a house or as big as a car or what?"

"As big as a car."

"Did the Great Silver Monster just walk in without thinking?"

"Yeah."

"And did you shut the door behind him?"

"He stayed in there."

"Did he say then, 'Let me out! I'll be good! I'll leave you alone!'?"

"Yeah."

"How long did you keep him in the Monster Trap?"

"Three days."

David thought the severity of the punishment was appropriate, "Gosh, after three days, anybody would want to get out!" David wondered how

Timmy had come to the decision to let the monster go: "In the end, did he say, 'Please let me out. I'll be good, I promise.'?"

"Yeah."

"Did you feel sorry for him in the end?"

"No."

"Where did you tell him to go after you let him out?"

"GO AWAY," Timmy shouted.

David wanted to know where Timmy had sent him: "Go away outside your house or outside Auckland?"

"Outside Auckland."

"Do you think he is bothering some kid in Hamilton now?"

"Yeah," said Timmy.

David supposed that with the monster gone Timmy's imagination would be in his own hands. "Did that mean you got your imagination back for yourself?" asked David.

"Yes!" Timmy exclaimed.

"And is that a good thing or a bad thing?"

"A good thing."

"Tell me, how you are using your imagination for yourself? Are you having fun with it?"

"Yep."

David wanted to know how Timmy was having fun with his imagination, but Timmy couldn't say exactly. So David turned to Alice: "Do you know any ways he has been taking his imagination back for himself?"

Alice had no trouble responding, "He has been drawing amazing things, but when he paints the Monster away, it is all in his mind."

David turned back to Timmy: "Do you remember how the world used to be black for you? Is it turning more gray or white or what?"

"More white."

"Is that a nice thing for you?"

"Yeah, pretty nice."

"Are you looking forward to spring now and more sunshine?"

"Yes," said Timmy.

The only question that remained now was whether Timmy had gotten back at the Great Silver Monster's ally, Sneaky Poo. He certainly had. "Really, what did you do?" David asked eagerly.

"I did the same thing I did with the Monster. I drew traps with my imaginary paintbrush."

"What did you do when you got Sneaky Poo in the trap?"

"I let him go after five days."

"You kept him for five days? Was he worse than the Great Silver Monster?"

"Yes."
"Did he say that he'd let you go to the toilet now?"
"Yes."
"Are you flushing him down the toilet?"
"Yep."

The myth of the perfect parent. Everyone in the family was delighted by what had happened in Timmy's life since the first meeting. There were some very important developments in Alice's life as well.

Alice had renounced her self-abasement. Her feelings about Timmy had "changed 100 percent," and her feelings about herself had undergone "a turnabout" as well. When David asked how this had occurred, she told him that she had found cause to call into question what Robert described as "trying to be a perfect parent." Apparently Alice had been subject to a lot of scrutiny and criticism from her family about her mothering for many years. Alice had tried not only to measure up to family expectations but also to go beyond those measures and impose perfection on herself.

During the interval between the meetings, Alice and Robert had joined together to revise their parenting ambitions. They now intended to refuse trying to exceed others' expectations of them. They did this by claiming their preference for their own expectations and choosing a new direction for their ambitions—delighting in their children and their "amazing imaginations."

Zack and Blade

In this case story, Dean provided consultation to therapist Karen Moore,[4] who discovered through expressive arts therapy an imaginary friend who had gotten seriously out of hand and was wreaking such havoc that a young man's life was threatened. If it weren't for Karen's aplomb, she could have easily been immobilized by the results of her careful and meticulous clinical assessment. Her concerns were the severity of Zack's suicidal and "psychotic" ideation, his "dissociative states," and his out-of-control "aggressive" and "self-destructive" impulses. If Karen hadn't been able to engage him in a mythic rite of passage that challenged him to use his physical prowess and imaginative powers for the good of himself and others, she might very well have found herself recommending his hospitalization.

When twelve-year-old Zack and his mother began their conversations with Karen, she heard about the havoc Blade was causing before she found out about Blade himself. Zack's mother came into the family session with Karen, very frightened. It appeared that Zack had kicked in the front door of their house. She was convinced that the son she knew and loved wouldn't do such a thing as trashing the house and lying about who had actually done it. But if it wasn't the son she knew and loved, who had done it? Who was this "son" who acted in such a wanton and destructive manner? She couldn't find her way out of this conundrum.

At that stage, Karen didn't know about Blade but she shared Zack's mother's sneaking suspicion that all was not as it appeared. Her suspicion was based on a drawing that Zack had brought in for her—a picture of an evil, fierce, and muscular warrior, half man, half animal. Karen decided to see Zack alone for half of the session and inquire about the picture. It was then that Zack revealed that this was Blade, who turned out to be a kind of imaginary friend or, more accurately, foe. She also found out that, according to Zack, it was Blade who had kicked in the front door! Zack told of how Blade then clapped his impressively strong hand/claw firmly over his mouth, got on the phone, and told his mother that burglars had knocked the door down. Of course, by the time Zack's mother and the police got there, Blade was gone, leaving Zack to face questioning by the police, and much worse, to face the music from his mother.

Zack told Karen that Blade was a fighting super-villain type, "part gorilla, part cheetah, part gymnast, part mutant, and part spider." Although Zack admired some of his qualities, he was furious with him for having gone too far this time. He had made his life impossibly miserable and had almost completely destroyed his relationship with his mother.

Zack explained to Karen that the incident that had taken place was in some ways typical: Blade always took over, did horrible things, told lies, and abandoned Zack to face the trouble. But in an another way the incident was significantly atypical: Zack was shocked at how far Blade had gone this time. Zack knew that Blade was getting too strong, violent, and dangerous. He wanted Blade dead and gone from his life, but he felt trapped because he thought that the only way to get rid of Blade was to kill himself! Zack was in a conundrum of his own—he didn't want to kill himself, but by the same token, he didn't want Blade ruining his life and hurting his mother.

Karen asked, "When does Blade take you over?" There were certain circumstances. "It happens," Zack explained, "when I am 5 percent angry, 5 percent upset, or whenever someone tries to push me around, even a little bit." To Karen's questions as to how comfortable these thresholds were for him, Zack replied that they were too low for his comfort "because when Blade takes me over, he makes me do crazy things." Although he had respected Blade in the past, Zack did not like his current relationship with him. Blade had betrayed him and had become "a cruel strong-arm dictator" of his life.

A week after this session, Karen told the story of Zack's relationship with Blade to the narrative team that Dean was supervising and to which she belonged. The entire team was both spellbound and terrified by this description of what was surely a perilous, life-or-death matter. The team expressed both its curiosity about Blade and its concern for Zack and pressed for more information about the two of them.

Some of their questions were: Where did Blade come from? Would Zack prefer to be able to get more angry or upset than 5 percent without Blade taking over? How did Zack hold Blade off for that 5 percent anyway? And what about Zack's mother? Had the incident with the door made her suspicious about Blade's secret existence? Did she think Blade and Zack were one and the same person?

When the team found out that Blade didn't come out when his mother was around, they wanted to know if Zack realized she was his ally. What would the future look like if Blade stayed around for the next five years? Could Zack revise his relationship with Blade or did it have to be a fight to one of their deaths?

When Karen returned to Zack with the team's questions, he was equally intrigued by their concern and interest in the two of them. He wanted to know exactly who they were and why they were so interested! After all, up until a few weeks ago, no one whatsoever had known that Blade had been in his life. Zack and Blade had been engaged for five long years in a secret and desperate struggle and guerrilla warfare. Now suddenly they found themselves battling under the fascinated gaze of half a dozen narrative therapists who wanted to learn about each of their alliances, tactics, and strategies.

In that session Zack did a lot of thinking and talking with Karen about the questions the team had asked him. He also filled Karen in on his history with Blade and brought her up to date on the status of their relationship. Blade had steadily been trying to gain total control over Zack, ever since the night, long ago, when he "came out of the clear blue sky" and attacked Zack in one of his dreams. Zack was only seven at the time, but he still carried the "scar" from that original attack, which had jolted him right out of bed. Since then, Zack's dreams had become a constant battleground. In the beginning the battle had been good for him because he had been able to develop his own strong warrior dream identity called "Storm Shadow," who was strong enough to fight back against Blade's family. He had managed to kill all Blade's relatives except for Blade's cousin Havoc.

After Zack's victory against his family, Blade had entered Zack's waking life and begun wreaking his revenge on Zack's relationships with his mother and his siblings. With the house trashing incident Blade had taken the upper hand in the war. Zack and his family were now alienated to the point where his mother was considering foster placement. Not only that, Blade reduced his anger threshold to 1 percent and made him do crazy things even though he wasn't "really mad."

Karen asked Zack about the times when Blade didn't take over. The only times Blade didn't were when Zack was sad or when there was "nice energy around." As a result of this knowledge Karen and Zack made an important discovery about Blade's "Kryptonite"—"nice energy" weakened Blade.

Karen asked if there were times Blade was of some assistance. In fact, there were. Blade gave Zack the power to climb up walls and trees, to do flips, and to hit hard in baseball. His flips were so good that Zack's friends were amazed by his gymnastic ability. Thanks to Blade, Zack had become one of the better players on the baseball team in a short time.

Casually, near the very end of the session, Zack surprised Karen. Despite the fact that Blade was taking him over much more easily these days, Zack related that he had walked away from a fight with a friend and on that occasion he "had 100 percent control over Blade." Although he found it impossible to explain, Zack knew "it was a physical act." He said he was under the threat of suspension at school and that he really didn't want to fight his friend, so he felt he had little choice but to physically stop himself from fighting. Karen knew this was a major accomplishment of willpower for him, as Zack was notorious throughout his school and his neighborhood for his uncontrollable temper.

When Karen reported the history as well as this recent event to the team, they had more questions for Zack about his relationship with Blade: Had Blade become a foe/companion to seven-year-old Zack? Had he helped Zack fight loneliness when his mother was at work? Had Zack attacked Blade's family to protect his own? Was Zack strong enough to deal with his temper without Blade? Had he outgrown Blade before he was willing to let Zack grow out of him?

They were also eager to know just how Zack had physically managed to control Blade: What had it initially felt like in Zack's body when Blade was coming to take him over? Where exactly did Zack feel power in his body when he exerted control over Blade? Zack said he had leapt off some steps before the fight had gotten out of hand: Did he use his gymnastic leg muscles to leap off the steps and jump out of Blade's way? The team was concerned about Zack using violence to meet Blade's violence. Was it one of Blade's tricks to keep Zack convinced that killing him was the only solution? Perhaps Blade was using a protracted battle strategy to entice Zack into an endless power struggle with him, to drain his energy and weaken him.

These questions were new and different for Zack and he gave them a great deal of thought. He had never considered how he kept physical control over Blade and he wasn't sure he had done it with any specific muscles. He agreed that controlling Blade was a great feat. After some consideration, Zack decided that he needed to kill Blade despite this startling turn of events and regardless of the benefits that Blade contributed to his physical being.

At the same meeting, Karen spent some time with Zack's mother. Although his mother still did not know of Blade's existence, she told Karen that she was sure there was something seriously wrong with her son and to this end she had decided to treat him differently and suspend all punishments against him. Even though his mother was unaware of Blade, Zack had at last found "a real life ally" in his life-and-death struggle.

Perhaps Zack's mother knew intuitively that "nice energy" made Blade weak. Perhaps Blade's family had been a "mean one" and never acted the way Zack's did. Whatever the case, she was certainly less vengeful than Blade was. It was starting to seem as if Blade might have overplayed his hand with his door bashing and lying about the burglars. Instead of getting Zack into more misery and trouble with his mother, this incident had elicited her concern!

It took another week before the Zack-Blade contest climaxed. It was then that Zack employed an influx of "nice energy" to decommission Blade's power to jump off high buildings. Then he was able to kill him in a dream battle. He explained the fact that he had gained strength and Blade had been mortally weakened by his mother's powerful "nice energy" barrage. In the wake of a months-long period of a "no toys restriction," she had surprised him with the present of a Super Nintendo. She had also taken him out to a family barbecue after he requested it. When he had asked her if he could go to that special event, instead of the expected "no" she had told him, "Anything you want to do, I am all for it." It was immediately after this that Blade was dispatched.

Karen had a final meeting with Zack after that epic battle. They reviewed his struggle together. The narrative therapy team had one last question: Had Zack learned anything more from the powerful Blade before he killed him off? At first Zack didn't think so, but he did concede that he had retained Blade's athletic prowess.

More important to Zack was that an abundance of "nice energy" was still around: Zack had actually spent some time just "hanging out" with his mother, which was much to his liking! He also said it was getting easier for him to be nice to his siblings as well. (Blade's cousin Havoc was still hovering around, but Zack told Karen that he was keeping a wary eye on him and keeping him away with a heart full of happiness.)

Karen was left with the strong impression that Zack's mother had helped him tremendously in his fight against Blade. Although Zack's mother never knew about this "imaginary foe," she had the wisdom to give Zack some special attention after Blade kicked the door in and lied about the burglars. She possessed the special wisdom that a parent can have—to know that her child's problem was one of those that punishments could not ultimately solve. Though she didn't know it at the time, she had helped Zack to kill Blade with her kindness.

Follow-up. Dean contacted Zack and his mother three years later to catch up on developments in their lives and to gain permission to publish their story. They were happy to give it in hope that others might be inspired by reading about Zack's journey. Zack had had some ups and downs but he was doing well in general. For example, he was eager to succeed at getting a well-paying job.

Interestingly, vanquishing Blade had not really been a satisfying long-term solution for Zack. Following the mighty imaginary battle, Blade had reappeared, but as the team had speculated Zack had found himself working out a productive relationship with Blade. Blade was still around to give Zack strength but couldn't take him over and wreak havoc in his life. With his imaginary foe no longer disrupting his relationships with constant cycles of attack and revenge, Zack was maintaining peaceful relationships with his friends, neighbors, classmates, and family.

111

PLAYFUL STORIES

CHAPTER 13

Jonathon:
"I Have Overcome That Much and I Don't Think I'll Be Able to Go Back"

The Lawson family is Pakeha (Caucasian New Zealanders) of English descent. The family members involved in the therapy are Jonathon, nine, Judy, his mother, and Ron, his father. They met together twice with David Epston over a month period. Sam, seven, and Jimmy, four, are also members of the family.

Let's say that in our conversations with a family an alternative story about the person-problem relationship has caught on and the counter-plot has begun to be thickened. However, it is still not time to relax and move on. An alternative story can need plenty of confirmation to really take hold and to survive the "hiccups," "backslides," and "come-backs" of a well-substantiated problem story. The problem story has the strength of repeated historical experience and of mental habit to back it up and make it endure. It is not a simple matter to help the child and family grow roots for a new story that are strong enough to allow it to take over and branch out into their future lives.

The following case first presents a playful approach developed between David and the Lawson family in the face of some serious fears. It goes on to demonstrate the painstaking and detailed work that follows an initial success. The therapist persists with queries to establish Jonathon's success in taking his life back from Fears, to explore and represent in language the "secrets" behind such an accomplishment, and to confirm Jonathon's historical and ongoing maturity and ability.

FIRST MEETING

Jonathon was nine years old when he came with his parents, Judy and Ron, to see David for the first time. It seems that Fear had entered the life of such a nice ordinary kid as Jonathon by pretty obvious means. While playing with a friend in a nearby park he had been savaged by a notorious guard dog that had been allowed to run free by its owners. No one would be expected to recover from such a trauma overnight. Jonathon's parents, along with other concerned neighbors, took legal action to ensure this would never happen again. (Jonathon was not the first victim of such attacks.)

Despite this action, Fear seemed to spread throughout Jonathon's life. First it opened the door for the appearance of fearful ghosts, who were especially horrible at night. Although Jonathon, by dint of his own courage, closed the door to such fearful ghosts, no sooner had he done so but fears of burglars took their place, threatening to enter the family home by way of windows and doors. As if this weren't enough for a young person to contend with, Fear went much further by convincing him that the police helicopter that was stationed not too far from his home was no longer conducting surveillance for lawbreakers but had sinister intentions to abduct him and take him he knew not where.

When David began to interview Jonathon, no one was surprised to learn that Fear had convinced Jonathon that he was younger than he really was and given him the impression that he was going backwards and downwards until he felt like "a five-year-old." Fear was far more compelling by night and left Jonathon fatigued, ragged, and distressed by day. Everyone observed that his lassitude was having severe effects on his schoolwork and his recreational activities. It had so interfered with his appetite that he found himself almost without one.

However, when asked by David about the nature of his and his parents' commitment to resist the Fear, Jonathon was only too willing to acknowledge that he was heartily sick of Fear giving him such a hard time. In doing so, for a moment, he broke free from his dispirited demeanor and spoke with a forcefulness that was to serve him well in the next few weeks.

Everyone agreed that Fear had taken his security away from him and made him depend on his parents, Judy and Ron, who had turned themselves inside out giving reassurances and taking any measures they could think of to provide him with security. Jonathon now stated his desire to win back his old sense of security. To this end, David proposed that he assume, on his own behalf and that of his family, the job of "Nightwatch-person" (Epston, 1986/1997).

Before getting down to the specifics of the job, David and the family spent a bit more time mulling over how the Fears worked. They reviewed the "Laws of Fear," which are:

1. Fears feed on avoidance; they increase in direct proportion to the time that they are not confronted.
2. Fears are weak; they need good friends to feed them.
3. Fears are infectious; they need to be isolated.
4. Fears are humorless; they cannot stand a joke at their expense.
5. Fears lurk in dark corners; they need to be exposed to the light.

These laws helped everyone see through some of the tricks Fears often employ in frightening the life out of young persons—and adults as well. By the end of this discussion, everyone was pretty disenchanted with the ways Fears operate in people's lives. A comradeship emerged, one in which David was only too happy to take a part.

Next David, Jonathon, and his parents tackled the job description for Night-watch-person. Considering the pickle the Fears had gotten him in, Jonathon might have wanted to fall back to a defensive position and continue to rely on his parents for vigilance and protection. Instead, Jonathon seized the opportunity to go on the offensive, to help provide security for his family, and to come back to being the nice, ordinary kid he had been before the trauma of the dog attack. Through questions from his family and David, Jonathon determined that he felt most brave and would mostly likely frighten the Fears if he went about his security work dressed in his baseball outfit, with his trusty bat and flashlight in hand. He was of the opinion that bi-hourly checks of all likely places (including doors and windows) by which an intruder might enter the home would be more than adequate protection. His parents generously agreed to accompany him on his rounds, but from behind so they wouldn't "get in the way of his courage." His father thought it would be a good idea for Jonathon to set a bedside alarm clock to rouse him so he could conduct his security round.

David felt at this point that it was fair to say they were already in breach of Law 4. He even took the opportunity to ask Jonathon how he thought Fear might cope with the high spirits and good humor that had entered their discussions. Jonathon found it hard to speak of; he was far more certain about the satisfactions he might experience by re-securing his home and his place in it. As a matter of fact, he thought such a prospect might be akin to revenge—or at least getting even with Fear. By the end of their initial meeting, the Lawson-Epston conspiracy against Fear was ready and able to test any further influence Fear might attempt to have over Jonathon's life.

SECOND MEETING

One month later, when the family returned for a second meeting, Jonathon looked like a nice, ordinary kid again. David invited Jonathon and his family to take the measure of their accomplishments over the past month, and to co-author a new story about Jonathon—one based on the courage and fortitude he had called on to take his life back from the Fears. Jonathon's new story is constructed through careful elaboration of the unique outcomes which might not otherwise have been fully integrated into his picture of himself and the pictures others might have had of him.

Jonathon's father reviewed their night-watching experience: "We got his baseball cap on, gave him his baseball bat. We put his jacket on. And then we went around and checked out a few things. Within a few days, we were walking further and further behind him."

Jonathon proudly recounted his own night-watching, "Me and Mum went around the side of the house and checked all the windows and doors. We only did it for a couple of nights."

"How come you decided to cut back on your work?" David asked him.

Jonathon replied thoughtfully, "Because I was learning that there are windows and doors and they can't be opened without making a real loud noise or breaking them."

David had to interrupt Jonathon for a moment to obtain his consent to record his remarks, so that they would be available should he be willing to consult with other young persons in the future who were considering embarking on night-watching in order to re-secure their lives. David began writing down what Jonathon and his family were saying.

Jonathon's mother Judy continued the account with relish: "We went around behind Jonathon. On the first night, he was convinced there was someone outside, so we went outside at 4 A.M. We had to check outside the gate and there was a man walking in the street." She turned to Jonathon and smiled, "We gave him a fright, didn't we?" Contagious laughter erupted. When equanimity was regained, David mock-seriously asked Jonathon, "Did you frighten some other person? Do you think that man is going to have to come to me about Fears?"

David then asked Jonathon's mother to take measure of Jonathon's change as a person, given that Fear had previously driven him backwards and downwards: "Judy, as you were standing behind Jonathon, did you know that he was getting a bit bigger as a person?"

Without any hesitation she replied, "Yes, he was. At first, I couldn't be more than a foot or two away from him and then I could be further away from him." Judy then recalled a remark that she had made to David earlier in this session—about how she and Jonathon had "laughed away" the last vestige of fear in Jonathon's life. She told David about a time this had happened. One night, Jonathon had wakened out of his sleep and then had run and jumped into his parents' bed. This had previously been a regular feature of their nocturnal lives. So much so that Judy had accustomed herself to just roll over and make room for him once she heard his feet hit the bedroom floor and start running. But on this occasion, she played a joke. She remained on the edge of the bed. Jonathon couldn't help but observe this. He started to laugh and so did she. Jonathon exclaimed in the telling, "Part of it was fun, wasn't it?"

Judy answered him, "And part of it was serious. So I agree that Fear doesn't like humor." She added to David, "We had quite a bit of humor. It was hard not to, really."

Jonathon's father informed David, "We tried rigging up the alarm clock for regular awakenings. It didn't work, but it really didn't need to work."

David then turned his attention to Jonathon and wondered if he was still going on his rounds two times a night as they had agreed on a month earlier. Confidently, he told David that he had stopped two weeks ago. David asked him how he had come to that decision. Jonathon replied with a tone of indifference in his voice, "Because it was getting a bit tiring. I knew no one was going to come and get me."

David told Jonathon that this was "certainly brave-sounding," but he still wondered, "How did you know no one would get you?"

Jonathon articulated his knowledge without much further ado, "The burglar fears had gone on for ages and ages and no one has robbed us yet."

David was given cause to reflect, "Does this mean that as you pushed Fear out of your life, Bravery came back?"

Jonathon assured him that this was the case.

David thought it would be prudent to review if the Fears were still playing havoc in two other significant areas of Jonathon's life. First he asked, "Are you getting a better night's sleep?" Jonathon reported that it wasn't so tiring but he was still waking up automatically in the middle of the night. David remarked that Jonathon might still have a left-over sleep problem. Jonathon thought so, too, but did not pay it much mind.

David then reminded Jonathon that a month before Jonathon had told him that the Fear problem had been turning his growing up backwards. He asked, "How old do you feel now?" Jonathon estimated, "About eight." David was impressed that Jonathon had regained about three years of his growing up in just a month's time.

David made a note of this chronology, since it is very important to measure progress. Then he asked Judy to confirm or deny this. Judy observed enthusiastically, "Yes, there has been a big jump with him. He has been doing far more independent things, like getting up and making his own breakfast for the last two weeks." Jonathon proudly added that he was cooking French toast. David immediately took the opportunity to record this fact and reiterated it, "Jonathon has been doing far more independent things, like making his own breakfast for the first time."

Judy continued, "He does everything. I don't do a thing. He gets the bowls out. Fries up the eggs. Turns the gas on. Cooks it up. Turns it all off. Very responsible."

David was impressed by the sheer independence of his independence, "I hope you don't mind me saying this, but that sounds like a ten-year-old thing. Do you think you have even gone ahead of your age?"

"Well, cooking myself breakfast, I think I have," Jonathon concurred.

David added to his record that Jonathon had gone ahead of his age in cooking breakfast.

But that wasn't the only way Jonathon had gone in the direction of independence. According to Judy, he was also setting the table and helping his brothers solve their problems. David wrote, "Helping brothers solve their problems."

APPRECIATING ONE'S OWN SUCCESS

David knew Jonathon was a modest type but he felt Jonathon warranted more pride for taking his life back so resolutely and in such short order. He thought it would have been extraordinary for a nine-year-old to have escaped the sense of shame for having been degraded by Fear to the level of a five-year-old! So that Jonathon might reevaluate himself accordingly, David asked, "Is it because you have solved this problem that you feel you are a bit of a problem-solving person?" This offered Jonathon another kind of description of himself apart from a "fearful" or "afraid" person. Jonathon hesitated and then said, "Not too much!" David asked him directly, "Do you think you solved this problem?" Jonathon had to admit that indeed he had. David pressed on, "Does that give you some kind of pride in yourself?" "Yah, a bit more than I used to have," Jonathon had to admit.

This was a very grudging admission, so David wondered if Jonathon might appreciate himself more pride-fully if he could see the pride with his own eyes. David held his hands up a short distance apart: "This is a little bit of pride." Then he spread his hands further apart: "This is a middle bit of pride." His arms now spread widely: "This is a lot of pride."

He asked Jonathon to show him with his hands how much pride he had achieved for having solved the Fear problem. David estimated Jonathon's hands-width at a "middle bit of pride." He then asked Jonathon to show him how much pride his mother had in him for solving his Fear problem. Without hesitation Jonathon flung his hands as far apart as they could go without discomfort. "So that would be a lot," David concluded. He then turned to Judy for confirmation. She looked admiringly at her son and said, "Yeah, there are a lot of things like the independence, getting breakfast, the way you are more mature with your brothers, that make me really proud of you."

David then backtracked to some of the other effects the Fears had on Jonathon only one month before. Recalling that the Fears used to spoil Jonathon's appetite, he wondered if this was still the case.

Judy exclaimed, "HE'S EATING MORE!"

David invited her to speculate, "Do you think Jonathon was scared sick?" Then he joked, "Judy, you are probably going to say 'I wish he would go back to being afraid so he wouldn't eat so much—it would be cheaper'!"

To Jonathon, David remarked, "Did you know that when people are scared they don't have a very good appetite?" Jonathon murmured his assent. "Have you got your appetite back? Did Fear rob you of your appetite?" Jonathon agreed.

"How much more food are you eating now than when your life was Fear-controlled?" Jonathon went over his typical breakfast: "Four pieces of French toast, Muesli and Sultana brand Wheetbix."

David marveled at his consumption, "You eat all that! If I ate that much I'd have to go back to sleep!"

"Now tell me," David continued, "because you are eating so much, do you have more energy?" Jonathon thought this over and recalled that he had been running faster, hitting more home runs, playing more sports, and in fact playing them better than before. David noted all this down and added Judy's observation, "He is doing his homework now, too!"

David then asked Jonathon how proud he guessed his father was of him. Jonathon guesstimated that his father was "a lot proud of me overcoming the Fears a bit more." David leaned forward and addressed Jonathon directly, being careful, as usual, about duplicating Jonathon's exact description, "Okay, here's the question. You said your Dad was a 'lot proud' of you for 'overcoming the fears a bit more,' but of all the things you have done besides, what do you think he is second most proud of you for?"

Jonathon pondered awhile, then replied, "Probably making my own breakfast."

Searching out the origins of such an innovative act, David asked, "Tell me, Jonathon, how did you get the idea to make your own breakfast? It's not a very usual thing for a person your age to do." In retrospect, David thought he might have added Jonathon's gender to the review of unusual behavior.

"I got it off Mum when she made French toast for us once," Jonathon said casually. His reply did not fully account for the independent nature of such an undertaking.

"Yeah, but hold on," David exclaimed, playing the Devil's advocate, "What you could have done was gone to your mother's room and said, 'Wake up! Make me some French toast!' How did you get the idea to make it *yourself?* Did you take some lessons from your Mum on how to do it?"

"Yeah, lessons!" Jonathon proudly replied.

As he couldn't help but assume there was more to it, David took his devilish advocacy a few steps further, "Weren't you scared the stove would blow up or that you would burn the food?"

Noting Jonathon's nonchalant expression, David exclaimed, "Look, I can't even talk you into Fear now! If I tried to talk you into Fear right now, would I get anywhere?"

"No, but . . . " Jonathon hesitated, but then the pride swelled up in him and he burst out, "NO, YOU WOULDN'T!"

"Why wouldn't I get anywhere if I tried to talk you into Fears?" David asked.

Jonathon advocated for his Bravery, "Because I have overcome that much and I don't think I'll be able to go back."

Slowly, and with considerable satisfaction, David recorded these comments in his notes.

PROBLEM COME-BACK PREVENTION

To reassure everyone that Jonathon's accomplishments would stand up to any come-backs that Fears might try to make in his life, David asked, "Tell me, Jonathon, is there any way Fear could drive you back?" With caution, Jonathon said, "I don't think so." David sought and gained Jonathon's permission to engage him in an imaginary dialogue with the problem, saying, "I know quite a bit about Fear because I have met quite a few brave kids. Do you mind if I be Fear?"

Assuming the role of Fear, David changed his voice to a slightly threatening tone: "Jonathon, what makes you think you are so brave, because I am telling you that there are some PRETTY SCARY THINGS that could happen to you?"

"Because I know a lot more about locks and sounds," he said in rebuttal.

The voice of Fear upped the ante, "Yeah, what about GHOSTS? Could I frighten you with a few ghosts?"

Jonathon refuted David again.

"What about MONSTERS?" David pressed.

David was rebuffed with a loud "NO!"

"Yeah, but I know some really scary monsters, some terrible ones! GREEN ONES!"

Now Jonathon clearly had the advantage, "They wouldn't work."

The voice of Fear pulled out its trump card, "What about VICIOUS DOGS?"

Jonathon reproved Fear with a definitive "NO!"

Jonathon was so authoritative that David began to worry about his going too far. He returned to his own voice: "Can I be me? I won't be Fear anymore! Now tell me, you aren't getting too brave, are you?"

"No . . . not too brave."

David then made a case for using fear for Jonathon's own purposes. "Some things are worth being a bit watchful of, like crossing the road, or climbing trees, right?"

Judy agreed wholeheartedly, pointing out that, "Our neighbor's eight-year-old Bruce has no fear at all and he has a lot of stitches from a baseball bat in the eye."

David wondered if Jonathon would be willing to assist Bruce. "Bruce is getting into trouble and having a lot more stitches and cuts than he really needs. You have outgrown some fears, a bit like old clothes, but there are still perfectly usable fears. Could you give him some of the old fears you don't need anymore?"

Somewhat confused by this idea, Jonathon said he "didn't know" and then added, "Bruce is a real hard person to talk to."

David proposed magic: "Could you invite him over for some of your French toast and then you could put your fears in between a sandwich of French toast and he would eat them and digest them?"

Jonathon did not respond to this vein of play, but David maintained his interest in Jonathon's expertise. David queried if Jonathon had been of any assistance to his brothers in the matter of fear. Sure enough he had.

It turned out that Jonathon's younger brother Sam had woken in alarm on one occasion. To no one's surprise this had to do with burglars. Although Jonathon did not give himself any credit for helping Sam, his father thought Jonathon might have done so, "Remember how Fears are contagious?" Ron reminded Jonathon, "By coincidence Sam had a fear of burglars, but he saw Jonathon dealing with it, so the fear hasn't come back to Sam."

David pressed Ron's point, "Jonathon, if you hadn't dealt with your Fears and your Fears were still dealing with you, do you think Sam would still be in the grip of Fears right now?"

Jonathon admitted that he probably would.

David then asked him if Sam owed him a thank you. Jonathon seemed confused by this prospect. "Look, how many nights sleep did you lose through Fears?"

"Six months."

"Do you think you saved Sam six months of sleepless nights?"

Jonathon replied, "Probably."

David went on to ask, "If I said to you, 'Would you like to have sleepless nights for the next six months?', what would you say to me?" Jonathon reassured David that he certainly would not. "And if I said to you, 'I'll show you the way to get around it,' would you be thankful to me?" Jonathon grinned with growing appreciation of himself. "Yup."

"If Sam could understand this and all he had to do was watch you, do you think he should be thankful?"

Jonathon's next "Yep" had an unmistakable air of certainty to it. All agreed that not only were matters restored but that Jonathon had gone ahead of himself during this six-month-long ordeal—an ordeal that had given him a mastery he might not have gained otherwise.

. . . .

CHAPTER 14

Tony:
"The Spiritual Boy Is Fine"

The Thompson family is African American. The family members involved in the therapy were Tony, ten, his sister Nicole, twelve, mother, Denise, and his maternal grandmother, Zelda.

FIRST MEETING

As his mother and grandmother told of their woes, Tony sat quietly, hanging his head slightly and staring off into the middle distance. Jenny could not tell whether he was listening or tuning out the conversation. She did learn that Tony was in a whole lot of trouble for a ten-year-old. He was getting suspended from school for acting up in class and getting in fights on the playground. He was being called into the principal's office frequently, which was a burden to his grandmother, who taught at the school.

The constant trouble came home with him as well, in the form of lying, stealing, destroying property, including his own toys, and using the phone to run up huge 900 number phone bills. He also had a reputation at home for being "unhelpful," "uncooperative," and "not listening." His mother Denise and grandmother Zelda were at their wits' end over these problems.

Jenny wondered if Tony's subdued demeanor was a matter of respect for his elders. Realizing that she should honor this, she put aside for the time being an attempt to get to know him apart from the trouble. Denise had made it clear to Jenny the importance of conveying how serious the situation was and how distressed she and her mother had become.

Jenny began to ask questions about the worry Denise and Zelda were feeling over Tony's welfare and future. She wondered out loud how much the worry had to do with raising an African American boy in a society where racism and injustice are pervasive.[1] Might it be easier to talk about these pressures with an African American therapist? After considering this, the women agreed that they would like to stay put. It turned out that the discussion of the social pressures on Tony and his family opened the door for a conversation that was to weave its way throughout the family's therapy.

After several family meetings, Jenny suggested an individual session in order to draw Tony out a bit. Belying his fierce reputation, Tony was shy and very polite, sitting quietly and gazing out the window. Jenny wondered if they could talk using puppets. Tony picked up a frog puppet and she picked up a snail puppet. Jenny's snail whispered to Tony's frog to tell her about Tony. When snail had been informed a little about Tony's interests, snail then asked frog what he thought Tony would say if he were given three wishes. Froggie thought for a while then whispered that Tony's wishes would be: (1) "To not be bad," (2) "to get along with other people in the house," and (3) "to have some Reeses Pieces."[2]

A TURNAROUND ON TROUBLE

Two weeks later Denise and Zelda returned for another family meeting. It seemed that the trouble was piling up both at home and at school. They focused with Jenny on the pressure, worry, and burnout they were feeling. Jenny realized that she, too, was very worried about Tony.

Late in the next meeting, fending off feelings of being overwhelmed by all the trouble, Jenny gathered a piece of news from Zelda: Tony had just had a relatively good couple of days at school. Grasping this small ray of hope, Jenny suggested another individual meeting with Tony. She wanted to find out more through the puppets about Tony's perspective on this good news. Perhaps together they could expand the meaning of this exception to the problem into a story of change.

Tony came in the next weeek. After finding out that Tony was interested in "turning around on trouble," Jenny discussed his success of the previous week—his two "trouble-free" days—in a thorough, detailed, and repetitive way. With some succcess under his belt, Tony found it easier to talk about "the Trouble." Before, the Trouble had so overwhelmed him that all he could say about it was that he felt he was "bad" and wished he were "good." Now that he had taken a few steps away from the Trouble, he was willing to reflect on its effects on his life and relationships with less guilt. Jenny's questions wove back and forth between contrasting how his life used to be when Trouble was tricking him, how it was now, and how it might be if he were to take some "more steps away from Trouble."

Jenny reviewed the recent developments in Tony's struggle with Trouble: "We were just talking about how your grandma said that in the last week she felt things were moving in a more positive direction. A few good things happened and a few bad things happened but she noticed that when she walked past the principal's office you weren't in there a lot, and she said the teacher called and said you had a good day and that was a nice change. She was pleased about that, and your sister Nicole agreed. You were telling me then about how you were working at turning it around. Could you tell me more about that?"

Tony was quick to reveal an important accomplishment: "The teacher told me to do something and I was doing it but my friend behind me was calling me and I don't listen to him. Then in silent reading time my friend was still calling and I don't turn around, I keep on reading." Jenny was impressed that Tony had been able to turn down such an invitation to Trouble. She ventured to guess how he might have been able to achieve this. "Did you just choose to ignore him?" Tony nodded. "How did it feel to do that? Did you feel strong?" Tony agreed emphatically, "Very strong!"

"What did you think about yourself for being able to do that?"

"I felt good," Tony said, as his face lit up.

"Did you notice that helped keep you out of Trouble? Or keep the Trouble away from you?"

"Yeah."

Interested in the details, Jenny asked, "Good, and what did your friend do after that. Did he stop?"

"Yeah, I ignored him and he kept on reading, too."

"Ah, so you really broke through that, didn't you? What would have happened if a friend tried calling to you in the old days before you started turning it around?" Jenny asked, seeking to contrast this event with the Trouble-dominated past.

"I used to just turn around and then I'd always get my name on the board."

Jenny wanted to contrast the feelings as well as the consequences: "Then you'd be caught in Trouble? How did it feel to have your name on the board?"

"Sad or mad," Tony said, quietly. There was a pause.

Knowing how important positive recognition was for Tony, Jenny followed, "I gather you didn't like that too much. I remember once you told me that you wanted to have your name on the board for reasons you could be proud of—you were hoping to become student of the week. Do you agree it's unfair for Trouble to trick you into getting your name on the board in a way that would make you mad and sad?"

"Yeah, yeah."

"When you felt mad or sad about seeing your name up there, was Trouble getting you put up or put down—you know, dissing you?"

Tony nodded.

"Hey, are you dissing Trouble instead now?"

"Yeah," said Tony with a grin.

"Were you surprised by your strength in ignoring trouble?"

Tony nodded. "And did you find out that you could still get along with your friends and be strong for yourself at the same time?"

"Yes."

"Did you decide you could catch up with them later, see them at recess?"

"Yes."

"Who do you think might respect you for doing that?"

"The teacher."

"Do you think I might have known you could do something like that?" Jenny continued her inventory of those who were part of the audience for a Trouble-free Tony. "Yeah," Tony concurred. Jenny continued, "Do you think that your family knew you were capable of something like that?" Tony flashed a bright grin and nodded his head in agreement.

"You seem pretty encouraged by that," Jenny noted. "Do you feel better about yourself this week?" Tony was still smiling his agreement.

While Tony was basking in some recognition, Jenny returned to an issue of great concern—his self-image. "Remember before, you made three wishes and one wish was that you didn't want to be bad? When you said that, I wanted to tell you that I don't think you're bad. Some-times you get pulled into Trouble. And you get into doing things that hurt you and even hurt your family, but just like your mama and grandma were saying, they think you're really a good person, but were getting tricked into Trouble. Do you know what we mean?" Tony was confused about this so Jenny queried him in smaller pieces.

"What do you think about yourself?"

"I'm good."

"Tell us the difference for you between being good and doing some stuff that's bad, like lying and stealing." Now Tony was clearly following and understanding. Seeing him acknowledge this difference between his image of himself and the behaviors that surrounded Trouble, Jenny turned to the prospective Trouble-free future.

"What do you think is going to happen now that you're turning this around? Perhaps in the next two weeks?"

"All the good stuff! Like I'll get some stuff and play with it, and ride the bike that I got from my sister's friend."

"Oh, so you think that now you'll have more fun?"

"Oh yeah!"

Jenny turned to a central issue for Tony and his family. His grandmother was a teacher at his school and her opinion of him was very significant to him. "Is it better when your grandma doesn't have to hassle you so much at school? When Trouble sneaks up on you, does she have to get in your face to take care of you?"

"Yeah, sometimes."

"How does that work?"

"The principal always finds out 'cause the teachers and her all have walkie-talkies and they use them to get the principal to come down, and then the principal tells Grandma."

"What does that feel like for you?"

"Makes me want to cry."

"Mmmm . . . does it embarrass you, too, in front of the other kids? Which would you prefer to have happen—have her have to hassle you or be more independent and then see her after school and enjoy each other?"

"See her after school."

Jenny knew that Tony's growing up was important to him. "Do you like being more independent . . . like being a bigger boy where the grown-ups don't have to look after you so much as they did when you were a little boy? You just turned ten now, right? Do you think it's a ten-year-old kind of a thing to be free of Grandma having to hassle with you?" Tony nodded, smiled wryly, and said, "Yeah." Jenny checked again: "Do you like that feeling of being a ten-year-old?" Tony was right with her, nodding.

Jenny invited Tony to compare: "How old does the Trouble and Temper make you feel?"

"Like a little boy."

"Do adults have to worry about little boys a lot?"

"Mmhmm."

"Do you feel you could just know Grandma's there at school and not have to see her all the time in trouble?"

"Yeah."

"So you don't need to have her in your business all the time anymore, like a little kid? Is it nicer to have Gandma pay attention to you when she's prouder of you? What does she say when she's proud of you?"

"It's good for me. She smiles at me," said Tony.

THE GODFATHERS

In spite of Tony's turning the corner in his personal efforts to escape from Trouble, Jenny noticed that Denise and Zelda were taking a very hard stand on Tony's behavior. They emphasized that they were still burned out from having had to deal with so much Trouble and that they did not want to "ease off" because they knew the risks that Tony could face if he continued to be in Trouble, such as an early death or incarceration. Jenny wanted to find a balance between their concerns about the risks facing an African American male and her worries about how a severe parenting approach might be affecting his positive view of himself.

Since she was not a member of a racial group that had to face these difficult choices from day to day, Jenny looked to an African American colleague to assist her in addressing the cultural considerations that were coming into play. With the family's consent, she invited her colleague and friend John Prowell and her husband Dean to form a reflecting team at the next meeting.[3]

Jenny initiated the team session by asking Zelda to recount the history of how Tony had come to attend the school where she worked as a teacher: "You work and teach at the same school where Tony is a student. The teachers have often turned to you when something's going on. You were talking about how you were dealing with those roles."

Zelda recounted the story: "Initially, when I went into teaching, I was thinking, 'This is an ultimate way to help rear Tony and Nicole. You can give them consistent attention, and let them learn they can't get away with things, because somebody's right there to tweak it, stomp it, and jerk the chain.' I asked Denise her thoughts about putting him in the same school when he was in first grade. We decided for it because Tony had been saying vulgar, violent things to adults since he was four years old. The plan was to change his environment. And things did change for two years. I mean, he was still antsy and bouncing off the wall and knocking on your door for attention but the violent behavior and talk stopped. But now it's resurfacing. It never got to the point where the principal and teachers were involved before. So, we've reached a saturation point where Denise meets with his teacher and the teacher is sending her little messages like, 'Have you thought about putting him in another school?' The teacher would rather not deal with that situation anymore. I jumped in with both feet—eyes open. Now I'm having second thoughts, whether it was the right thing to do."

"I'm trying to grapple with what you're up against," Jenny responded. "What I've heard from you all is that you've put a lot of time and energy and care and concern into raising this family. We're talking about a lot of trouble, right? And you are facing some special challenges in raising a boy, you said, since there have been several generations of girls only." Zelda and Denise nodded.

"And to let Dean and John know, I gather that the whole family feels that he has some unique abilities—as you put it, 'there's something really special about him.' When I talked with Tony, I found out more about how smart he is. He knows how to do his work and he's a talented artist. I also think he's got a good imagination."

"We know there's a lot of talent there. We're trying to weed out all the other stuff," Zelda clarified. Denise continued, "He's got some honest concerns and desires about what he would like to do for other people. But things keep getting in his way."

"Denise, there was something really important in the first discussion we had together," recalled Jenny, wanting to recap the substance of previous discussions. "You spoke about how different it was raising this boy than raising your daughter and that you were really worried about raising an African American boy in an unjust society. You've had a lot of worries that Tony might 'go bad.' You ask yourselves, 'What if his behaviors don't get contained? Where might he land? What are the risks and pressures for him?' We talked about the frightening statistics for African American boys. What supports a young man to grow and deal with his behavior while avoiding those risks? And then there's Tony's internalized self-image. We're all concerned that he thinks he's really bad—not that he knows he's engaged in bad behaviors, but that he's worried that he is bad. Can these worries take all of us over in some way? Is it obscuring the talents that we're talking about?"

Denise was nodding and murmuring her assent as Jenny spoke. Jenny continued, "Are some of these cultural and social pressures so intense and insidious that they exert extra pressure on you? Do they encourage an overload of worry for you to deal with? For example, when an African American boy steals a bit of money or misbehaves, isn't it more charged with worry about him turning toward a criminal lifestyle than if a Caucasian boy did it?"

Zelda and Denise were in agreement with Jenny's estimation of the extra burden placed on them by these factors. Zelda added, "A parent has to try to analyze things to the nth degree so they can figure out what needs fixing." She reflected on parenting Denise with regard to her knowledge of the negative outcomes that any African American child faces. "I think to myself: 'I've traveled this road before and I can tell you.' But telling a child something is not the same as them learning for themselves. So I just have to say, 'Okay. When you find out for yourself, you come back and tell me, and then let's discuss it.' That's the way I raised them."

"Do you feel that in the long run, you have a pretty close relationship with your daughter?" Jenny asked. She turned toward Denise when she heard her agreement. "It has happened, hasn't it, like your mother said? Have you come back to your mom and talked about stuff that you've reflected on?" Denise laughed and said warmly to her mother, "A lot, hey?"

"So there's some real good communication happening."

Denise replied, "We're a close-knit family. That's what she's always called us, a close-knit family, and we really are. We are always there for each other. And right now everybody is focused on Tony."

Zelda wondered out loud about Denise's observation: "And that's probably causing him a whole lot of stress—too much focus."

This dovetailed with other questions and dilemmas that Jenny wanted help from the family and the team to reflect on: "How do you raise an African American boy and support his independence, spirit, defiance, and assertiveness in a society like this, in a way that's not going to expose him to harm? Does all the worry and pressure drive you sometimes to come down hard on him—seeking to protect him? But if you don't come down on him hard enough, do you worry he's likely to get in trouble out there? What will encourage him to have spirit but not expose him to the risks he faces by virtue of his color? How do you condemn behavior that will get him in trouble while still supporting his unique identity?"

Denise described her perspective: "I want him to know I love him with all my heart, but I do disapprove of a lot of things that he does. We share tears. We hug, we tell each other, 'I love you,' and everything."

Zelda shared her thoughts on the issues: "Well, everything that you raised makes sense, and I'm trying to approach this problem with Tony in a loving, kind way. It doesn't mean that he's bad, it's just not okay to do those things. The spiritual boy is fine. It's all that other impulsive, activity-driven stuff that gets our tempers flared."

She considered the dilemma of just how much support a child should receive when he or she engages in bad behavior: "I'm thinking that some of this positive approach might work on TV, but in real life it doesn't work. On TV the kid's in some dilemma and they're all sitting around the kitchen table grinning and laughing. I've got a problem with that. It looks so easy when they do it. Maybe we need to go get on TV. But I guess that's what we need to learn. I want prevention. We need to just back up, slow down, and think."

Jenny asked, "Can you think of an incident where prevention has worked?"

"Where prevention actually worked?" repeated Zelda to herself. "All I can think of are incidents where I thought I'd laid the groundwork and it didn't work. We'd have a question-and-answer session with Tony beforehand, like, 'Guess what this is made out of. It's made out of plastic. What happens if you push or poke it with something sharp? It's going to break. Is that what we bought it for? No.' From my experience with him I know that Tony is intelligent enough to feed back every single correct answer. I'm thinking, 'You've got it!' But when impulses take over—boom—oops, then we've got a problem."

"Is your sense of what comes between him and his intelligence—his impulses?"

"Yes, because he can answer every question. Logically, he understands it, but I don't know why it doesn't work," Zelda continued. "To me, going over those questions and answers was the prevention part."

"You know, that makes me think," Jenny mused. "I think there's another insidious pressure in our society—to blame yourself as a parent or as a grandparent, you know?"

"I've been through that. And I've gotten to the point where I don't care who's to blame. Let's fix it."

"I hear that."

"I would say I've shed all the tears I'm gonna shed, and I've felt bad when I'm supposed to feel bad. We're talking about something else now."

Although it had been discouraging to hear that Zelda's prevention efforts with Tony had failed, Jenny appreciated that all could hear of Zelda and Denise's determination to make changes with Tony.

As the first part of the interview drew to a close, these issues had been touched:

- How could the family best accomplish the goals of protection and prevention?
- What was the balance between punishment and praise?
- How could Tony and the family free themselves from worry about the frightening outcomes that face an African American boy?
- Had those worries influenced them to overfocus on Tony to the point where he thought he was bad?

These difficult questions soon became the focus of the reflections of the "therapy godparents," John and Dean.

The issue of prevention was raised again when John Prowell gave his reflections: "I'm wondering how much of Tony's behavior is really about protesting something that's going on in the system? If we leave out the effects of culture, we might more or less give it the name—bad behavior. But, on the other hand, what is his message? Are we able to interpret that message in a way that doesn't minimize what is trying to shine through? I heard lots of wonderful qualities about him, and yet, these are not really coming through in the way I think he would like to have them come through. I'm also wondering how responsible he has to be for the legacy of being an African American male? How much negative identity has he internalized? Does he feel that somehow he has to crusade in a way that will give him more space in the world—like some of the great African American athletes have been able to do?"

"Let me comment on that," interjected Zelda, "and maybe we can break into what you're getting at. On occasion, I know I have used terms like: 'If this behavior goes on and you get to be an adult, are you gonna be one of those people that's sitting over there in prison? Is that what you want to be?' I know I've said that, to make a point. 'You've got to make different decisions because you don't want to end up like that.' So how has he internalized that? I'm not sure."

"I'm wondering, does he see it that it's his task to make a broader window to operate in?" mused John.

"Well, he could," replied Zelda, "and then there was another incident with the boys down the street. They were giving him the wrong advice about how to operate with drugs. So we're always giving him advice that's saying you can't fit into that category. Let Denise tell you about that."

With that introduction, Denise began to tell a story that showed prevention none of the therapists could have anticipated.

"Tony told me something very shocking," Denise began. "I figure in the '90s, nowadays, most kids wouldn't tell their parents something like this. He came running up the street one Saturday afternoon and he said, 'Mommy, you know what? Little Mike and So-and-so and So-and-so are smoking weed and snorting cocaine.' These boys were right down the street, the oldest is thirteen. I think the youngest is ten, and the other's eleven. I was really shocked. My jaw just hit the floor, and I thought, 'Excuse me?' I said, 'How do you know that's what they were doing?' He said, 'Well, they put something white on their hand. And they did like this.'" She demonstrated sniffing. "Now, I didn't expect this to come out of his mouth!

"I'm really glad he told me," she continued. "I had told him just two weeks before, 'I don't even want you down the street hanging with these kids anymore.' Then two weeks later, he tells me this. And I'm thinking that any other child wouldn't have told their parents this because they never know how their parents might react.

"But I'm thinking, I'm glad he told me, because one thing he knows is that I don't do drugs. I don't allow them and I don't tolerate anybody around us that does them. I was just in shock. That's something kids should just not be getting the idea that they can do. The only way I could figure out to prevent him from trying it was to keep him from going down there. He might still go down there, but the only thing I can stress to him is—don't do it. I don't care how much they say, 'Here, do it, Tony, it's not gonna hurt you,' I stressed to him that I wish he wouldn't. Because he's never seen me do it, he will never see me do it."

Zelda jokingly told everyone about the kid's attitudes about drugs and alcohol: "Tony and Nicole harangued the devil out of me about a beer with no alcohol in it!" Denise mimicked the tone of their response to smoking: "Oh, my God, once I smoked cigarettes—they had fits. I stopped smoking on December 31st 'cause my kids were having a fit. So I said, 'Okay, fine.' And I told Tony, 'That's not the best thing for you either. And if you're doing drugs, you can never get anywhere in life.' That's what I want him to know, drugs will kill you, drugs will make you hurt your family and do all kinds of things that you never thought you would do. I tell him, 'Don't indulge in anything that takes control over you. You always have to be in control.'"

"I'm wondering if Tony was acknowledging his own wisdom, too, by coming to tell you about the boys down the street," John asked thoughtfully

"Well, we discussed that," Denise replied. "I told him, 'I am glad you brought this to my attention.' Because I thought, had it been any other child, they might have not have known how to come to their parents with that. But I look at it like this. We talk about everything. Whatever my kids want to know, I tell them. And a lot of people fault me for that. They say, 'Well, you know, they're kids, why do you tell them stuff like that?' Because it's reality—sometimes reality might hurt you. That's what I told my mom on the way here. Tony and I hugged and everything, because I was just so shocked that he told me. I told him, 'I'm glad you told me this.' This is letting me know he trusts me a lot, enough to tell me this kind of stuff."

"What does that point to about the communication in your family?" Jenny asked. "And what does that say about Tony when he shows the wisdom to separate himself from drugs in spite of whatever pressures he may have to face?"

Denise answered, "When he ran in the house saying, 'Mama, you know what?' I thought, 'Oh, my God. What have those boys done?' That's not what I expected he would do."

"I wonder if that speaks to the prevention that you try and work for?" asked Jenny.

Everyone agreed that it had.

At this point Dean shared his reflections about the conversation that had taken place during the session: "I have two things I'd like to reflect on before we run out of time. There were some expressions you used that I took off on as metaphors. One was when you said that Tony was healthy in spirit but that you had to weed out the bad behavior. Weeding, in my view, can be a pretty merciless process. You've got to be pretty cold. Like when you prune a tree. You've gotta prune it right when the spring starts, when it's growing the most. You can't be timid about it. You've really gotta cut. And when you're pulling out a weed, you've got to pull out every single root under the ground, or else you're gonna be seeing those weeds again. And I thought that when Zelda said, 'I felt like going back to the old style of discipline.' I thought maybe part of the old style should be returned to. But how do you do this in a way that it weeds out the bad behavior without convincing the child that he is basically bad?

"I heard two different metaphors that show how this family is able to accomplish this. One is the one I just mentioned about weeding in the old style. The other one came to me when I heard you say the family is close-knit. Knitting requires careful attention to putting each stitch in place. You just can't do things without that care because you'll knit something that just falls apart, or you will make mistakes that cause hours of extra work to take mistakes apart and redo them for the result to be durable and beautiful.

"I think that's the other side of the weeding coin, where Tony is seen as a person and in spirit. Like you said, he's not bad; the things that he's doing are bad. You try and weed out the person from the behavior and you value him as person and knit him into family love and appreciation. Is this the way that this family is struggling with how to put together the weeding style—where you pull hard or you cut firmly—with the knitting style, where you pay attention and you work with care and gentleness?"

"Oh, yes," Denise agreed. Zelda was nodding.

"Both of those work together?" Dean wondered. "Do you feel that either one of these styles alone will not satisfy this family, or work for Tony? I was thinking about this in terms of prevention. For example, there was one story where Zelda talked about explaining everything to Tony in advance, and hoping he would use his intelligence, but it seemed like the impulses took him right over. So the new style alone didn't work there. Then there was the other story, where Tony came and told his mama about the drugs because he felt enough closeness and he didn't fear his mama so much that he wouldn't tell her that there was a danger down the street. Was that an example of the knitting style at work—he had a close-knit relationship with his mom so he could come to her with the trouble? Is there a struggle to put the right style on the right thing?"

"I'm impressed," Denise replied. "Because I like exactly the way you said that and exactly what you just said. I'm very impressed, because basically, we have the close-knit part, but then we also have the prevention. It's exactly what you said. And I never thought of seeing it that way. We're trying to prevent, but then all the time we're still close-knit as far as getting us together. I've never looked at it like that. The danger is down the street, but still, he's being Tony."

At the end of this meeting, Dean and John declared how much they had enjoyed getting together with the family. Zelda expressed that she had enjoyed meeting Dean and John. She said the family feeling made things easy. While talking about how much everyone would like to keep in touch about how things were going with Tony, John suggested that he and Dean might serve as "godfathers" for Tony on his journey. Denise and Zelda laughingly agreed that this would be fine. The idea was proposed that John and Dean would stand in the wings, be caught up on developments and called in as needed. "Would that work for you?" Jenny asked Tony. "Yes," he said, smiling shyly at John and Dean.

A LETTER: "THE SPIRITUAL BOY IS FINE"

Jenny sent the following letter to the family after the team session:

Dear Denise, Zelda, Nicole, and Tony,

The team enjoyed meeting with you and learning about your family. We discussed how, although the "spiritual boy is fine," Tony has encountered a "pull into some trouble" and may have internalized some negative identity. The whole family has been affected by worry over Tony, and is very aware of the challenge of raising an African American boy in an unjust society.

There were two components we talked about in your family: the close-knitting and loving, and also the pruning and limit-setting. You seemed to have worked hard to cover these. Denise and Zelda, we wonder to what extent the pressure of worry could have taken over and stressed you, clouding your perspective on your actual success in protecting, loving, and getting through the values you want to Tony? We were impressed to learn about how Tony had encountered some dangerous drugs and how he not only had the good sense to stay away, but came home and talked about it with his mama. Denise, did you learn how much you are getting through to him after all? On reflection, what else do you think this says about you as a close-knit family?

At my last meeting with Tony, I learned that Tony has been coming through on his intention of turning around on trouble. He told me, "I work at turning it around." Did you realize he had so much determination to weed his own behavior? He said that in school that week, he had tried to "listen to the teacher and do what she said," and instead of getting thrown off by his friends, he had practiced "not listening" when they were calling to him and distracting him. He said that when he does this he "feels strong," the teacher likes it, and he "feels Grandma feels better about him." I am very pleased to hear this, since Tony's first wish was to "not feel bad." Is Tony choosing to knit himself to his family and teacher and weeding out so called "friends" who are headed towards Trouble?

Tony's second wish was "to get along with other people in the house." Tony, I was pleased to see both your wishes starting to come true, because of your determination. I could tell the second one was coming true because Nicole told me, "Before he used to bother me. Now he's stopped kicking the door and tripping me in the hallway. He's minding his own business more, and letting me mind mine. It helps me to get more work done."

Nicole, now that Tony is minding his own business more, does this make you feel differently towards him? Do you see him respecting you more? Does this give you more respect for Tony? You said, "He's starting to get along with others." Is he knitting himself back with you, returning to being the brother you have seen and loved in the past?

Looking forward to learning more about Tony's abilities.

Jenny, John, and Dean

THE SUMMER LIST

There were several more meetings over the summer. Tony's turnaround held course and he came up with more positive surprises for Denise. Wanting to keep track of these developments, Jenny kept a list of Tony's accomplishments.

1. Tony met his goal to "be good all summer," earning himself special presents, a bike and a truck.
2. He did well at summer camp and even slept outside in a tent, showing his bravery and maturity.
3. Tony listens better.
4. He is talking and sharing with Denise especially, and being closer-knit again He is hanging out with his mother in a fun way, talking, watching TV together, and relaxing.

5. Denise feels that he is less stressful to be around. He is not fussing anymore the way he used to.

6. Tony is helping out at home and is taking responsibility for keeping his room clean.

7. Denise and Zelda notice that he is able to think of things to do and is thus more independent. Denise has new perspective on "how he's capable of doing it."

8. All agree Tony is bringing peace to his household.

9. Tony seems to be experiencing more freedom as he is becoming more independent.

10. He has been doing his homework for summer school, doing it well and getting through the corrections.

11. He has overthrown and turned his back on old behaviors that Trouble used to get him into, like fighting, throwing rocks at windows and cars, and stealing. In class he has quit throwing paper and talking out of turn. Watch out Trouble, here comes Tony!

12. Tony seems "happier, goofier, sillier and more relaxed," and his family can tell he is enjoying his happiness and confidence in himself.

13. At school now, Tony likes to help out, for example by volunteering in the cafeteria.

14. A measure of his freedom from Trouble: Mr. Heller at the front office almost forgot his name!

15. He used to not be allowed in music class; now his music teacher has commented that he's much better.

16. Tony got a new dog, Jewell, and is helping to feed and look after her.

THE GODFATHERS ARE KEPT INFORMED

All had agreed that it would be a good thing for the Godfathers to be kept informed. Jenny continued to apprise John and Dean of developments with Tony and carried their reflections back to the family. Jenny pulled together her notes and the team's reflections and wrote the following summary letter.

Dear Denise, Zelda, Nicole, and Tony,

John and Dean were delighted to have an update on the news. Last time we met we added to the chronicle of Tony's remarkable turnaround.

Tony, with the love and support of your family, you have achieved and held onto a remarkable turnaround on Trouble. You said you had "gotten tired of Trouble," and that you had "found courage to be brave." You said you looked up to Denise as an example. As you put it, "Mommy has a lot of courage. Mommy taught me to stand up to other people, she have faith in me."

Tony, you are discovering your independence and self-pride now instead of being made to look as if you are younger and a follower. You reported, "I stopped thinking that I'm bad. My new friend thinks I'm smart. My teacher smiles at me now." You said that your mother and Nicole are happy "cause I stopped going to the office." And if Trouble tries to tempt you? "I'm gonna say, I'm not down for Trouble no more." Some examples of the anti-Trouble techniques you used are: "walking away from teasing and fighting" and changing some friends.

When we touched base in July you, Denise, were happy to say that Tony had been listening and helping out at home during the summer. You thought that he seemed "happier with himself." When you would say to him, "I need to get this done," Tony would listen and take the initiative to do the job. One time, you even came home and found Tony vacuuming the house! You were so surprised to see him and hear him say, "I didn't want the house to be messy when you came home." It seems that initiative has made a major reappearance in Tony's life, with your steady encouragement.

Nicole, you said that Tony is distracting you a lot less, so you can relax and work better. Your grades have improved this year. You used to have to look after him a lot more at home, and protect him at school. Nicole, you said that "He's helping to do stuff when I ask. Before he didn't want to do nothing anybody told him to do. I think he's learning to respect people more." We remember Denise saying how important it was for her children to know respect for others, and self-respect. Nicole, we think you showed your love and generosity to your brother when you said, "I feel happy for Tony." The adults have noticed that you have stopped saying "you're dumb" to him. They also notice that he's sticking up for himself better, so you don't have to worry so much about defending him.

Zelda, you pulled things together at school to provide the best environment for him there. You have been taking steady steps to support him at school and find you are not "putting out fires anymore." Tony is avoiding the fires instead. Instead of following in Trouble's footsteps he's put himself out of Trouble's way. Now, Zelda, you said you appreciate that you can "concentrate on my own work because he's concentrating on his."

What a turnaround! We are all very impressed. Tony, members of your family who knew you better knew that you were capable of this. Your mother loves you and has a lot of faith in you. Zelda, who loves you too, was confident things would change, "with the right kind of focus."

Denise and Zelda, your collective decisions and concerted efforts have supported this turnaround. Providing all this support has not been an easy task. You have been very aware of facing the challenges and worries of raising an African American boy in this unjust society.

Tony, now you are making efforts to help your family. We all look forward to keeping in touch with your growth. We three would like to meet together with you and *your family to celebrate your accomplishments so far, and encourage you to keep up your freedom from Trouble in the future.*

With our respect and very warm wishes,
       Jenny, and the "godfathers," John and Dean

Jenny sent a draft of the letter to John, for him to give his final okay. John wrote his own letter for Jenny to pass on to the family:

Dear Jenny,

I am ecstatic about Tony's triumph over Trouble. I think that his ability to notice the attributes of his grandmother, mother and sister, and to use them as a model is absolutely remarkable.

I would definitely like to meet with Tony and his family and ask questions about how he was able to see through Trouble and that Trouble was not to be trusted. Also, I want to know more about how he was able to outsmart Trouble. I am impressed with Tony's awareness about how Trouble was not his friend, and only caused him to have difficult relationships with people who cared about him. I have many more questions to ask Tony about how he was able to see his family as his friends and that they were to be trusted over Trouble.

I am grateful that you shared Tony's accomplishments with me. I always believed that Tony had the right stuff. I believed that he had the capacity to overcome trouble and therefore am very pleased to have been a member of his team. I remain a team member for Tony on his future endeavors.

With respect and best wishes,
      John Prowell

FOLLOW-UP

Over twenty months have passed since the date of these letters and their final meeting. Denise, Zelda, Nicole, and Tony have kept in touch, always with news that has warmed the hearts of Jenny and the godfathers. During the latest phone call, when Jenny was checking about including their story in this book, Denise let her know that Tony was doing very well at school. He had received a positive report card; not only that, he had made the honor roll! She was delighted about his behavior at home, finding him to be helpful and a pleasure to be with. In fact, she said, he continued to amaze her. But it made her happiest of all, she said, to see Tony's pride in himself.

CHAPTER 15

. . . .

Jason:
"I'm Lighting My Own Lantern Now"

The Bloom family is of Jewish descent. The family members who met with Jenny include Jason, age eleven, Kim, his mother, and Elliot, his father. The family met with Jenny six times.

FIRST MEETING

Elliot and Kim began by telling Jenny about Jason's insomnia and fears, which paralyzed him and prevented him from engaging in all kinds of typical eleven-year-old activities. These problems had plagued Jason most of his life. By now they were all exhausted, worn out from endless nights of disrupted sleep. As they spoke, Jason blushed under his dark hair, squirmed in his seat, and finally took to hiding himself under the couch pillows, muttering "I don't know" in response to Jenny's questions. Based on her past experience with shy eleven-year-old boys, Jenny wondered silently if "I don't know" was going to be Jason's consistent reply to questions throughout the therapy. It looked like this was going to be a challenge.

Concerned about Jason's apparent embarrassment and the risk of the problems defining how he might experience his introduction to her, Jenny suggested interviewing Jason "aside from the problems." Asking his parents about his interests and abilities, she learned that he was a talented artist and juggler, involved with short-wave radio, and good at dominos. Overhearing this, Jason started to peek out from under the cushions.

Eventually, when the conversation returned to the unfortunate effects of the problems, Jason could at least state his interest in freeing himself from Fears and being able to sleep in peace. Having learned that Jason was an artist, Jenny asked if he might be interested in using cartoons to show his relationship with Fears. He started right to work and completed a few panels by the time the meeting ended.

SECOND MEETING

Jason arrived with his cartoon portfolio at the ready. In it, he demonstrated how Fears took over at night and had him working on his security by turning on his light, turning up the radio, and having his parents regularly check on him. Then Jason made the momentous and surprising announcement that this was what "used to happen." He affirmed Jenny's guess that he was taking ground back from Fear.

Jason's parents confirmed that he had slept through many nights during the past several weeks. He had had only one brush with Fear during that entire time. In a daring experiment, Jason had turned off the blaring radio and blazing light that he had been using to protect himself. Delighted to hear about this experiment and all it implied, Jenny was tempted to jump up and down and cheerlead with sweeping superlatives. She managed to contain herself somewhat and decided to gather as much detail as possible about how he had made these changes.

"Did you surprise yourself or did you know you had it in you all along?"

"Well, I guess I knew," said Jason.

"So who's got who on the run? Do you think that Fear's got you on the run or do you think you've got it on the run?"

"I've got it on the run," he grinned.

Before getting more details from Jason, Jenny turned to his parents; "What do you two think about that?"

Elliot responded thoughtfully, "I think we're making a really good start. There was only one night when he didn't think he could go to sleep, so I thought we were going to have one of those nights that we talked about. But I said, 'You're just overtired,' and he went right to sleep. I think my not checking on Jason and helping him free himself of being checked is really reinforcing a good behavior that lets him go to sleep when he wants to and in a way that is easier than how he was able to do it before."

These comments made great sense to Jenny. "Now that you have the wisdom of hindsight, do you think that the Fear hoodwinked you into 'feeding' it by checking on it? Is there almost an implicit implication that if the Fears need so much checking and protecting against, then they must be pretty scary?"

Elliot nodded knowingly as Jenny continued, "Sometimes Fear can get you to do stuff, subtly, and you don't even realize you're playing into its hands. When you told Jason he was overtired, do you think that was supportive of Jason and undermining of Fear? Or the other way round? After all, Fears are extremely cunning, aren't they!"

"Yeah, I was impressed with that too," Elliot agreed, "because he did go right to sleep after that, which is very unusual. He usually gets into a cycle. When he says he can't get to sleep, everything usually reinforces that."

Kim addressed Jenny's question next, "His determination can work in many ways. When he's determined that he can't sleep, then his determination can feed that. Because he is a very determined person, especially when he decides he's going to do something." Jenny could see her point, "It seems like it's important what kind of path his determination gets set on." She turned and addressed Jason, "Which way is it going now?"

Jason considered this, "Well, one of the ways that I sort of changed, well a lot of it was the way that mum talked about—trial and error."

Jenny wrote and spoke simultaneously, *Trial and error*, "Trial and error is an important principle?" Jason nodded. "So, how have you been applying trial and error?"

"Well, I tried with my light off, and it worked, and then I tried with my radio lower, and tried with it lower, and then finally I turned it off."

"What did you discover? Were you on the edge of your bed, so to speak . . . thinking . . . wondering what would happen when you turned it off . . . or were you already feeling comfortable?"

"Well, first I turned it off, then I was sort of like going like this (Jason demonstrated this by fidgeting nervously), then I kept on looking back at it, putting my hand out ready to turn it on any second."

"So your hand kept getting drawn back to it?"

"Yeah."

"You've got me on the edge of my chair! What happened, did you somehow relax it?"

"Well, I don't think I turned it on!"

"Really! Did you discover something? Was fear tricking you by saying, 'If you don't keep it on I'll come and get you'?"

"After I did it I felt prouder of myself!"

"You felt prouder of yourself? Did you feel yourself growing up a bit more?"

"Yeah," said Jason with a smile.

"What did your Pride tell you about yourself that you didn't know before?"

"Well, that I didn't need the radio on."

"Could I quote you in writing? 'I found out I didn't need the radio anymore.' Were you surprised by that?"

"Sort of."

"Sort of and sort of not at the same time? Did you sort of take it in stride? What did it make you think about yourself? Did you think 'I'm braver than I thought'? Any ideas like that?"

At this point Jason let Jenny in on how this had all started following their first meeting together: "Well, I don't know, a lot of it told me that I can do pretty much anything I set my mind to, because on the way home from the last session I announced that I was gong to try it with my radio off."

"Oh, you did. Oh, really?"

"Yeah, I just did," Jason continued. "So I just did—at one point I really wasn't sure about it but I decided to go through with it."

Jenny continued to write and speak, *"Not sure, but decided to go through with it.* What gave you confidence when you weren't sure?" Jason gave this question a good deal of thought. Finally he concluded, "I just tried to keep my mind off the fear. I tried to ignore it, you could say."

Jenny decided to tell Jason some of her between-session thoughts: "Well, you know I came up with some ideas, just in case you didn't have any. I thought a bit about what it might take to cut through Fears like that, and I was going to suggest some ideas this time, but I'm afraid that you've already figured it out."

Kim laughed, "A lot of it!" But Jason didn't want anyone to go too far "Still not all of it," he added "I might still need to come back sometime . . . "

"Yeah," Jenny reassured him, with a wink. "You don't have to do it all at once! You could slow down. I don't want you to go too far all at once." Jason grinned from ear to ear. "Take your time and do a good job," Jenny added.

THIRD MEETING

The third time Jason and his parents met with Jenny they had made further important discoveries about how the Fears invited Fear-watching. Elliot shared his insight, "I remember we had a ritual where Jason would say 'Will you check on me?' This was the language that we used. For example, 'Check on me in twenty minutes' was categorical. Jason really expected it and he enforced it. You know, it felt like it was trapping—an 'entrapping language' I guess. Now he has changed it. Now he'll say, 'Will you stop back in if you're in the neighborhood?' I think he still expected us to be in the neighborhood, but it was not in the same 'entrapping language' he used to use."

Jason joined his father's recollection, "Well, a lot of it was foreshadowing, because you know how at first it started out with checking me every ten minutes, then fifteen, then twenty, then thirty." This jogged Elliot's memory, "Oh yeah, that's right, Oh brother!" He sighed out loud, but smiled too. "We tried, but I don't think we were ever able to extend it beyond thirty."

Kim joined in, "The checking sort of fed the sense of distrust. Jason would say 'Check in thirty minutes,' and at twenty-nine minutes and thirty seconds—boom! 'Where are you?' and there would be a sense of alarm, and everybody would get worked up. He'd get worked up 'cause we weren't there exactly, punctually. We'd get worked up because we thought this was kind of silly." Elliot concluded, "He couldn't get to sleep if he got worked up. It was really bad! It was a downward spiral of alarm."

Kim contrasted this with the current situation. "Once in a while when we checked on him recently, he'd just be dozing off, and we'd wake him up. "Right up!" exclaimed Jason in the midst of everyone's laughter. "Now I can admit it I suppose," he added. Kim reminded Jason, "There were lots of times you'd wait up for us. Now you're not looking at the clock. You're not waiting for us to come in at a certain time."

Jenny was interested in the idea of entrapping language. "So it sounds like it's not so tense now, like the entrapping language was. There's something really different about the language you're using now. Is it a friendlier or more relaxed language? Like if Jason used to say 'Check on me in 20 minutes,' would the Fears trick him into thinking that if it didn't happen exactly on time something terrible was going to happen?"

Jason understood exactly. "Well, that happened a lot of the time, but then it just became a habit!"

"I'm really excited about this discovery that you've made about a new language!" exclaimed Jenny. "I think that's so intriguing. Did you make that up yourself or did your parents talk about it with you?"

"No, I just made it myself," Jason answered proudly.

"How did you do that? How did you find a more freeing sort of language to use for yourself? Did it just happen, did the words just come out, or did you think, 'I don't like the way I'm saying this?'"

"Well, the words just came out."

"Do you think they came with a different sense—a sense of confidence?"

"Yeah!"

"Was it a cool, more relaxed, more casual language, like, 'Hey you know, if you're around, stop by'?"

"Yeah, something like that."

"So what did that language tell you about yourself?"

"Well, that I wasn't as scared anymore."

Jenny wrote as she spoke, "'That I wasn't as scared anymore.' Could I ask your parents what it said to them?"

"Okay, sure."

Jenny turned to Jason's parents, "What did it communicate about him to you? What did that new language, that more relaxed or casual language, say to you?"

Elliot answered first, "Oh gee, it really said that he had really understood what we were talking about and had made a great effort at altering his behavior. He was trying to be casual or relaxed about it, to make it sort of almost optional. I don't think it is quite optional yet, but it's like, Okay, when we can . . . so I was really impressed."

Jenny saw that there was more latitude between "Come when you can" and "exactly thirty minutes," "Does that give you more freedom— you're not so pinned down, having to jump through hoops in the same sort of way?" Elliot was quick to agree.

"I imagine that must make you feel pleased about his being more of his eleven-year-old self," Jenny reflected.

"Absolutely. Oh yes," Elliot concurred.

Jenny turned to Jason, "That means your parents can have some of their own space too. I imagine there would be a lot more relaxation in your household like that." Jason agreed there already was.

Not only was Jason creating a new language with his family, but he was busy making cartoons too! After he had brought out and showed his cartoon work-in-progress, Jenny had an idea, "Well, you know what, I really like this cartoon that you're doing. I'd love to see if you could keep going on it. It looks like the beginning of a history. Could you add more captions about some of the other things that the Fear was getting you to do? Could you add another sheet that shows the ground that you've taken back from Fear?" Jason seemed interested, so Jenny added, "You know, if the Fear tries to get the better of you, and you get the better of it instead—can you make a panel about it and show how you got the better of it? 'Cause the Fear's probably embarrassed you a lot and this is your chance to come back, and embar . . . "

Jason interrupted, "Embarrass the Fear!"

"You can get even don't you think? Does that idea appeal to you or is that just my idea?" Jenny wondered. Jason obviously relished the idea of getting even.

"Well, I'll tell you something that I've noticed," Jenny confided in a conspiratorial whisper. "Fear doesn't like fun. Do you notice that?"

"Sort of, yeah."

"I don't think Fear likes to hang around lots of humor or fun or confidence. Have you noticed that? It's very hard for Fear to be itself where there's relaxation around. That's why I'm so happy to hear about this more casual, relaxed atmosphere, and your atmosphere of confidence, with all your family joking with each other. I think those are really great signs of taking a whole bunch of ground back from fear, don't you think?"

Kim chimed in, "Yeah, some of those midnight hours that we've had together have *not* been fun . . . we've had more fun during the day."

Jenny considered this, "Well, it would be nice to make the night a friendlier, more fun place, too, wouldn't it. It doesn't have to be a scary place. That's just Fear's idea. You can have your own ideas!"

FOURTH MEETING

When Jason arrived with Kim for his fourth meeting he had an announcement to make. He had gone on an overnight field trip with his class, had "slept great," and, he exclaimed, "I had the most fun I ever had!" Jason set the scene for this new accomplishment by explaining that he had tried to stay away from home once before and it was so disastrous that he had been afraid to ever take another chance. They had all been apprehensive that morning when he left, but they got over it. This seemed especially significant since, from Jason's point of view, the inability to stay away overnight had been one of Fear's most crippling restrictions. Jenny was about to go to town on this, but Jason continued with his revelations. He added that the night he was away he had had an asthma attack but he had controlled it and not even told his parents about it! Amazed by his courage, Jenny asked how he had managed the attack by himself.

"I suffocated it," he said matter-of-factly.

"I never heard someone put it that way! That's a really creative way of putting it! You suffocated asthma, instead of letting it suffocate you?"

"Yep," he smiled, "and not only that, ever since I've been back, I've been on this spring schedule where I'm going to sleep at 8:30 and waking up at 7 . . . I've just been sleeping great, and I haven't waked up!"

Jenny was totally intrigued. "Do you sense a new power growing, or are you just reclaiming your power?" He nodded with an excited look on his face. Jenny guessed that Jason was agreeing to both possibilities. She turned to Kim, "Do you, too, see Jason's power growing, or see rather the reclaiming of his power?" Jason excitedly interrupted Kim's response to reveal a special ability that was known only to him up to that point.

"Well, I've been doing something that Mom doesn't know about," Jason shared in a hushed tone.

"Do you want me to know about it?" his mother asked.

Jason was ready to let the cat out of the bag, "Yeah, well, I've been trying to get the Chi stronger inside of me for a long time."

"What have you been doing to strengthen your Chi?" Kim asked, curious.

"Meditation." Jason couldn't stop his giggles; "Meditation and exercises." He giggled some more, then paused more reflectively. "I've been practicing slowly . . . I've been doing Tai Chi."

"Have you really?" Jenny asked, sharing looks of wonderment with Kim. "Have you been developing this on your own? When have you been using your Chi in strengthening yourself recently? Does it have something to do with what you've accomplished?" Jason concurred, "The meditating part has. It's made me feel more confident, it's relaxed me when I'm scared. That's what I'm doing at night—I'm meditating because it relaxes me."

Jenny was very curious to know exactly how Jason's special ability worked and what its history was: "How did you come across that knowledge and how have you been developing it? Jason revealed that he had "learned stuff from my Dad." It turned out that these teachings had been very helpful and that Jason had been developing his "mental energy" on his own. Kim and Jenny were both intrigued. "Could you help explain that more to us?" Jenny asked. "It seems like a rather unique or special thing for someone your age to take something like that and practice it without being in a class."

"Well, there's two ways I have," Jason explained carefully, "One of them is this—I call to my thoughts and I think of perfect thoughts, like a beach with the waves rolling up on the sand." Everyone sat quietly and breathed for a pause. "My other way is, I'll take a word that has two syllables in it, but it's short, like 'Sony.' Then, when you breathe in, you say 'So'; then when you breathe out, you say 'ny' like this, 'So . . . ny.'"

Just listening was so relaxing that Jenny couldn't help but join in, "So . . . ny," she sighed. "Does that calm your mind? What times of the day or night do you do this? Before you go to sleep or when you wake up?"

"Yeah, a lot of the times before I go to sleep."

"I'm curious because you've made such a turnaround on the Fear and Insomnia and gained so much freedom from them, I'm wondering if these are ideas or practices that you've just been using lately, or have they been building up for a while?"

"Well, two years ago, I was way more violent—I was just like walking around punching and kicking wherever I went. But now, the only time I do it is like when I'm in my room, and I just start to train, and stuff, I guess."

"Was Jason taming or destroying his problems?" Jenny wondered aloud

to Kim, offering a choice of metaphors. Jason raised his fist and affirmed, "I'm strong but I'm under control."

Jenny thought back to their first meeting when Jason was taken over
by the "I don't knows." "Well, is he a constant surprise to you as he is to
me?" Jenny asked Kim. "Did you know he was taking this so seriously
and applying himself?"

"No! I did not. He's full of surprises!"

Jason added his own observation, "Most of these sessions, Mom learns
something about me."

FIFTH MEETING

When Jason walked in with his mother, Jenny noticed that he looked
keyed up. "What are you interested in this time?" she asked, "I have a
feeling that you have something in mind."

Jason wished to take up a suggestion from an earlier meeting to make
two sandtrays. They would show "an idea of how Fear was conquering
me, and then how it all turned around." Jenny noted to herself that he
seemed to be using some of the adult language from previous sessions as
a bridge to his own creative ideas.

Jason made his first sandtray quickly and with great absorption (Figure 15.1), while Jenny and Kim talked. Then he turned to them and
announced, "Okay, I'm done."

"This is all symbolic, so don't get any ideas," he warned Jenny and
Kim as they looked together at the sandtray full of figures.

"Well, are you ready to show us?" his mother asked.

Jason pointed to the Star Wars figure of Yoda. "See, this is me. Don't
get any ideas. This isn't what I look like in my dreams!" he exclaimed,
giggling with embarrassment. His mother was struck by a coincidence,
"Can I say one thing though? When you were a baby what did we call
you? Before you were cognizant, we called you Obi One Kenobi, but
what we really meant was Yoda!"

"You're kidding!" exclaimed Jenny.

"No, we used to call him Obi One."

"Okay," Jason interjected, wanting to get on with his description, "so
I'm running through the tunnel—I'm trying to escape—I'm running
through the tigers and they can't follow me into the tunnel, but I go into
this side and these guys (fighting figures) are after me, so then I just run
and I stay in the tunnel, . . . and I stay in the tunnel and then I light a
lantern, and I walk out and everything's okay." Jason paused. "So then,
that's how Fear felt for me."

Jenny and Jason's mother took this in slowly and carefully.

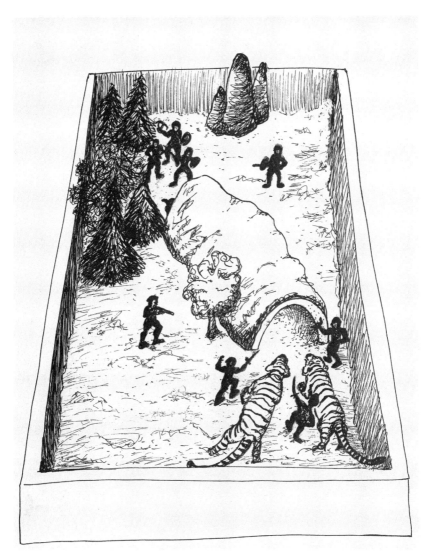

Figure 15.1 Yoda trapped by the Fears, peeks out of the tunnel.

"With all these Samurais attacking the tunnel?" Jason's mother asked. "I said this was just symbolic!" Jason emphasized. "I understand," Kim reassured him. He relaxed a little.

"Was it like you were on the run?" Jenny asked.

"Yeah," he agreed, "so I tried to avoid it and then Fear just kept coming back to me."

"What happened next?"

"Okay, well I was being chased by tigers, which I was afraid of, so I tried to avoid it by thinking of something else. Then I just got new ideas which lead to new Fears, and then I tried to escape those and then I got new ideas which lead to new Fears. Then when I was in the tunnel, I called on Mom and Dad and they turned on the light and then everything was gone."

Jason's mother understood what Jason was getting at. She smiled warmly at him. "You seem to be able to light your own lantern now, because you don't call on us in the middle of the night anymore to light the lantern."

"What a lovely comment!" Jenny said, seeing the light herself (so to speak). "I must admit I was trying to think of something like that to say, myself."

Following Kim's lead, she asked Jason, "You used to depend more on your parents to light the lantern . . . are you able to light it yourself now, and at the same time have their support?"

"I'm lighting my own lantern now. Mmmhmm yep!" Jason exclaimed exuberantly.

"That seems like it changes a lot of things. Do you have Fears even more on the run now instead of their chasing you? Is it like when you light a light, the shadows disappear?"

"Before I used to have all of this," Jason said, spreading his hands over the whole sandtray. "After the Fears came they took over."

"Were you driven into the tunnel?" Jenny followed him back into the world of the sandtray.

"Yes, I was trapped, and since I was trapped, my mind kept flashing back to the Fears and I just stayed in the tunnel. So then what I did was just sit up and think, sometimes waiting for Mom to come in, or I would go get them."

Suddenly Jenny entered Jason's dark tunnel in her mind, feeling as if she were having her own flashback of his experience of being in his room alone at night. She realized that Jason felt safe enough now that he could let her and his mother in on this scary time. Jenny wondered whether Jason, by developing his competence in dealing with night fears, had gained a vantage point from which he could acknowledge and articulate his old relationship with Fears. "That really gives me a sense of what it was like in your room," Jenny said pensively. "Your story gives me a real sense of that and of the transformation that occurred when you began to light the lantern for yourself."

SIXTH MEETING

When Jason returned again with Kim for their final meeting, which Elliot was unable to attend, he was keen to report more success staying overnight at his cousin's place. As he was really solidifying his reputation with himself as a good sleeper and tamer of Fears, Jenny and Jason decided to complete his entry in the *Fear Facer's Handbook* (Figure 15.2). He contributed an illustrated poem and shyly agreed to be interviewed about his knowledge. The interview wove back and forth between his old and new relationship with fear.

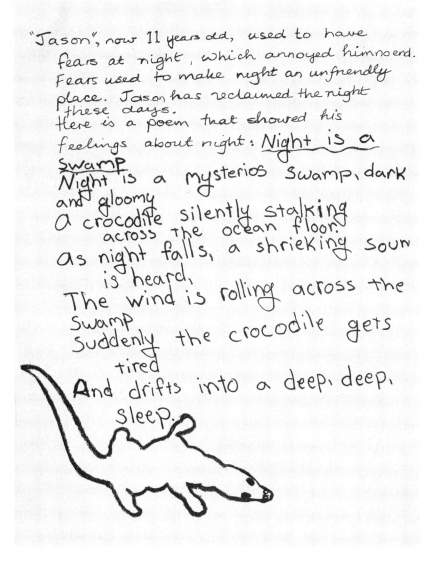

Figure 15.2 Night is a swamp.

Jenny began, "What have you learned about yourself in this process?"

"I've learned, let's see, that I can do more than I thought I could, and that Fear was getting the best of me."

"What is it like now?"

"Now I'm getting the best of Fear."

"Are you getting the best of yourself for yourself too—like your imagination? Did Fear used to take over your imagination? Do you have more imagination for yourself, and less for Fear?"

"Not that much at all for Fear really."

"What does it make it possible for you to do in the future? Anything you couldn't have imagined?"

"I can imagine more thoughts, like scary thoughts, and not get any freaked-out ideas about them."

After the interview was completed, and by way of saying farewell to his Problem, Jason created his second sand-tray (Figure 15.3). As Jason, Kim, and Jenny stood gazing over it together, Jason, pointing, began his symbolic narrative: "Well, in my imagination the tigers didn't become so big . . . they lost a lot of space till all they had was this part. Then I gained more space. I felt better about myself, so I used my imagination and turned it around. I gave myself an army to fight them with, till all they had was the tunnel."

Jenny could see that the tables had been turned. "You backed them into the tunnel?" she asked.

"Yeah, so they're all fighting to get into the tunnel, and all of them are retreating into it," Jason responded.

"But they don't look nearly so dangerous," Kim noted.

"Yep!" Jason agreed, "so all of them are turning back, and they're going into the tunnel. Before they were chasing me into the tunnel but I used my imagination! I got an army, and now they're all trapped in the tunnel."

While studying the tray Kim noticed the reappearance of Yoda. "He's in the chariot!" Kim cried out when she saw him. "Yep, that's me!" Jason enthused. "What's he doing . . . what's he up to?" Jenny wondered. "Just looking at the tigers and smiling," Jason said.

That made Jenny smile, too. "If he's smiling does that mean he's having more fun now with his imagination?"

"Yep!" Jason agreed easily.

"He turned it into a fun thing?" Jenny asked. "That's pretty impressive."

As Jason continued to answer questions about different details in the scene he had portrayed in the sand, Jenny began to reflect on his use of a battle metaphor. She decided to inquire further into what relationship Jason preferred to have with the Fears. "Is this a final battle, or does it go on and on? Is it more fun to keep going? To have a sense of an ongoing

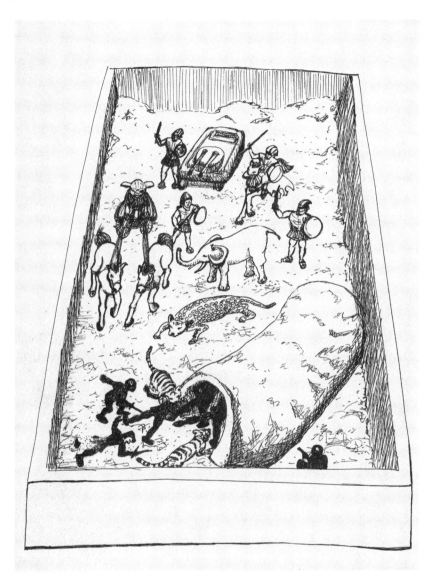

Figure 15.3 Yoda and his army drive the Fears into the tunnel.

play relationship with the Fears and their mates?"

Jason grinned, "Well, now they're just trapped in the tunnel, but sometimes they come out just for a peek, and my army chases them back." Jenny had the feeling that Jason was in fact having fun playing cat and mouse games. Rather than trying for a simple win, he seemed to be trying to find a balance of power.

Jason set out his long-term relationship with his fears in his own way:

"Maybe when I get older and I get really, really used to being in charge of the Fears, I can go hang gliding."

Jenny was amazed yet again by his vision: "Gosh, you've got a lot of ambitions!"

Kim was surprised too: "I didn't know about the hang gliding. I learn so much in here!"

Jason had yet another surprise up his sleeve: "Didn't you always know I wanted to go skydiving? I've just told Dad my plans. When I'm twenty-one, I'm going to skydive into college."

The image of her son skydiving into college struck Jason's mother as more amusing than fearful. "It's okay with me, Jason!" she said laughing.

CHAPTER 16

. . . .

Sophia:
"I Won't Make a Place for You in My Heart,
But I'll Make a Place for You in My Skin"

The Bielski family is Pakeha (Caucasian New Zealanders) of Polish and English descent. Sophia was thirteen at the time of their sole session with David Epston, which she attended along with her mother, June, father, Walter, and ten-year-old sister, Jennifer.

The following consists of a highly detailed interview conducted by David with Sophia and her family. It illustrates the elaborate work that can go into explicating a complex relationship between a person and a problem. Sophia was suffering from severe eczema. Sometimes a problem like eczema, asthma, or chronic pain cannot be eliminated but can be prevented from controlling a person's consciousness. This kind of problem is one that has a compelling physiological reality, yet David discovers that Sophia has certain abilities that can be used to encourage a more empowered relationship with the eczema. The relationship between body and mind is taken into account, as David works to externalize "The Itch," something that Sophia has some control over, and to develop her powers of mind in relation to it. In the interview he invites Sophia to enter into a dialogue with the Itch and to negotiate a new arrangement in which she ascertains that she can gain some control and relief from its relentless effects.

Sophia's mother had requested an urgent appointment, since matters had reached crisis point. Sophia had always had eczema, but conventional medicines had kept it under control. Four months earlier, however, Sophia had been teased by a classmate in a physical education class when some irritated flesh was visible below her gym shorts. From there on her eczema went out of control.

A month-long hospitalization ensued and remedied the medical situation. However, Sophia "ripped herself to pieces" almost immediately on returning to school. She was unable to sleep more than an hour or two a night and found herself too fatigued to attend school even if she wanted to.

Now Sophia's parents had to stay awake at all night in order to secure Sophia's hands so she could not do further damage to her own flesh. They sought another admission to the hospital but the doctors acknowledged that her medications were nearing toxic levels and that sooner or later Sophia would have to return to school. It was their opinion that sooner would be better. They suggested a referral to David, who has had a long association with the Children's Hospital in Auckland.

THE MEETING

As his interview with Sophia and her family got underway, David noticed that she was obviously dealing with the problem in front of his eyes. Sophia informed David that she had "a fair bit of itchiness on both her arms." David immediately observed that she was not sitting on her hands, so she must be using her mind to stop herself from itching. He asked how she was defeating IT in their presence. "Am I right in thinking you've got a good mind?" he asked. Responding to Sophia's affirmation, he queried, "What's good about your mind?"

"I'm determined. Once I start something, I like to finish it off, battle it out."

David asked Sophia if he could confirm this with the rest of the family. All agreed that Sophia was "determined." David checked with Sophia's younger sister about whether Sophia's determination was, from her point of view, a good determination . . . after all, it could turn sour." This was not the way Sophia's younger sister saw it. Her opinion was that it was a true and worthy determination.

David immediately gained the impression that Sophia was a loved sister and daughter and wondered out loud whether that was the source of her determination. He commented that Sophia would need a lot of determination because she would have to fight a problem that is both persistent and intermittent, qualities which could, as he told her, "weaken a young person's hopes—you think you've won and it still comes back."

GETTING TO KNOW THE PROBLEM'S WAYS

Using his knowledge of this particularly oppressive aspect of the problem, David asked, "Say, if you went free of it for a while, would you be able to predict when the Itch would get particularly bad again?" Sophia could make such a prediction. In fact, she could time its return to within a half-hour. She detailed the daylight hours in this manner. Then her mother asked her about the night. Sophia replied that her nightly "Itch time" would typically be between 9 P.M. and 1 A.M.

David observed, "That's nasty that it is so unrelenting at night." He checked again with Sophia: "Can I ask you, if you were determined to go to sleep—and that sounds odd because you don't usually determine yourself to go to sleep, that's something you usually allow to happen—do you think that if you slept from 9 P.M. to 1 A.M. you would bypass the Itch and give it the slip?"

"It would still be there but not as viciously," she replied.

David checked with the rest of the family as to whether they had observed the "viciousness" of the Itch and they all agreed that night Itches were indeed the most vicious. David reiterated, "So if you could sleep from 9 P.M. to 1 A.M., you would escape the viciousness?" Sophia thought that indeed she could.

David continued to gather some important knowledge about the Itch and about Sophia. He was interested first of all in what "fed" the Itch. He found out that anxiety was "pro-Itch." Then he found out, that although the Itch died down after 1 A.M., it was still worse than during the day. He hypothesized about this: "Is it that during the day you are so busy having fun and learning that essentially your mind is somewhere else? And when you go to sleep you think about it—it is the time of turning off the busyness and it then tricks you into itching?" Sophia agreed that this was so but with the caveat that the Itch could still overpower her in the day, too.

David returned to the observation that she was not scratching as they spoke. He learned more from Sophia about the ways by which she was capable of "putting mind over matter" to prevent the Itch in the moment. Sophia confirmed that she could make a mild Itch die down even though it would not totally disappear. "How do you imagine you are doing that?" David asked. Sophia seemed to misunderstand his question as "How do you know you are actually doing that?" instead of, "What are you doing to accomplish such a feat?" She reiterated, "How do I know I am doing that? Because as I'm doing that when I have a mild Itch, it begins to die down." She then added, "But if I start thinking about the Itch again, it will come back." David interjected, "Oh, your mind is powerful here?" This brought Sophia to thinking about how she accomplished the lessening of the Itch: "Well, I have to keep thinking that I haven't got an Itch."

David wondered, "So to some extent you are tricking your mind by making your brain listen to you rather than listen to your body? You are separating your body and your mind?" Sophia agreed. David was busy developing an idea about her special ability to use her powers of mind. He attempted to "type" her ability by comparing it to abilities of other children. David introduced Sophia to the stories of two other children he had met that had similar abilities.

David read Sophia this letter from the mother of Michael, eleven, describing his relationship with a severe genetic skin disorder.

Dear David,

It took Michael awhile to acknowledge he had any special abilities but a few months after he received your letter he came up with the following:

When Michael was two, I taught him deep breathing to relax, and he knew then that being relaxed was far less painful than tensing in pain.

I also realized he could take things far further because if an injury was too painful for him to use breathing to overcome pain, he would run for his sheepskin rug and put himself to sleep with blood running from a wound. As a younger child he had a maturity beyond his years. I had put this to his constantly having to endure pain, especially as a preschooler.

Now I've noticed Michael often plays his best sports while injured, as if his concentration away from his sore feet increases his determination elsewhere.

Hoping this is some assistance to you here.

Regards,

    Michael's mother.

There was also a letter from Michael:

Dear David:

Thank you for contacting me with your letter. Sorry I have not contacted you earlier. I find it quite difficult to answer your questions because I'm not aware that I have special abilities to control pain.

In answer to your questions:

1. *Mainly I can block out pain to my feet but I can also fall asleep if I have a headache.*

2. *If I have really bad pain, I look around and try to concentrate on something else. When I'm lancing blisters and I know it's going to hurt I try deep, slow breath-*

ing and make my foot relaxed and floppy. I carry on deep breathing while I watch TV.

3. *Yes, from thinking about it now, I think Mum has taught me good things about pain control.*

4. *I know I would have felt heaps more pain in my life if I didn't have my pain relief tactics.*

5. *I turn off feeling from my knees down when I concentrate on other things, mostly when I am playing sport. In-between times, when I'm not needed by the team, I limp, but when I'm involved, I will not feel anything. When I'm feeling very irritable or feel sick, or have a headache, I can cut off the feelings by closing my eyes, relaxing, and going to sleep. If I wanted to, I could feel a pain in my feet by thinking about that pain.*

I have had trouble thinking about replying to your letter, because until now I had no idea I was controlling pain.

Regards,

   Michael

Sophia resonated with Michael's experience of pain relief. David asked Sophia to name her ability. She called it "distracting myself." He then tried to detail how it worked: "Where does your body go and where is your mind? Do you feel your Itch has gone away or have you gone from your Itch?" This was an important distinction because it opened up both possibilities—one for Itch elimination and the other for Itch management. David then learned that Sophia felt that she took her mind away from the Itch and that she did that by getting it on a "train of thought" that led away from the Itch. Sometimes a pain cannot be eliminated but it can be prevented from controlling a person's consciousness.

David was impressed by this ability and chose to pursue Sophia's control of the situation by looking at it in both directions at once, getting the Itch better and making the Itch worse. "Say you wanted to be mean to yourself, could you recall your Itch and make it even worse?" Sophia replied that she could. David asked, "How would you do that?" He checked with Sophia about pursuing this line of inquiry: "Do you mind me talking about this? I don't mean to be doing it in a harsh way." It was okay with her. She showed him that she could scratch just once and bring back the Itch. David remarked, "One scratch will reunite you with the Itch? Do you have any particular thoughts that would be itchy thoughts?" "It looks very red," Sophia replied.

David found out that the power of the Itch to get stronger with a single thought made Sophia quite angry and frustrated. David asked her to share her preference, "If, by any chance, you got angry at your Itch

and saved your skin, rather than getting angry at your skin and supporting your Itch, which one would be better from your point of view?"
Sophia looked at him quizzically. David gave voice to his protest against
the pain the Itch was causing Sophia and her family: "This isn't fair. I
don't consider this fair at all, fair to you or anyone else, but least of all
you."

Sophia understood and concurred that getting angry at the Itch
was preferable. David continued, "Say you knew you were frustrating
your Itch by refusing to scratch it, would that give you satisfaction
and revenge?" Sophia thought carefully about this and decided it would
not because simply not scratching would only make the Itch stronger.
David refined his question and asked, if she found a track away from
the Itch in her mind, would that give her satisfaction? Sophia agreed.
David found out that such satisfaction would strengthen her determination and that having the Itch ruin her sleep would weaken her determination. Sophia reckoned that she usually would only get one and
a half hours sleep a night, and lack of sleep kept her from going to
school. The whole family agreed that this was an accurate account of
the typical scenario for Sophia and that they were all getting a bit
"scratchy" about it!

David reviewed the state of affairs with Sophia, now that he knew a
bit about her and a bit about the Itch, all the while knowing that she
had been defeating the Itch as she sat there in front of him for the past
twenty minutes: "Look, right, you are an intelligent young woman with
a special ability. This ability may have something to do with your intelligence, or it may have something to do with having to suffer under this,
and I know it's really unfair and I feel awful about it. However, it is nice
to have an ability and it is nice to take advantage of it. How do you
think you've taken advantage of that ability right now to separate yourself from the Itch? I've been watching you and I knew you were doing
something and I just thought to myself, 'I'll keep talking in a relaxed
way, in an interesting way, because I learned that you like being distracted from the Itch.' Do you have any understanding of how that
worked for you?"

Sophia replied, "I just tried to put the Itch at the back of my mind and
involve myself in the conversation."

David's curiosity was piqued: "How did you put the Itch from the
front of your mind to the back of your mind?"

"My train of thought wasn't on my skin," Sophia replied.

David wanted to clarify Sophia's evaluation of her ability and checked
with her if in fact she did consider it an "ability." Sophia felt it was a "bit
of an ability."

Because David differed in his evaluation of her ability, he wanted her permission to feel differently about it. "Do you mind if I think it is a lot of an ability?" David asked. "Do you mind me being a little bit ahead of you on this? You wouldn't consider me unpleasant?"

"No," replied Sophia.

David was ready to lay out his ideas on how to help Sophia: "Do you think in any way if we worked together to develop and strengthen this ability of yours and make it more available to you to use whenever you wanted and for whatever you wanted it for—and I would argue that you save some of it for other things too, like studying or having good dreams, or relaxing to put yourself to sleep—if we increased your awareness of whatever it is that you do and this success you are having now, could it be better?" Sophia readily agreed that it could.

"And would you resent getting better at this in any way?" David checked.

"No," replied Sophia.

David carefully evaluated where Sophia saw herself in concrete terms: "What percent do you think you are good at it now?"

"About 30 percent."

"Would you say that's pretty good?" David checked.

"Yes, but not on a strong Itch, just if it's small one."

"An Itch has to start small, right," reminded David. "To attack, you've got to start somewhere."

Sophia's mother, June, added that she thought Sophia would "be good at jumping on top of it before it got big." Sophia informed them both that "It can work both ways, I can fight it and get stronger against it or it can be stronger against me. Everytime I give into it, it doubles!"

David had an idea that he thought might put a new twist on things: "Do you ever think, 'Look, I really have been defeating you (the Itch) a lot lately and I feel you should score the odd goal on me, so I think I will scratch you, but scratch you in a nondoubling way?"

Sophia knew David's "twist" already, so she went further with one of her own: "If I am thinking that way, I might fall for Itch's trick and think that when I am scratching it will give me relief. When I've got that in mind, I do scratch it, but then I think to myself, 'It's not giving me relief.' "

David was happy to be in conspiracy with Sophia against the Itch. He wondered if Sophia's refusing to believe that she was getting relief from the Itch was a form of revenge against the Itch. Sophia explained that it was her "determination" coming out. David summarized that if Sophia were not tricked by the Itch, then that would determine her determination. David wondered if undoing eczema's trick, as she just had, gave her satisfaction and made her even more determined.

"YOU BE THE ITCH AND I'LL BE YOU."

At this point in the interview David felt he had a good beginning knowledge of the wiles and the power of eczema and Sophia's special abilities and determination. He felt that Sophia knew the Itch pretty well, but that maybe she might benefit from seeing her skills through David's eyes. He contrived a conversation in which she could take the role of the Itch and he would play her. "How about you be the Itch and I'll be you," he proposed playfully. Sophia accepted his invitation.

DAVID (as Sophia): Well, look, you have given me a pretty hard time a lot of my life and I really think I'm going to have to ration my itching of you. I will only itch you to my satisfaction, not to yours, and you will have to like or lump it!

SOPHIA (as the Itch): I'm sorry but I am in charge of your skin right now and unless you want some discomfort, you'd better scratch me.

DAVID (as Sophia): I've fallen for this many many times before, Itch. You always promise that if I scratch you, you'll be satisfied. I know that every time I do, you double the price! I'm getting a little bit sick of this trick. I'm a young woman now and I can't be fooled by your trick. What makes you think you can fool me?

SOPHIA (as the Itch): Why don't you scratch me a little bit harder. I'll prove to you I won't get any worse.

DAVID (as Sophia): I've heard that one before. You think I'm a sucker! I've seen through it. I've seen the light! I'll tell you what, I'll compromise, I'll get an ice cube from the refrigerator and soothe you or I'll put a little bit of soothing cream on you. But that's all you're getting from me, that's all you deserve.

SOPHIA (as the Itch): You can do that for now but it's only going to dull me partly. I'll be back in twenty minutes and then I'll haunt you again!

DAVID (as Sophia): Okay, try me. But your twenty minutes is okay because I know you can't do a deal with a Devil.

SOPHIA (as the Itch): You just try putting ice or cream on me but I'll still be there in the back of your mind. There'll be an Itch there!

DAVID (as Sophia): Oh sure, but you are in the back of my mind, not in the front of my mind. When you are in the back of my mind I can put a lot in the front of my mind. I know that if I get involved with a conversation or my imagination you'll stay in the back of my mind. I know I've got to live with you, but you're not my boss. You're just like a flat-mate. You've got to play by the rules!

SOPHIA (as the Itch): I can accept that, but you've got to understand that I control you to a point where I can make you scratch me or give you discomfort.

DAVID (as Sophia): Well, I think you are a bit arrogant. I don't know where you got that idea. I think you have lost touch with me and the person I've become. Haven't you been realizing that I have been scratching a lot less or itching a lot less? Haven't you realized that I am getting more mature? You are starting to bug me and I have started to be more active and take control in my own life and you are going to have to fit in with that!

SOPHIA (as the Itch): I don't know.

DAVID (as Sophia): Well, Itch, that's the first time I've caught you without words. I'm telling you I'm just getting smarter than you are. I know that when I was a little girl you had it all over me. Well what could I do? You were taking advantage of a four-year-old. I couldn't fight back. Now I have mind power. You may have my body but I've got my mind.

SOPHIA (as the Itch): I feel that you have strengthened up and that's making my job harder.

DAVID (as Sophia): Well, that's your lot in life. Would you have preferred to get me weaker so you could dominate me and destroy my happiness? Is that what you want?

SOPHIA (as the Itch): Yes.

DAVID (as Sophia): Well, I've got a name for someone like you but I don't dare say it! Just tell me what your plans for me are.

SOPHIA (as the Itch): You'd probably stay mostly discomforted as you are now. I might ease off you because I know you will get stronger and eventually fight me off. But, I'd at least give it my best shot.

DAVID (as Sophia): So you don't want to go easy, you will go hard. You don't know who you are playing with, do you? Do you know me that well? Or, do you just know the four-year-old me? You don't know that I've been gathering strength in my mind because you just know my body!

SOPHIA (as the Itch): I can dominate your mind sometimes.

DAVID (as Sophia): What do you think about the times that you can't?

SOPHIA (as the Itch): I get annoyed.

DAVID (as Sophia): Guess what? That pleases me. You are going to be getting a lot more annoyed. Do you think you should go get some therapy for the way you are going to be feeling as I get my mind strong? I'm feeling a bit sorry for you now. I suppose there is some other child's life you could wreck. Do you want to move off?

SOPHIA (as the Itch): I don't mind if you get therapy but I won't leave because I'll always be there, but I will weaken off.

Another relationship with the problem

DAVID (as Sophia): I don't mind you hanging around as long as you keep your place and respect me. I could live in harmony with you. But you can't wreck my pride! I'll tell you that. I won't permit it.

SOPHIA (as the Itch): Okay, I'll strike that deal with you.

DAVID (as Sophia): What's your deal? You can hang around me and be in my life, but how are you going to operate on me?

SOPHIA (as the Itch): Well, now and then, you have got to accept that sometimes I am hungry for a scratch and you've got to satisfy me, but most of the time I'll try to keep down.

DAVID (as Sophia): What, one day a week? What do you think would satisfy you? A half-hour here and there?

SOPHIA (as the Itch): Say if you get upset or get worried then I might get a bit worked up and get a bit aggravated them. And then I would need a bit of calming down.

DAVID (as Sophia): Ah hold on, so when I am worried or upset, then that's when you get a little bit worked up yourself?

SOPHIA (as the Itch): A little bit.

DAVID (as Sophia): I see. If I learned to calm myself, relax, and learned to worry in an anti-worry way, then there wouldn't be such a need for you to be scratched, would there? Is that okay or would you feel neglected?

SOPHIA (as the Itch): That's okay, as long as you know I'm still there.

DAVID (as Sophia): Okay, I'll always make a place for you . . . . I won't make a place for you in my heart but I'll make a place for you on my skin.

SOPHIA (as the Itch): Yeah, that's okay.

DAVID (as Sophia): Is that a deal? Can we rest easy with each other? Can we sort of cooperate? So what do you want from me?

SOPHIA (as the Itch): I want you to accept that I'm there.

DAVID (as Sophia): Okay, you're there.

SOPHIA (as the Itch): And that when I do need to be scratched quite badly, you would.

DAVID (as Sophia): Okay. But what about this thing about doubling when I give in and scratch you? That's not a very good deal for me. "Scratch me this hard," then double the price.

SOPHIA (as the Itch): Well, if I stick to my side of the deal, then I'll calm down, then my powers won't double so much.

DAVID (as Sophia): Okay, so you'll calm down, and I'll calm down. What do you think about me going to sleep tonight? Do you mind if I get a good night's sleep and would that calm you down if I calmed myself down? Do you feel all right about that tonight? Or should we fight? Do you think you could give me a night off tonight? We could fight tomorrow night.

SOPHIA (as the Itch): Well, I think I need some time to accept that I've got to calm down because it would be a pretty big change for me.

DAVID (as Sophia): Say you did calm down, is there anything you'd like to ask of me? You have been very fair in your negotiating. You've compromised. What would you ask of me?

SOPHIA (as the Itch): That you don't do things that you know will aggravate me.

DAVID (as Sophia): What aggravates you the most? I'm getting a lot more sympathetic toward you, you know. I feel a lot closer to you. You are being very reasonable.

SOPHIA (as the Itch): Like eating too much sweet foods.

DAVID (as Sophia): That's going to be hard for me. I love sweets. Eating too much sweet food. Like what?

SOPHIA (as the Itch): Chocolate.

DAVID (as Sophia): What about Mars bars? Can I eat them?

SOPHIA (as the Itch): You can eat them but only to the extent that you want to check that I'm still there. Or else I'll bite back and show you that I really am still there.

DAVID (as Sophia): So chocolate in moderation. What else?

SOPHIA (as the Itch): Not overdoing things like PE (physical education), not overdoing it too much because you get hot and that causes the itching.

DAVID (as Sophia): Yeah, overdoing it. Heat isn't too good, is it?

SOPHIA (as the Itch): No, it isn't, but summer can be okay, like going to the sea and things, but the heat gets pretty uncomfortable.

DAVID (as Sophia): You really wouldn't want to live in the tropics too much, would you?

SOPHIA (as the Itch): Not really.

DAVID (as Sophia): What other things would you ask of me? You know, keeping cool. Is that emotionally cool or . . . ?

SOPHIA (as the Itch): Both, don't put things on me that you know have aggravated me before.

DAVID (as Sophia): Like what?

SOPHIA (as the Itch): Creams, or I'll show you again that they have aggravated me. I won't ever like them.

DAVID (as Sophia): Do you feel that I am showing a bit more respect by going along with you a bit? Do you feel I've grown up and become your equal?

SOPHIA (as the Itch): Yep.

DAVID (as Sophia): I'm getting a different idea about you, quite frankly, because I thought you were just out to make my life a misery. I can see now that you have your own concerns. I never thought of your position much. I only thought about mine. You get older and you start thinking about other people's feelings. You've got your own thoughts and your own needs. So if I take you into account, you'll take me into account?

SOPHIA (as the Itch): Yes.

On the way out, Sophia's parents asked if they might have a few words with David. He looked forward to this, since despite their apparent tiredness, they looked blissful as they dried their tears. Speaking sotto voce, Sophia's mother said, "She is an inspiration to us," as her father nodded his agreement.

FOLLOW-UP

David received a joyous phone call late the next day from Sophia's mother. Apparently Sophia had fallen asleep the night before and she had gone to school that morning. However, she had started to itch and had gone to the nurse's office and phoned her mother. Sophia's mother told David that she was very busy that day at work and had told her daughter that she was unable to pick her up.

This was the first time Sophia's mother had not picked Sophia up after such a call. When she did so at the end of the day she found that Sophia had returned to her classes and "had the best day at school in months." Sophia's mother remembered what an inspiration her daughter was to her. She told David that her new confidence in Sophia supported her decision to not pick her up when she called from the nurse's office.

After that day several phone conversations confirmed that Sophia was more in control of her eczema than ever before and that further meetings were unnecessary. David felt that both he and Sophia had gotten to know the Itch better—what helped and hurt—but most importantly they had explicated in satisfying detail Sophia's maturity and a new version of her life with eczema.

CHAPTER 17

Terry:

"So after a Long Time in Horror
I Live in Peace Again"

Terry's family is Pakeha (Caucasian New Zealanders) and of Irish and Welsh descent. The family members involved in the therapy were Terry, twelve, and Dorothy, his mother. They met with David Epston eight times over an eight-month period.

FIRST MEETING

"He's overloaded with guilt," Dorothy summarized after sharing her concerns about her son, Terry. She had just told David of Terry's hand-washing, excessive worrying, daily vomiting on the way to school, and hysterical responses to viewing people kiss on TV and to "dirt" in general.

Dorothy, still undecided about its merit, told of an attempt that she and Terry's older sister had made to disrupt his screaming demands to put cushions over their eyes when people on TV were kissing. They had, with exaggerated good humor and a bit of teasing thrown in, refused to comply with his demands. Their policy behind such a practice was that "it was better to be open with him so he felt okay about it." Terry nicknamed their tactics as "teasing"; when asked by David if he considered such "teasing" to be benevolent or malevolent, he assured David that it was "benevolent."

David asked what effect "benevolent teasing" had on the problem. Terry was quick to say, "I'm making some headway with the compulsions and it (benevolent teasing) has been helping me along." David speculated, "Your mum and your sister could have thought they were upsetting you rather than strengthening you?"

"Not really," replied Terry.

David asked for further information. "You knew it was for your own good? How?"

"Yeah, they were laughing and they weren't shouting. They didn't have frowns on their faces."

David wondered aloud to Terry, "Do you think that you saw the joke of it all? Do you think Guilt and Compulsions don't like to be made fun of?"

Terry replied sagely, "Yeah, but I like them to be made fun of because then it is a lot easier to talk about them. And you just think, 'They are silly thoughts and I can fight them off.' "

David, thinking that everyone had stumbled onto something outstanding, asked a question to confirm this and to contribute to his ongoing process of reviewing his ideas, "When your mother and older sister benevolently tease you—you can fight off the thoughts and be stronger?" Terry answered in the affirmative.

Picking up on Dorothy's initial comment that Terry was "overloaded with guilt," David double-checked with Terry, "Is it okay for me to call it Guilt?" When Terry concurred, David took the liberty of personifying the problem: "Do you mind my saying that Guilt has a voice and kind of speaks to you?"

"No," said Terry.

"I'm asking you this because Chris, who had a run-in with similar sorts of problems—he was sixteen at the time by the way—gave me his consent to tell you what he found out—that Guilt talked to him and told him to do things," David continued. "What does Guilt say to you, Terry?"

Terry replied by speaking through the voice of Guilt: "You have to be perfectly clean. Your hands have to be all nice and clean. They're not meant to be dirty."

David couldn't help getting angry hearing Guilt's demands on Terry's hands, and could not stop himself from telling Terry about his feelings: "I get quite angry just thinking about it!"

Terry went on in further detail about the demands, still mimicking the voice of Guilt: "The thoughts you are having at the moment are nasty and malicious. You are not meant to have them. You are strange and inhuman. You are the only one who has them. You are abnormal!"

Earlier David had promised Terry that he would not get overly excited or angry about things, so he had to control his rising anger at the ludicrous lies that Guilt was telling Terry.

SMARTER THAN GUILT

David formed the opinion that Terry was "quite a smart character" and his mother smiled and nodded her agreement. He assumed that Terry was, in fact, a smarter person than Guilt was taking him for. So he asked him, "Why do you think Guilt lies that way? What are its purposes in having you spend all your time obsessed and compelled?"

Terry replied thoughtfully, "Well, it's trying to help me get my mind off things I don't want to think about—that I'm scared of thinking. It's trying to help me not think about things, but it is hurting me really."

This answer confirmed David's opinion about Terry's overall smartness and his knowledgeable relationship with the problem. It reminded him of the similarly knowledgeable thoughts of Chris. David read out loud a letter he had written to Chris, which Chris had donated to the "archives" of The Anti-Habit League for just such a purpose.

Dear Chris,

Chris, you told me you aren't worrying so much about your schoolwork. I marveled at this. You told me that "worrying isn't helping" and for that reason you dropped it and yet your effort level has stayed the same. Chris, do you think your compulsions have tricked you and almost betrayed you into their grip? What promises did they make to suck you in? Did they promise you everlasting happiness if you wiped your bum clean, or washed your body spic-and-span? Do you think these are childish ideas or do you think there is any truth in them? Before, you thought, "They were just weird things I did." Now it seems you are seeing through the tricks that Guilt was playing on you.

OVER THE EDGE

Setting the letter to one side, David turned back to Terry: "How did you see through the tricks Guilt was playing on you?" Terry pondered the question for a moment: "Mum said you shouldn't wash your hands all the time. A lot of it was my father's compulsion-ism of being clean." (Terry's father was living in another country at the time.) "And cats, because we have three cats at home. I can handle them a lot and stroke them."

Terry assumed the authoritative and disapproving tone of the "voice" at this point and railed, "They're dirty and filth-ridden. Dust and everything is dirty!" He then resumed his normal tone. "I suppose my suspicions . . . well, I got them off Dad so I am heavily suspicious of stuff."

David asked, "Did you realize this was going too far?"

Terry promptly nodded, "Yes, over the edge."

David wondered if Terry's recognition that he was going over the edge had led him to take a stand against the Compulsions. It turned out that it definitely had. David wanted to hear exactly what had happened the first time it did.

Terry recalled, "It was gnawing at me all the time. Then I would wash my hands after a while. I just went longer and longer until I didn't have to."

Reviewing this discussion, David asked, "Do you think Guilt was taking advantage of your mind rather than you using your own mind?"

Terry, with a small measure of relief, responded, "Yeah, it was taking the use of my mind to the verge of a breakdown. I felt . . . I felt I was falling to pieces and was going to crumble. My personality was going to crumble and I was going to become a nervous wreck."

"Well," David responded, after taking a deep breath, "I am glad you did what you did and that was formidable. Are you a little bit, middle bit, or large bit proud of yourself for what you've done?"

Terry's modesty restrained his reply: "Sort of middle proud of myself."

David gently contested this: "Do you mind me being more proud of you than you are proud of yourself? Is that okay with you?" Terry accepted David's discrepant opinion.

David pursued his line of inquiry further: "Did you have any sense you could drive these thoughts out of your mind? Or you can drive them out when they start bugging you?"

Terry acknowledged that "some of them I can but some are strong and persistent."

David's bias showed in his choice of the next question: "Can you tell me about the ones you have kicked out of your mind, the ones you seem able to subdue, boss around, and order out of your mind rather than being bossed and ordered around by them?"

"The ones about washing my hands," Terry informed him. "Some of the thoughts for people my age—adolescent thoughts. The small ones about myself and that."

"Terry, which is your favorite opponent? Which one are you winning against pretty regularly?"

"Washing my hands."

"What qualities have you possessed for a long time that would have made me guess that you could have done this if you were heading in the right direction?"

"Having a short temper. I got fed up with them. If something gets in my way, I kick it away!"

David turned to Dorothy and asked, "Are there any other signs that told you he was getting stronger as a person and more courageous?"

Dorothy replied, "Last year at school he's done really well. The teachers have said what an outstanding sort of person he is. He did well academically, and he has a great sense of justice, too."

David, seizing on Terry's sense of justice, asked, "Terry, do you think it's just or fair that your life be wrecked at this age? That your personality should disintegrate?"

Terry's reply was very considered: "If it's going to disintegrate, I think it should be when I'm older." Then he became more assured. "Yeah, it was going to wreck my life so I wouldn't be able to enjoy it to the fullest. When I'm old and feeble at least then I wouldn't have much to look forward to, but at a young age I've got nothing to look forward to—just misery."

David turned to Dorothy to seek some evidence for an alternative history of Terry's life: "Dorothy, when you think back to Terry's life before this, what qualities did he have that would have predicted that he could do this? Has he had to overcome other adversities so far in his life?" Dorothy gave an account of how Terry had fought "his way out of vomiting in the gutter every day."

Summing up Terry's new relationship with the problem, David asked, "Did you figure out your compulsions weren't like a friend, but more like an enemy?"

Terry nodded vigorously, "Probably!"

SECOND MEETING

Terry came into the next meeting and immediately told the news: "The thoughts that were bothering me are now all gone!"

"Am I right in thinking that you got these thoughts outside of yourself and eyeballed them?"

"Yes," replied Terry.

David was curious. "How do you imagine you did that—because you must have thought they were inside your head, that they were your thoughts?"

Terry thought about this for a moment and replied, "Well, I just watched programs on TV and I gradually put up my own fight! I imagined a tough, malevolent person standing there—really big. But the thoughts were weak rather than tough. I got to thinking they were weak."

"Now that's pretty different, as you used to see them as strong and persistent," recalled David. "It sounds as if you got a different idea about these thoughts, that they were tough on the outside but weak on the inside." Terry and Dorothy agreed that this described a bully perfectly.

"How did you formulate these ideas that allowed you to stand up to this bully?" David wondered. "Were they from a dream, vision, or an invention of yours?" Terry identified the source of his inspiration to be a cartoon show he had watched. "Did you do this in the privacy of your creative mind?" asked David. "Do you think you have special abilities in any way?" Terry somewhat uneasily admitted, "I guess I am a bit inventive."

David wanted to know more about Terry's inventions. He told Terry that he wanted to know about this and he wanted to satisfy his curiosity about how Terry's mind worked. David mused that it was refreshing to get to know Terry's mind with the obsessive thoughts cleared to the outside of it. David was excited by the prospect that, if Terry could drive the hand-washing thoughts out of his mind, his mind might be "flexing its muscles" with inventions. Terry readily agreed that there were many more inventive thoughts going into the space those other obsessive thoughts had preoccupied. "They've gone away and all of a sudden other stuff, like fantasy and science fiction writing, is flowing in!" he exclaimed.

"Does it make you happy or sad that those thoughts aren't in your mind and you've got your own mind filling up the space?" asked David.

"VERY HAPPY," Terry exclaimed.

David asked Dorothy if she had been aware of Terry's newfound happiness. Dorothy let an amazing cat out of the bag: "David, he hasn't had a headache for about three weeks and that's a MIRACLE!" Although startled for a moment by this revelation, David recovered enough to shake Terry's hand and offer heartfelt congratulations.

When the dust settled it turned out that Dorothy hadn't considered it worthwhile to tell David about the headaches at the first meeting because, as she put it, "Terry has had a headache every day for eight long years!" After consulting numerous specialists, she had forced herself to accept this as something Terry would have to live with.

"Do you think these thoughts were aching your head?" David asked. Terry immediately nodded.

"As you take over your mind, are you giving yourself a fair bit of pleasure and fun?" he continued. "Do you think in a manner of speaking that these thoughts were giving your head a bit of a pounding?"

"Very much so," agreed Terry.

"How much of your mind do you think you have regained and what percentage foothold do these thoughts still have in your mental territory?"

Terry replied that he had 99.9 percent of his own mind.

FREE AT LAST

While David's mind was reeling from this statistic, his thoughts turned to Brett, who, as David told Terry, was going to be very interested in this indeed. Brett was also twelve years old and he was in a life-or-death struggle with "Anorexia and Perfection," which he considered to be "a married couple." Brett and his family had been exchanging their video-taped sessions with others through David.

"Now tell me, Terry, this is quite an achievement," David began, "but I know you are pretty uncomfortable when I get too enthusiastic so I will try to keep calm here. Will you allow me to share some of your ideas with Brett so he can hear how you keep these thoughts from tak-ing your mind over again? Surely these thoughts tried to convince you that you weren't in the right and that they should be occupying your mind. When you started to push them away, what did they do?"

Terry replied easily, "They didn't put up much of a fight. They gave up the towel quite easily. Then they tried to come back and there was a little bit of a spat, but with one flick of my finger, they were gone."

"Really!" exclaimed David. "What are your thoughts about the fact that your mind is now free from guilt, worry, and compulsions and head-aches, too?"

"Free at last," sighed Terry. "I can do my own thing instead of having those thoughts in the back of my mind telling me what to do, like, 'You can only have so much fun.' I was only able to act like I was having fun because deep inside I was worried."

David wondered how the thoughts actually tried to convince Terry of this. Terry mimicked for him, "You are not meant to have fun; you are meant to have a limit of it."

David was shocked. "Oh, isn't that mean! When you tell me that I get quite angry. Do you think that it is a mean thing to say to a young person? I mean, these are supposed to be some of the best years of your life and it's telling you not to have fun! What do you think about that? Doesn't that make you question the morals and ethics of these voices— taking away a young person's pleasures?"

"They do that," explained Terry. "I have friends that have fun together, enjoy themselves and laugh but I am back there in the junkyard of empty space."

"Is that what you call it—the junkyard of empty space?" quipped David. "What have you been filling up your mind with now that they are gone? Some good experiences, some creativity? What about friendships? My guess would be that there is more of you to be friends with now."

"I have started to make friends and put up with some people that I was really intolerant of last year." Terry explained to David that in the past he couldn't tolerate mistakes, his or his classmates. When they were enjoying themselves, he would think that they were good and deserved fun, and because he couldn't enjoy himself, he must be bad.

"I'm glad to hear that you are free of this torture," David told him.

Terry explained to David that freedom wasn't the issue. The thoughts had been trying to protect him.

"Do you think they were overprotecting you?" David asked.

"No," Terry continued to explain, "the Guilt was power-corrupt. Because it realized, after it helped me avoid things I didn't want to think about, that it could control my mind and manipulate it. And then it realized that it could control my mind so completely that it could get my mind to keep the Obsessions there so they wouldn't die away."

With these brilliantly perceptive remarks about the way Guilt and Obsessions take over and inhabit a young person's mind recorded for Brett, Terry and David's second conversation ended.

THIRD MEETING

A month later, a third meeting took place. Terry began the session by reading aloud a story he had written:

> Once my mind was plagued by guilt. I was forced by my mind to conduct a series of rituals such as hand-washing. My life was like a bowl of dust blowing away in the wind. I had hardly any activities or clubs to go to. My life usually centered around my schoolwork. I didn't have many friends, and if I did, I would usually argue or get nasty with them, as they were happy. My life was going down the drain.
>
> Then one day, a day in which freeness would finally invade the "infected" areas of my mind, my mother decided, after seeing me go through a time of pain and guilt, to take me to see David Epston. After only one visit, the shell of guilt that had covered me crumbled and light and freedom came to me again. I started making new friends and with my old friends started tying the tethers back together, which over time had been left to rot and slowly decay. So after a long time in horror, I live in peace again.

After a pause pregnant with appreciative silence, David congratulated Terry for his passionate account of freedom and peace. Terry asked David to keep it for other young people he might meet in the future and for people like yourselves, dear reader.

David then sought to catch up with Terry's recent developments, guessing there would be a lot. "How has your life been going? Has Guilt put up any obstacles to you taking back your life and mind?"

"Lately I've been having so much fun, I'm getting tired," Terry observed. "I guess my body isn't used to it. I used to sit around and mope all the time."

Dorothy was concerned that, although Terry had been doing great, he had gotten grumpy several times. "It has to do with his schoolwork," she explained. "He is a real perfectionist. If he can't get it right the first time, he gets angry about it. There was a little bit of that."

In the meantime, Terry had been watching videos of the meetings between David and Brett (with Brett's permission), where Brett had contested "the curse of the idea of Perfection." Terry and David reviewed Brett's comeback from Perfection and Anorexia.

David asked Terry, "What do you think the rock singer Sting meant when he sang, 'Perfection is all very well, but don't be surprised if your life on earth is hell'?" Terry interpreted the lyric readily: "You will always be imperfect; you will never become perfect. Your mind always creates something to say it's imperfect, even if you think it's perfect. The night before it's perfect, then the next day it's not."

David asked Terry, "Can you tell the difference between 'good enough' and the 'curse of the idea of Perfection'?" Terry slowly shook his head from side to side.

David wanted to be helpful: "Do you think we should work out which idea you want to live your life by?" David tried to give Terry a clear example of this: "Say you decided to join a club called 'The Curse of the Idea of Perfection Club.' Look ahead ten years and tell me, would that be a life of happiness or a life of misery?" Terry caught on to this readily. "Misery, because I wouldn't have much self-esteem. The curse would always say, 'You are imperfect. You have to make yourself perfect. You are just a piece of trash in the rubbish heap.' I wouldn't be good for anybody or anything. I would probably fail every job because my mind would be saying, 'This job is too imperfect for you, or it's too perfect for you, or you're too imperfect for it.' "

"What would it do to your relationships with other people?" asked David. "I would try to get them to be perfect." Terry clarified this: "I wouldn't listen to other people because my mind wouldn't let me listen to them because they would be perfect in my mind's eye and I would be imperfect. So since I wasn't perfect, I would have failed."

David knew that if Terry could project the consequences of Perfection into a hypothetical future as well as he had, he could certainly do the opposite. "So, Terry," David continued, "if you were to oppose Perfection in your everyday life, how would you go about it?"

"By setting reasonable goals and not going to extremes. Instead of trying for a 100 percent, I would probably go for the 80's."

"Look, I don't know if I should be charging you money for these conversations. You have all these good ideas. I learn a lot from you."

David had a feeling that Terry knew what he was talking about from experience, so he asked, "Can you think of any incident lately where you could have been driven by Perfection but you decided to be 'good enough'? My guess is that it is creeping into your life just by what you are now doing."

Terry didn't hesitate: "Today! In art. I was drawing pictures and I kept making heaps of mistakes I decided I didn't have to get it right but just to give it my best go."

David knew the power of the curse. "You didn't destroy it?"

"No, I didn't rip it out of my book," Terry reassured him.

Hearing of this incident triggered Dorothy's memory. "He did it last night, too!"

"Congratulations!" David exclaimed, "So what did you do instead of ripping it out the book?"

"I said to myself, 'Hey, I'm giving it my best. If I can't draw it, I just can't. I'm not Leonardo da Vinci.' "

David was impressed, "Did you know that when you were doing that you were taking a stand against Perfectionism in your life?" Terry was uncertain.

"When I first met you, Guilt and Perfection had been telling you that you were a 'second-rate' person," observed David. "Do you think you've graduated yet into being a 'first-rate' person?"

Terry gave this some serious thought. "I guess I have," he ventured, "but some bits are still sticking to the old ways. But my restless bits are starting to move. There is a big battle going on inside my head. It's a bit back and forth with that bully."

David was impressed with Terry's maturity and knew that he was really taking on the bully now. "There's quite a lot going on in your head," David mused. "Is there any way your mum and I can get in your corner?" David then thought about the efforts that Terry had made on his own and added, "Or is it enough just to celebrate your victories and let you know we think that what you are doing is important?" Terry chose the latter option: "It is important to celebrate with me."

"Do you think your life is better the way it's now going?" David asked.

"Yes, because I can communicate with people my own age. I used to think I was too high and they were immature, but now I'm playing with them."

"Have you got too many friends? Have you gone from Mr. Loneliness to Mr. Popularity?"

"Yeah."

"What suits you better, loneliness or popularity?"

"I suppose popularity because in some aspects my life is becoming good, but in other aspects, it's draining away a bit."

"Too much activity?"

"Well, it's only recently I've figured out this Perfection thing and I'm a lot freer now. The thing was that I spent so much time on my work but now I'm freer."

At this point Dorothy interjected with the continuing miracle of Terry's recovery from headaches: "He's only had two headaches since we first met you. That's unbelievable. He used to have them all the time for the past eight years."

"Is it pleasing to you that your head isn't being ached by Perfection?" David asked. Terry considered the connection between Perfection and headaches: "I can think more. I can enjoy my life more without having to worry, if I do this, I'll get a headache and be sick."

David wondered at Terry's freedom from the tyranny of worrisome headaches: "From what you tell me, your life sounds a lot freer in general. Would you agree or am I making too much of what you have told us today?"

Terry responded quickly, "I've become not only freer but more free-willed, but aspects of my life have gone into overdrive and other aspects have gone into reverse."

"What's gone into overdrive?"

"Making friends, enjoying life to the full."

"Do you want to keep going or do you think you've caught up on all the fun you missed out on?"

"I've got a long way to go on that." Little tears glistened in the corner of each eye as he recalled the utter misery of his life up until the present.

"Do you want to keep in overdrive in the friendship area even if it might mean you have to reverse in some other areas of your life?"

"Yes, I want to drop back to a normal level in my schoolwork so it's not all go. I don't want to be like a ship floating up in the air."

"Are you putting less effort into your schoolwork?"

"Yes. If I keep going, I could get punished."

When David heard this it gave him an idea for a further revolt against Perfectionism: "I know Perfection would really hate you getting a detention, but do you think you could get a detention on purpose? You would find that hard to do, wouldn't you?"

As Terry nodded, David checked with Dorothy: "Is this okay with you, Dorothy—just once?"

"Fine," Dorothy replied with a laugh.

"What could you do, Terry?" David continued.

Terry had an idea: "Forget about doing my homework."

"Yeah, that would be a good one," David agreed. Then he suggested a modification: "Or if that is too hard, do it, but flush it down the toilet and say you didn't do it." When David saw Terry hesitate he added, "I'm not suggesting you be outrageous, just forgetful. Do you think you can do that or is it too hard yet?"

"I would get a little upset."

"What about making some mistakes on purpose and seeing if you can stand up to it?"

"I could do that."

Seeing some mischief crossing Terry's face, David asked, "Have you got any ideas? Your ideas are always better than mine. Any anti-Perfection tricks?"

"I could have a special book where I make lots of mistakes and smudge it a lot and pretend my teacher is looking at it."

"When you do that, let me know how you feel about mocking Perfection. I'll hope to hear about it next time we meet," David requested. He then checked with Dorothy, "Is this a good tack we are taking here?"

"Oh yes," she assured him, her eyes crinkling with mirth.

FOURTH MEETING

David, Terry, and Dorothy met again one month later on a day that came to be known as "freedom day." The following letter summarized their conversation.

Dear Terry and Dorothy,

Terry, today was your "freedom day" and what a day it was for all of us. You informed us that you "didn't get upset when I make a mistake. I just carry on and cross out the mistake." In the old days, "I would have tried to rip the page out and start over again, even if it was near the end." When I inquired as to how you made this happen for yourself, you said you spoke back to Perfection in the following manner:

"I'm not going back to the way I was, I'm going to get out of this mess."

And when I asked if you had, you gave an imperfect answer, "99 percent out." There were some other instances of defying Perfection. For example, when all the other kids were playing Space Invaders on their computers instead of doing their homework, you said to yourself, "Who cares! I'll play a game too!" You then went on to inform us that you are getting busy with kids your age. You put it rather quaintly, "I bounce like a frog from lily pad to lily pad." And you have found some kids are quite interesting whom you had previously believed were "boring, boring." You are even starting to come to some conclusions about what you might want in a friend. Here are some of the qualities you cited: "patience, understanding, honesty, cheerfulness."

When I asked you both to assist me in designing an anti-Perfection "program," you came up with the following "map":

1. *First, "get someone else to talk to so you can express your victories; otherwise, Perfection will put you down and make you ignore them." You said one needs some "sideline cheering." And you warned people, Terry, of what tricks Perfection would employ to put you down; "It will say it's not a good enough victory, and that you've got to work harder, that your victory really was a waste of time." Dorothy, you said affirming Terry seemed to mean a lot to him. You tried holding or squeezing his hand and that seemed to work well or "telling him he had done fine."*

2. *Teasing: Terry, you thought it was critical "to bring things out in the open." Dorothy, you thought you had pulled Perfection's leg. We all agreed that a mischievous attitude rather than a deadly serious attitude was the way to rout Perfection.*

3. *Terry, you suggested doing the following: "Think of yourself in the future if you follow the Perfection path, but then look at the path you want to follow, and see what side has green grass on it." Terry, you said that when you did this, you realized that your brain had been "hand washed" rather that "brain washed."*

4. *Dorothy, you thought, too, that people shouldn't wait too long before they start their resistance to Perfection.*

5. *Terry, you recommended people "make a list in your mind of all the things you do that other people don't do. Then oppose the big ones first and work your way down the list, one at a time.*

6. *You recommended, Terry, that therapists have a "positive attitude, cheering me on."*

7. *Terry, you thought getting revenge on Perfection was a very good idea once you get the better of it. You have been taking revenge by being more "care free." You said, "I'm a person of the present and am enjoying my life more. I'm not worrying about my future so much now."*

8. *In general, you offered the following advice: "Don't listen to Guilt. Go for the top in a non-Perfection way. Don't be driven by Perfection. If you do, you can never have an achievement."*

Brett and I are now working on your diploma in Imperfection (Figure 17.1). Dorothy, you thought it should have "Well done, Terry!" on it and, Terry, you thought it should have "I walked through hell of despair to the Garden of Eden" on it. Well, I guess you will both have to wait and see.

Yours impurfectly,
    David

FINAL MEETING

Terry took up "free-spiritedness" and "naughtiness" both at home and school. He felt able to talk in class instead of being quiet all the time

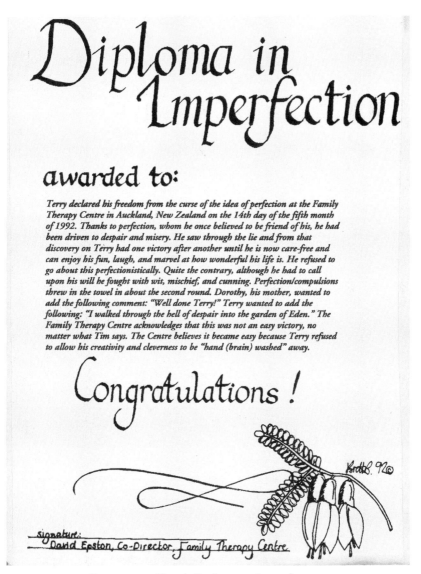

Diploma in Imperfection

awarded to:

Terry declared his freedom from the curse of the idea of perfection at the Family Therapy Centre in Auckland, New Zealand on the 14th day of the fifth month of 1992. Thanks to perfection, whom he once believed to be friend of his, he had been driven to despair and misery. He saw through the lie and from that discovery on Terry had one victory after another until he is now care-free and can enjoy his fun, laugh, and marvel at how wonderful his life is. He refused to go about this perfectionistically. Quite the contrary, although he had to call upon his will he fought with wit, mischief, and cunning. Perfection/compulsions threw in the towel in about the second round. Dorothy, his mother, wanted to add the following comment: "Well done Terry!" Terry wanted to add the following: "I walked through the hell of despair into the garden of Eden." The Family Therapy Centre acknowledges that this was not an easy victory, no matter what Tim says. The Centre believes it became easy because Terry refused to allow his creativity and cleverness to be "hand (brain) washed" away.

Congratulations !

signature:
David Epston, Co-Director, Family Therapy Centre.

Figure 17.1 Terry's Diploma in Imperfection.

and on a few occasions he "mucked around instead of working all the time." He had even played some "naughty tricks" on Dorothy, like "spilling stuff on purpose" and "doing stuff I'm not meant to do."

Previously he had always been frightened to go to sleep at night. He had "prayed to avoid nightmares." Now his dreams had turned stranger and more adventurous, including such epics as "going to school and being extremely naughty." In fact, the dreams, according to Terry,

"were guilt-free," whereas before he had "worried about the consequences of thinking like that."

Terry described some of his internal developments over this period
of time. "I just really feel happy. Now I express my feelings openly. If I
feel grouchy, I let people know by expressing it. In the old days, I bottled
it up and got headaches." Terry critiqued the idea that he was only allowed so much happiness (20–40 percent maximum), because otherwise "guilt would have become redundant." He then expressed his
newfound wisdom about the role of Guilt in a person's life. "Guilt needs
a certain amount of misery if it is to grow into an uncontrollable force in
a person's mind." Dorothy agreed that Terry's "confidence level is much
higher. He'll give things a go. He meets things head on and is courageous. He is no longer sick of his headaches. He feels more worthy of
the good things in life and believes in himself."

From thereon in, the "problems" did make some comebacks on Terry
"once in a blue moon." But he always found ways to "repel" them. For
example, he said, "I'm still frightened that if I don't wash my hands just
before I go to bed, the dreams will run amok at night." He discovered
that this only happened when he was "off guard, sleepy, and couldn't be
bothered thinking." To outwit sleepiness, he'd "go behind the fear and
scream at it. 'This is not going to really happen!'" This assertive approach gave him so much relief he "completely forgot about the fear."
He also employed one of his "mum's techniques" which was to imagine
"walking in a nice big garden with hundreds and hundreds of flowers,
especially cosmos flowers." He saw that even if such "bouts" returned,
"they were becoming shorter and shorter; in the old days, they used to
engulf me and last at least two or three weeks."

In fact, Terry had been appreciating his imagination and putting it to
good use. "My wondering just comes when I'm fed up with the real
world." Terry informed David that he used "his wondering" to "redirect
my thoughts and organize my dreams." At school, he had decided "to
go with nerds and minorities" and had made a close friend who was
"always interested in reading books and good to listen to "but he is himself." Terry likewise determined "to be abnormal, to have some special
ability." "I am not your average citizen" was the way he expressed his
individuality.

Terry's last words to David were "I am so happy to just get everything
off my back. I am not putting up with hand-washing. If I hadn't stopped
hand-washing, I would have been depressed, miserable, or irritable."

FOLLOW-UP

David and Terry met four more times over the course of the next year. Terry assumed the duties of the presidency of the Anti-Habit League of New Zealand, consulting to other young people. He and the vice-president decided on the application of a young man, Ben, twelve, about a year later.[1] Ben had reclaimed his life from a Mr. O (obsession). A videotaped application interview of Ben and his parents had been sent to Terry by David for his opinion. David considers this to be the most convincing follow-up of his work with Terry that a person could have:

Dear David,

I was greatly impressed by Ben's battle with Mr. O. When I read your letter how he was before he was hospitalized and then seeing him on video, I noticed his great change. He has really changed. I do believe he has worked hard enough to receive the New Zealand Diploma of Impurfection.

At the moment life is good for me. I'm in the top class in third form and have recently turned fourteen. The only bad thing has been the death of my grandfather some time ago and I am just about over it. And as for Perfection, my borders have been closed to him. Mr. O, as you called it, has not visited.

Best wishes,

　　Terry

Concluding Thoughts

· ·

If you read something that sounded like a "miracle cure" in our case stories, we didn't mean to imply that the problem always went away and never came back. In some of the more difficult predicaments we describe, the child's being released from the hospital, putting a stop to a destructive habit, or being welcomed at school instead of being expelled was a desirable and specific outcome. However, when we contacted families to ask for their consent to be in this book, several told us about new problems that arose or talked about how the old ones continued or resurfaced in milder forms. Such feedback from family members included statements such as: "Well, he's still dealing with some fears, but I guess he doesn't let them stop him from living his life. He has more ways to deal with them now." "We feel we have more tools now for communicating about our disagreements." "Well, he still gets angry but Temper doesn't take over, and he reminds us to be cool ourselves." "He wakes up at night sometimes, but he doesn't wake the whole family up and create an uproar."

Our understanding of these comments is that in most situations it is a child's or family's relationship with a problem or the relationships they have with each other in the face of a problem that is made available for therapeutic revision. In order to diminish the effects of the problem, we have found it beneficial to delve less into the problem itself and concentrate more on what occurs when these relationships are restoried.

An alternative story may involve leaving the problem behind to be stored in the dusty archives of memory. More often than not, however, it is the living relationship with the problem that is transformed. We are more likely to think of problems as being resolved rather than solved. When we looked up "resolve" in the dictionary, the musical definition struck us: "the progression of a dissonant tone or chord to a consonant tone or chord." Analogously, the dissonance of problems can be brought into an unexpected harmony through narrative. The resolution, if approached with a lightness of heart, humor, or playfulness, is dynamic.

The narrative structure of a book or a therapy can imply a clear beginning or a settled ending in every case story. We ourselves are tempted to resolve the complexities of life's dissonances into such clichés as a "happy ever after" ending. But of course, life stories are always in the making. Some problems are messy and complex (indeterminate in duration and multifactorial in cause). This doesn't mean that relationships with them are not resolvable—and some resolutions are spectacular.

As narrative therapists we hope to convene a forum to critique the effects of problems and their limiting sociocultural prescriptions, generate a richer palate of new possibilities and rehabilitate old ones for choice making (in the present and in the future), and co-author preferred stories. To accomplish these tasks we (a) engage in externalizing conversations that invite the active participation and responsibility of all concerned parties—even those beyond the bounds of the immediate therapy; (b) value the preexisting abilities of all parties regardless of age or position, especially those abilities that were previously considered inadequate or irrelevant; (c) expand the definition of who is "qualified" to offer new skills or value old ones beyond those considered to have professional credentials; and (d) reach out to diversify those seen as knowledgeable and helpful to include extended networks and relevant communities of concern.

What we find has changed, by the time the family is ready to celebrate and confirm their accomplishments, is that the search for who was to blame has been called off, the knowledge and skill inventory has grown to encompass the "taken for granted" and the fantastical, and the resources for new understanding and help have become more bountiful.

We leave you with a poem written by Jenna at age thirteen. (Her story is told in Chapter 8.)

> *Jenna's Prayer*
>
> I hope that in the future people after me will see
> A world green with beauty and blue, limitless skies.
> That pollution will be the evil queen in a fairy tale.
> I hope that sickness will only be a cold
> And diseases with no cure simply myths,
> Or scary stories told on Halloween.
> I hope poverty and crime will be a bad dream
> That someone had centuries ago.
> That "homeless on the street" will be an unknown phrase.

I hope "war" will be an alien word,
Or one of the many ways to say "world peace."
That the "isms" will be only fossils of past hatred.

I hope in the future the world will be green and healthy,
But not paradise—
That would be boring.
Instead the future should be like my life.
Not perfect,
But really great.

Notes

• •

CHAPTER 1

1. Since only one case story in this book mentions work with child sexual abuse, we refer the reader who is interested in narrative approaches for therapy with child sexual abuse to Adams-Westcott and Isenbart (1990, 1996), Laing and Kamsler (1990), and Roberts (1993).
2. See Epston (1993), Gergen (1994).
3. See also Dickerson and Zimmerman (1996).
4. When play in therapy is referred to, it is not meant to be separated from verbal discussion. They go together hand in hand. One of the main features of narrative therapy is verbal play. The practitioners represented in this book, among others in the field, vary widely in their style as to how much of an interview is taken up in conversation and how much verbal conversation is woven through other modes of communication, such as symbolic play with sandtray, dollhouse, or puppet theater.
5. Regarding children and schooling, see the special (1995) issue of *Dulwich Centre Newsletter: Schooling and Education: Exploring New Possibilities.*

CHAPTER 2

1. Leon's "Squirmies" would typically be diagnosed as attention deficit hyperactivity disorder. For further discussion on this topic see Nylund and Corsiglia's (1996) article: *From deficits to special abilities: Working narratively with children labeled ADHD.*
2. During the first meeting David, Maggie, and Gregory talked about the divorce. However, we skim over this aspect of the conversation to illustrate the collaboration between Gregory and David, with a focus on Gregory's special ability.

CHAPTER 3

1. See de Shazer, 1991.
2. See Gilligan, 1982; Hancock, 1989; Pipher, 1994.
3. While we hold the fundamental assumption that our point of view is not assumed to be objectively fixed or ultimately correct, we do not intend to wholly depart from the notion of objective truth or to engage in moral relativism. For example, the tendency to organize our lived experience into meaningful narratives is an ethological hypothesis that has yet to be disproved and thus may considered to be objective (Bruner, 1990). Most importantly, every viewpoint taken by an observer has moral and ethical implications for those over whom the observer has power and influence. Lengthier discussion of these significant issues is beyond the scope of this book; suffice it to say we find it very important to underscore the notion that our point of view should be thoughtfully chosen and that ethical obligations, responsibilities, and values arise from that choice.
4. See Roth and Epston (1996a, pp. 153–154) for a training exercise that offers "a lively and potent introduction to the transformative power of engaging in problem-externalizing conversations."
5. See Madigan and Epston, 1995.
6. See Epston, White, and "Ben," 1995; Zimmerman and Dickerson, 1994.

CHAPTER 4

1. Please assume that the term *parents* may be interchangeable, where applicable, with grandparents, foster-parents or other persons assuming a primary caretaking role for children. The term *family* assumes that the family may consist of children with sole parents, same-sex couples, or parents who live separately, as well as extended family groupings.
2. We feel it is sometimes appropriate to see children individually and tend to respect a family's wishes when this request is made. While there are no fixed rules, we inquire about the family's interest in individual therapy for the child and discuss it with them.

   We have found that when a child is recovering from trauma and her current environment is safe and settled, it may be helpful to work individually with her. On the other hand, when sexual assault has been disclosed, Margaret Roberts (1993) argues cogently in her paper "Don't Leave Mother in the Waiting Room" for joint sessions with mothers and children wherein their intimate relationship (which has been disturbed by the offender) is reauthored while the offender's role is made visible.
3. As Michael White (1993, p.132) comments, "I am thinking of a solidarity that is constructed by therapists who refuse to draw a sharp distinction between their lives and the lives of others, who refuse to marginalize those persons who seek help; by therapists who are prepared to constantly confront the fact that, if faced with circumstances such that provide the context of the troubles of others, they just might not be doing nearly as well themselves."

4. For an in-depth discussion of men who are abusive in relation to partners and children, see Alan Jenkin's (1990) book, *Invitations to Responsibility*, as well as the interview with Michael White by McLean (1994) and Waldegrave (1990).

5. This segment is a narrative version of a transcript that was published previously by Epston and Brock (1989, pp. 99–100).

6. Michael suspects that the preference for a Tasmanian Devil animal identity may very likely be restricted to Australian children.

7. The Leslie Centre is a child and family agency in Auckland, New Zealand that is sponsored by the Presbyterian Support Services.

8. It is important for North American readers to know that "tea" should be translated to "dinner" rather than "a cup of tea."

CHAPTER 6

1. For a comprehensive description of the use of letters in narrative therapy, see *Narrative Means to Therapeutic Ends* (White & Epston, 1990b).

CHAPTER 7

1. Waldegrave (1992) has made a compelling case for the ethical obligation of a therapist to articulate mental health issues in the sociopolitical sphere. Lobovits, Maisel, and Freeman (1995) provide a discussion of the ethics of collaborative practices in therapy.

2. A method of questioning, called internalized-other questioning (Tomm, 1989) is especially suitable for interviews with this kind of audience. In this approach, the client plays the role of the "internalized other," who is then interviewed as if he were in the room, For example, if Tommy's grandma were no longer alive, Tommy could be asked to imagine what she would say, and to speak as if he were her. The therapist might then ask Tommy (as grandma), "So, grandma, what made you the most proud about what Tommy did this week at school?" Tommy replies (as grandma), "Well, I'm most proud of how he defended that boy who was getting teased. I always knew he would stick up for what's right."

3. See Freedman and Combs (1996), Friedman (1995), and White (1995) for detailed discussions and descriptions of the use of a narrative reflecting team.

4. See also Freeman and Lobovits (1993) and Wood (1985).

5. For examples of certificates and letters see White and Epston (1990b).

6. To subscribe to *REVIVE: The Magazine of the Vancouver Anti-anorexia Anti-bulimia League*, write to: REVIVE, 1168 Hamilton Street, Suite 207, Vancouver, B.C. Canada V6B 2S2.

CHAPTER 8

1. While we prefer to offer a culturally appropriate referral to such a family, this may not be possible or even desired by the family.

2. In a parallel vein, Melissa and James Griffith (1994) have discovered in deal-

ing with somatically based problems (e.g., so-called "somatoform disorders") that "unspeakable dilemmas" may make verbal communication unsafe and even impossible. They have found that, before the condition can be resolved, the dilemma needs to be addressed both in awareness of the body's posture and movement and though safe verbal expression.

3. Jenny's active interest in including Gene was partly informed by Michael White's (1988b) paper "Saying Hullo Again: The Incorporation of the Lost Relationship in the Resolution of Grief". This article offers the metaphor of "saying hello" as well as the more commonly favored one of letting go or saying good-bye as a means of resolving grief over a loss.

   She was also reminded of her experience living in the heart of an Asian community, where altars to the ancestors are kept in many households. When something important is happening, family members will light incense and then sit in meditative prayer in front of a photograph of their loved one, who is "informed" and "consulted" in the imagination about events.

4. It is important to note here that (as part of the therapist's discussion of safety rules and etiquette) we may want to put forth a "pass agreement"— where any member of the family has the right to pass on responding to any particular question or suggestion to try an expressive arts activity (Chasin & Roth, 1990; Rogers, 1993).

5. To get the benefit of colorful visual representation while in the process of "mapping the relative influence of person and problem," Jenny has experimented with the technique of mind-mapping (Buzan, 1976). Anyone familiar with this method of accessing knowledge in visual form might enjoy experimenting with narrative applications of it. The problem can be placed in the middle of the page and different colored tangents drawn off it with sub-tangents for related activities and ideas, in order to brainstorm everything known about its operations, effects, plans, etc. Another map can then be created with the alternative story/outcome/solution in the center, to brainstorm about inspirations, unique outcomes, and so on.

6. Some creative work has been done in combining dramatic enactment and narrative therapy. See, for example, Barragar Dunne (1992), Chasin and Roth (1990), and Chasin and White (1989).

7. Sandplay is involved here in the context of narrative therapy, in quite a different way from by the Jungian (Kalff, 1971) and English schools (the "world technique" developed by Lowenfeld, see Bowyer, 1976). While Jenny also uses the sandtray in open and exploratory ways, here we limit ourselves to its specific use in a narrative approach.

CHAPTER 9

1. Sculpey is the brand name (in the U.S.A.) of a modeling clay that has a consistency similar to plasticine, but can be baked to harden.

2. Kevin follows in the well established footsteps of Rupert the Bear, who

has regularly consulted to Michael White. David first met Rupert in Adelaide, Australia, in 1981. One might speculate that over these last fifteen years of service an unlicensed therapist like Rupert might have burned out, but if anything he is more afire than ever. Rupert came into Michael's practice thanks to Sophia Vogt, who had this to say: "I invest a part of me in Rupert. Love went into his creation. Because of this, he is not some stuffed inanimate object but a little creature who has evolved a special set of characteristics, just like people do. He has his own stories to tell and to hear these all you have to do is listen properly—not from ears, but from the heart. If you can communicate with him in this way, you will find that he gives so much."

CHAPTER 10

1. This story is a revision of Epston and Betterton's (1993) article, "Imaginary Friends: Who are They? Who Needs Them?"
2. Taylor, Cartwright, and Carlson (1991) report that "imaginary companions are surprisingly commonplace. The most recent research shows that as many as 65 percent of preschool children have imaginary companions (
3. David would like acknowledge in particular Suzie Snyder's grandfather Ross for his contribution to this list.

CHAPTER 12

1. Popular books in children's literature draw on this theme; such as in *There's a Monster in My Closet* (Mayer, 1968), a story in which a boy who is terrorized by monsters goes on to tame and befriend them.
2. For ideas for imagination warm-ups, see de Mille (1976) and Oaklander (1978).
3. This idea was based on C. G. Jung's technique of active imagination in relation to dreams, explicated by John Sanford in his (1978) book: *Dreams and Healing: A Succinct and Lively Interpretation of Dreams.*
4. Karen Moore prepared the initial draft of this case story. At that time she was a doctoral fellow at Xanthos Counseling Center in Alameda, California.

CHAPTER 14

1. See Boyd-Franklin (1989) and Pinderhughes (1989).
2. For our non-American readers, Reeses Pieces are small disks of peanut butter covered with chocolate.
3. Dean, a Caucasian, and John, an African American, formed a partnership to offer culturally accountable and diverse perspectives to the family and their therapist (Lobovits, Maisel, & Freeman, 1995; Lobovits & Prowell, 1995; Tamasese & Waldegrave, 1993; White, 1995).

CHAPTER 17

1. David's work with Ben is described in detail in Epston, White, and "Ben" (1995).

References

....

Adams-Westcott, J., & Isenbart, D. (1990). Using rituals to empower family members who have experienced child sexual abuse. In M. Durrant & C. White (Eds.), *Ideas for therapy with sexual abuse* (pp. 37–64). Adelaide, Australia: Dulwich Centre Publications.

Adams-Westcott, J., & Isenbart, D. (1996). Creating preferred relationships: The politics of recovery from child abuse. *Journal of Systemic Therapies, 15*(1), 13–30.

Axline, V. (1987). *Play therapy.* New York: Ballantine.

Barragar Dunne, P. (1992). *The narrative therapist and the arts.* Los Angeles: Possibilities Press.

Bowyer, L. R. (1976). *The Lowenfeld World technique: Studies in personality.* Oxford, England: Pergamon Press.

Boyd-Franklin, N. (1989). *Black families in therapy: A multisystems approach.* New York: Guilford.

Brems, C. (1993). *A comprehensive guide to child psychotherapy.*
Boston, MA: Allyn & Bacon.

Brooks, P. (1984). *Reading for plot: Design and intention in narrative.* New York: Knopf.

Bruner, E. (1986). Experience and its expressions. In V. Turner & E. Bruner (Eds.), *The anthropology of experience.* Chicago: University of Illinois Press.

Bruner, J. (1986). *Actual minds/possible worlds.* Cambridge, MA: Harvard University Press.

Bruner, J. (1990). *Acts of meaning.* Cambridge: Harvard University Press.

Buzan, T. (1976). *Use both sides of your brain.* New York: Dutton.

Carroll, L. (1989). *The complete works of Lewis Carroll.* London: Nonesuch Press.

Carter, B., & McGoldrick, M. (1988). *The changing family life cycle: A framework for family therapy* (2nd Ed.). Boston, MA: Allyn & Bacon.

Case, C., & Dalley, T. (Eds.) (1992). *Working with children in art therapy.* New York: Routledge.

Chasin, R., & Roth, S. (1990). Future perfect, past perfect: A positive approach to opening couple therapy. In R. Chasin, H. Grunebaum, & M. Herzig (Eds.), *One couple, four realities: Multiple perspectives on couple therapy.* New York: Guilford.

Chasin, R., & Roth, S. (1994). Externalization linguistic key to a new approach in family therapy. *Psychiatric Times,*

Chasin, R., & White, T. B. (1989). The child in family therapy: Guidelines for active engagement across the age span. In L. Combrinck-Graham (Ed.), *Children in family contexts: Perspectives on treatment* (pp. 5–25). New York: Guilford.

Combrinck-Graham, L. (Ed.) (1989). *Children in family contexts: Perspectives on treatment.* New York: Guilford.

Cowley, G., & Springen, K. (1995, April 17). Rewriting life stories. *Newsweek,* 70–74.

Damasio, A. (1994). *Descartes' error: Emotion, reason, and the human brain.* New York: G. P. Putnam & Sons.

de Shazer, S. (1991). *Putting difference to work.* New York: Norton.

de Mille, R. (1976). *Put your mother on the ceiling: Children's imagination games.* New York: Penguin.

Dickerson, V. C., & Zimmerman, J. L. (1993). A narrative approach to families with adolescents. In S. Friedman (Ed.), *The new language of change: Constructive collaboration on psychotherapy* (pp. 226–250). New York: Guilford.

Dickerson, V. C. & Zimmerman, J. L. (1996). Myth, misconceptions, and a word or two about politics. *Journal of Systemic Therapies, 15*(1), 79–88.

Durrant, M. (Autumn, 1989). Temper taming: An approach to children's temper problems revisited. *Dulwich Centre Newsletter,* 1–11.

Durrant, M. (1995). *Creative strategies for school problems.* New York: Norton.

Epston, D. (1986/1997). Nightwatching: An approach to night fears. *Dulwich Centre Review,* 28–30. Reprinted in M. White & D. Epston, *Retracing the past: Selected papers and collected papers revisited.* Adelaide, Australia: Dulwich Centre Publications.

Epston, D. (1989a). *Collected papers.* Adelaide, Australia: Dulwich Centre Publications.

Epston, D. (1989/1997). Guest address, Fourth Australian Family Therapy Conference. In D. Epston, *Collected papers.* Reprinted in *Retracing the past: Selected papers and collected papers revisited.* Adelaide, Australia: Dulwich Centre Publications.

Epston, D. (1991/1997) Benny the peanut man. *Dulwich Centre Newletter,* 1, 12–14. Reprinted in D. Epston, *Catching up with David Epston: Published papers (1991–1996).* Adelaide, Australia: Dulwich Centre Publications.

Epston, D. (1992) Temper tantrum parties: Saving face, losing face, or going off your face. In D. Epston & M. White, *Experience, contradiction, narrative, and imagination: Selected papers of David Epston & Michael White, 1989–1991.* Adelaide, Australia: Dulwich Centre Publications.

Epston, D. (1993). Internalizing discourses versus externalizing discourses. In S. Gilligan & R. Price (Eds.), *Therapeutic Conversations* (pp. 161-177). New York: Norton.

Epston, D. (1994). Extending the conversation. *Family Therapy Networker, 18*(6), 31-37, 62-63.

Epston, D., & Betterton, E. (1993/1997). Imaginary friends: Who are they? Who needs them? In D. Epston, *Catching up with David Epston: Published papers (1991–1996).* Originally published in *Dulwich Centre Newsletter, 2,* 38-39.

Epston, D., & Brock, P. (1989/1997). A strategic approach to an extreme feeding problem. In D. Epston, *Collected Papers*. Reprinted in M. White & D. Epston, *Retracing the past: Selected papers and collected papers revisited*. Adelaide, Australia: Dulwich Centre Publications.

Epston, D., Morris, F., & Maisel, R. (1995). A narrative approach to so-called anorexia/bulimia. In K. Weingarten (Ed.), *Cultural resistance: Challenging beliefs about men, women, and therapy* (pp. 69-96). New York: Haworth.

Epston, D., & White, M. (1992). *Experience, contradiction, narrative, and imagination: Selected papers of David Epston & Michael White, 1989-1991*. Adelaide, Australia: Dulwich Centre Publications.

Epston, D., White, M., & "Ben" (1995). Consulting your consultants: A means to the co-construction of alternative knowledges. In S. Friedman (Ed.), *The reflecting team in action: Collaborative practice in family therapy* (pp. 277-313). New York: Guilford.

Freedman, J., & Combs, G. (1996). *Narrative therapy: The social construction of preferred realities*. New York: Norton.

Freeman, D. (1979). *The anthropology of choice*. The Presidential Address of the Anthropology, Archaeology and Linguistics Sections of the 49th. Congress of the Australian and New Zealand Association for the Advancement of Science in Auckland New Zealand. Author's reprint.

Freeman, J. C., & Lobovits, D. H. (1993). The turtle with wings. In S. Friedman (Ed.), *The new language of change: Constructive collaboration in psychotherapy* (pp. 188-225). New York: Guilford.

Freeman, J. C., Loptson, C., & Stacey, K. (1995). *Collaboration and possibility: Appreciating the privilege of entering children's narrative worlds*. Handout from workshop presented at the "Narrative Ideas and Therapeutic Practice" Third International Conference, Vancouver, BC.

Friedman, S. (Ed.) (1995). *The reflecting team in action: Collaborative practice in family therapy*. New York: Guilford.

Garbarino, J., Stott, F. M., & Faculty of the Erikson Institute (1992). *What children can tell us: Eliciting, interpreting, and evaluating critical information from children*. San Francisco, CA: Jossey-Bass.

Gergen, K. (1994). *Realities and representations: Soundings in social construction*. Cambridge, MA: Harvard University Press.

Gil, E. (1994). *Play in family therapy*. New York: Guilford.

Gilligan, C. (1982). *In a different voice*. Cambridge, MA: Harvard University Press.

Goffman, E. (1961). *Asylums*. Garden City, NY: Anchor Books.

Griffith, J. L., & Griffith, M. E. (1994). *The body speaks: Therapeutic dialogues for mind-body problems*. New York: Basic.

Hancock, E. (1989). *The girl within*. New York: Fawcet.

Hillman, J. (1994, May 13) *A desperate need for beauty*. Titus Workshop, Lesley College Graduate School.

Imber-Black, E. (1988). *Families and larger systems: A family therapist's guide through the labyrinth*. New York: Guilford.

Jenkins, A. (1990). *Invitations to responsibility: The therapeutic engagement of men who are violent and abusive.* Adelaide, Australia: Dulwich Centre Publications.

Kalff, D. M. (1971). *Sandplay: Mirror of a child's psyche.* San Francisco, CA: Browser Press.

Kerr, J. (1968). *The tiger who came to tea.* Glasgow: Collins.

Knill, P., Barba, H. N., & Fuchs, M. N. (1995). *Minstrels of soul: Intermodal expressive therapy.* Toronto: Palmerston.

Laing, L., & Kamsler, A. (1990). Putting an end to secrecy: Therapy with mothers and children following disclosure of child sexual assault. In M. Durrant & C. White (Eds.), *Ideas for therapy with sexual abuse* (pp. 159-181). Adelaide, Australia: Dulwich Centre Publications.

Lobovits, D. H., Maisel, R., & Freeman, J. C. (1995). Public practices: An ethic of circulation. In S. Friedman (Ed.), *The reflecting team in action: Collaborative practice in family therapy* (pp. 223-256). New York: Guilford.

Lobovits, D., & Prowell, J. (1995). *Unexpected journey: Invitations to diversity.* Paper from workshop presented at "Narrative Ideas and Therapeutic Practice" Fourth International Conference, Vancouver, BC.

Loptson, C., & Stacey, K. (1995). Children should be seen and not heard? Questioning the unquestioned. *Journal of Systemic Therapies, 14*(4), 16-32.

Madigan, S. (1991). An interview with Chris Beels. *Dulwich Centre Newsletter, 4,* 13-21.

Madigan, S., & Epston, D. (1995). From "spy-chiatric gaze" to communities of concern: From professional monologue to dialogue. In S. Friedman (Ed.), *The reflecting team in action* (pp. 257-276). New York: Guilford.

Mayer, M. (1968). *There's a nightmare in my closet.* New York: Dial.

Maisel, R. (1994). *Engaging men in a re-evaluation of practices and definitions of masculinity.* Paper presented at "Narrative Ideas and Therapeutic Practice" Third International Conference, Vancouver, BC.

McLean, C. (1994). A conversation about accountability with Michael White. *Dulwich Centre Newsletter, 2 & 3,* 68-79.

McLean, C. (Guest Ed.) (1995). Schooling and Education: Exploring new possibilities. *Dulwich Centre Newsletter, 2 & 3.*

McLean, C., White, C., & Hall, R. (Guest Eds.). (1994). Accountability: New directions for working in partnership. *Dulwich Centre Newsletter, 2 & 3.*

McLeod, W. (1985). "Stuffed" team members. *Dulwich Centre Review, 57-59.*

McMurray, M. (1988). *Illuminations: The healing image.* Berkeley, CA: Wingbow.

Mills, J. C., & Crowley, R. J. (1986). *Therapeutic metaphors for children* and the child within. New York: Brunner/Mazel.

Milne, A. A. (1957). *The world of Pooh.* New York: Dutton.

Moustakas, C. (1973). Children in play therapy. New York: Ballantine Books.

Nylund, D., & Corsiglia, V. (1996). From deficits to special abilities: Working narratively with children labeled ADHD. In M. Hoyt (Ed.), *Constructive therapies* (Vol. 2, pp. 163-183). New York: Guilford.

Nylund, D., & Thomas, J. (1994). The economics of narrative. *Family Therapy Networker, 18*(6), 38-39.

Oaklander, V. (1978). *Windows to our children.* Moab, UT: Real People Press.

O'Hanlon, B. (1994). The third wave. *Family Therapy Networker, 18*(6), 18-26, 28-29.

Paley, V. G. (1990). *The boy who would be a helicopter: The uses of storytelling in the classroom.* Cambridge: Harvard University Press.

Parker, I. (1995). *Deconstructing psychopathology.* Thousand Oaks, CA: Sage.

Pinderhughes, E. (1989). *Understanding race, ethnicity, and power: The key to efficacy in clinical practice.* New York: Free Press.

Pipher, M. (1994). *Reviving Ophelia: Saving the selves of adolescent girls.* New York: Ballantine.

Popper, K. R. (1986). *Objective knowledge: An evolutionary approach.* Oxford: Clarendon.

Ranger, L. (1995). *Laura's poems.* Auckland, New Zealand: Godwit.

Roberts, M. (1993). Don't leave mother in the waiting room. *Dulwich Center Newsletter, 2,* 21-28.

Robbins, A. (1994). *A multi-modal approach to creative art therapy.* London: Kingsley.

Rogers, N. (1993). *The creative connection: Expressive arts as healing.* Palo Alto: Science and Behavior Books.

Rosenwald, G. C., & Ochberg, R. L. (Eds.) (1992). *Storied lives: The cultural politics of self-understanding.* New Haven: Yale University Press.

Roth, S., & Chasin, R. (1994). Entering one another's worlds of meaning and imagination: Dramatic enactment and narrative couple therapy. In M. F. Hoyt (Ed.), *Constructive therapies* (pp. 189-216). New York: Guilford.

Roth, S. & Epston, D. (1996a). Consulting the problem about the problematic relationship: An exercise for experiencing a relationship with an externalized problem. In M. Hoyt (Ed.) *Constructive therapies* (Vol. 2, pp. 148-162). New York: Guilford.

Roth, S. & Epston, D. (1996b). Developing externalizing conversations: An exercise. *Journal of Systemic Therapies, 15*(1), 5-12.

Seymour, F. W. & Epston, D. (1992). An approach to childhood stealing with evaluation of 45 cases. In M. White & D. Epston (Eds.), *Experience, contradiction, narrative, and imagination: Selected papers of David Epston & Michael White, 1989-1991.* (pp. 189-206). Adelaide, Australia: Dulwich Centre Publications.

Smith, C. & Barragar Dunne, P., (1992, November 8). *Therapeutic loving and empowering choices: Narrative psychology, constructivism, and drama therapy.* Workshop presented at National Association of Drama Therapy Thirteenth Annual Conference, San Francisco, CA.

Stacey, K. (1995). Language as an exclusive or inclusive concept: Reaching beyond the verbal. *Australian & New Zealand Journal of Family Therapy, 16*(3), 123-132.

Tamasese, K., & Waldegrave, C. (1993). Cultural and gender accountability in the "Just Therapy" approach. *Journal of Feminist Family Therapy, 5*(2), 29-45.

Tapping, C. (1993). Other wisdoms, other worlds: Colonisation and family therapy. *Dulwich Centre Newsletter, 1,* 1-40.

Taylor, M., Cartwright, B., & Carlson, S. (1993). A developmental investigation of children's imaginary companions. *Developmental Psychology 29*(2), 276-285.

Tolkien, J.R.R. (1965). *Lord of the rings.* Boston: Houghton Mifflin.

Tomm, K. (1987). Interventive interviewing: Part II. Reflexive questioning as a means to enable self-healing. *Family Process, 26,* 167-183.

Tomm, K. (1988). Interventive interviewing: Part III. Intending to ask lineal, circular, strategic, or reflexive questions? *Family Process, 27,* 1-15.

Tomm, K. (1989). Externalizing the problem and internalizing personal agency. *Journal of Strategic and Systemic Therapy,* 8(1), 54-59.

Tomm, K., Suzuki, K., & Suzuki, K. (1990). The Ka-No-Mushi: An inner externalization that enables compromise? *Australian & New Zealand Journal of Family Therapy, 11*(2), 104-107.

van Gennep, A. (1960). *The rites of passage* (Trans. M. B. Vizedom & G. Caffee). Chicago: University of Chicago Press.

Waldegrave, C. (1990). Just therapy. *Dulwich Centre Newsletter, 1,* 5-46.

Waldegrave, C. (1991). *Weaving threads of meaning and distinguishing preferable patterns.* Lower Hutt, New Zealand: Author's reprint.

Waldegrave, C. (October, 1992). Psychology, politics and the loss of the welfare state. *New Zealand Psychological Society Bulletin, 74,* 14-21.

Walters, M., Carter, B., Papp, P., & Silverstein, O. (1988). *The invisible web: Gender patterns in family relationships.* New York: Guilford.

Weller, J. S. (1993). Planting your feet firmly in Emptiness: Expressive arts therapy and meditation. *Journal of the Creative and Expressive Arts Therapies Exchange, 3,* 104-105.

White, M. (1984/1997). Pseudo-ecopresis: From avalanche to victory, from vicious to virtuous cycles. *Family Systems Medicine,* 2(2). Reprinted in M. White & D. Epston, *Retracing the past: Selected papers and collected papers revisited.* Adelaide, Australia: Dulwich Centre Publications.

White, M. (1985/1997). Fear busting and monster taming: An approach to fears of young children. *Dulwich Centre Review.* Reprinted in M. White & D. Epston, *Retracing the past: Selected papers and collected papers revisited.* Adelaide, Australia: Dulwich Centre Publications.

White, M. (1986/1997). Negative explanation, restraint, and double description: A template for family therapy. *Family Process, 25*(2), 169–184. Reprinted in M. White & D. Epston, *Retracing the past: Selected papers and collected papers revisited.* Adelaide, Australia: Dulwich Centre Publications.

White, M. (Winter, 1988a/1997). The process of questioning: A therapy of literary merit? *Dulwich Centre Newsletter,* 8–14. Reprinted in M. White & D. Epston, *Retracing the past: Selected papers and collected papers revisited.* Adelaide, Australia: Dulwich Centre Publications.

White, M. (Spring, 1988b/1997). Saying hullo again: the incorporation of the lost relationship. *Dulwich Centre Newsletter,* 7–11. Reprinted in M. White & D. Epston, *Retracing the past: Selected papers and collected papers revisited.* Adelaide, Australia: Dulwich Centre Publications.

White, M. (Summer, 1989/1997). The externalizing of the problem and re-authoring of lives and relationships. *Dulwich Centre Newletter,* 3–20. Reprinted in M. White & D. Epston, *Retracing the past: Selected papers and collected papers revisited*. Adelaide, Australia: Dulwich Centre Publications.

White, M. (1991/1992). Deconstruction and therapy. *Dulwich Centre Newsletter, 3*, 21–40. Reprinted in D. Epston & M. White, *Experience, contradiction, narrative, and imagination: Selected papers of David Epston & Michael White, 1989–1991*. Adelaide, Australia: Dulwich Center Publications.

White, M. (1993). Commentary: The histories of the present. In S. Gilligan & R. Price (Eds.), *Therapeutic conversations* (pp. 121-135). New York: Norton.

White, M. (1995). *Re-authoring lives: Interviews and essays*. Adelaide, Australia: Dulwich Centre Publications.

White, M., & Epston, D. (1990a/1997). Consulting your consultants: The documentation of alternative knowledges. *Dulwich Centre Newsletter, 4*, 25–35. Reprinted in D. Epston & M. White, *Experience, contradiction, narrative, and imagination: Selected papers of David Epston & Michael White, 1989–1991*. Adelaide, Australia: Dulwich Centre Publications.

White, M., & Epston, D. (1990b). *Narrative means to therapeutic ends*. New York: Norton.

Wilson, J. Q. (1993). *The moral sense*. New York: Free Press.

Wood, A. (1985). King Tiger and the roaring tummies: A novel way of helping young children and their families change. *Dulwich Centre Review*, 41-49.

Zimmerman, J. L., & Dickerson, V. C. (1994). Tales of the body thief: Externalizing and deconstructing eating problems. In M. F. Hoyt (Ed.), *Constructive therapies* (Vol. 1, pp. 295-318). New York: Guilford.

Index